Also by Dr. Shana Clark:

"My Money's on the Turtle"
Published in 2010

TAMING *the* DRAGON

MANAGING MENTAL ILLNESS

SHANA WIBBERLEY CLARK, M.D., DR. P.H.

COVER ILLUSTRATIONS BY JOHN ED BON FED

BALBOA PRESS

A DIVISION OF HAY HOUSE

Copyright © 2014 Shana Wibberley Clark, M.D., Dr. P.H.

All rights reserved. No part of this book may be used or reproduced by any means, graphic, electronic, or mechanical, including photocopying, recording, taping or by any information storage retrieval system without the written permission of the publisher except in the case of brief quotations embodied in critical articles and reviews.

Balboa Press books may be ordered through booksellers or by contacting:

Balboa Press
A Division of Hay House
1663 Liberty Drive
Bloomington, IN 47403
www.balboapress.com
1 (877) 407-4847

Because of the dynamic nature of the Internet, any web addresses or links contained in this book may have changed since publication and may no longer be valid. The views expressed in this work are solely those of the author and do not necessarily reflect the views of the publisher, and the publisher hereby disclaims any responsibility for them.

The author of this book does not dispense medical advice or prescribe the use of any technique as a form of treatment for physical, emotional, or medical problems without the advice of a physician, either directly or indirectly. The intent of the author is only to offer information of a general nature to help you in your quest for emotional and spiritual well-being. In the event you use any of the information in this book for yourself, which is your constitutional right, the author and the publisher assume no responsibility for your actions.

Printed in the United States of America.

ISBN: 978-1-4525-9001-1 (sc)
ISBN: 978-1-4525-9003-5 (hc)
ISBN: 978-1-4525-9002-8 (e)

Library of Congress Control Number: 2014900546

Balboa Press rev. date: 01/29/2014

CONTENTS

Preface ix
Introduction xiii

Chapter 1   What Is a Psychiatric Problem and What Is Not 1
Chapter 2   Is Mental Illness Inherited? 13
Chapter 3   The Phenomenon of Transference 32
Chapter 4   Types of Mental Illness 38
Chapter 5   Choosing and Changing Providers; What Therapy Is
            All About 58
Chapter 6   What a Reasonable Person May Expect From
            Psychotherapy (Talk Therapy) 70
Chapter 7   Attitudes to Psychopharmacotherapy (Medication) 84
Chapter 8   What a Reasonable Person Can Expect from Medication 92
Chapter 9   How to Save a Buck (or Two) 108
Chapter 10 The Skinny on Side Effects 119
Chapter 11 Medications in Schizophrenia 134
Chapter 12 How to Talk so Your Provider Will Listen 145
Chapter 13 How to Tell Your Story 159
Chapter 14 It's Your Life 176
Chapter 15 How to Manage Your Provider 193
Chapter 16 Motivation and How to Enhance it 208
Chapter 17 Effort is Necessary for a Full Life 221
Chapter 18 Controlling Your Moods 235
Chapter 19 "Getting Stuck"; Professionalism for Patients 258
Chapter 20 Responsibility in Mental Illness 269

Chapter 21	Attitudes of Providers	279
Chapter 22	How to Make a Geographic Move without Running Out of Your Meds	304
Chapter 23	How to Talk to a Mentally Ill Family Member	314
Chapter 24	Particular Situations	342
Chapter 25	What Form Does Your Wealth Come In?	355
Chapter 26	Ending Treatment	364
Chapter 27	Hopes for the Future	380
Chapter 28	Summary and Farewell	387

To All those who Dream of being free of upsetting illness, this book is dedicated

PREFACE

I have been working in the field of psychiatry for over twenty years, in which time I have treated over ten thousand people spread over the eastern half of the United States. I have treated this many people because most of the work I have done has been by contract, usually from four to eight months in a given locality. I have also been a consumer of mental health services for over forty years as I write this in the spring of 2013. So I am well acquainted with both sides of the professional desk (the patient's side and the provider's side).

The purpose of this book is to help patients and their families navigate the sometimes bewildering world of being a mental health consumer. I remember when I started on my career as a patient, how puzzling it all was to me. I am going to show the reader a little of what goes on in the mind of the provider, as well as some tips so my readers may be smarter consumers of psychiatric services.

I will begin with a discussion of what is a psychiatric disorder and what is not. This is because not everybody who gets a 'bump' in life (by 'bump' I mean some negative eventuality or loss – a person loses a job, undergoes a divorce, sustains the death or significant illness or disability of themselves or of an important family member) – not everyone who undergoes such a happening is unable to carry on, thank God. Many people excuse their bad feelings as entirely understandable given the external events just mentioned. And indeed, that is a reasonable point of view, <u>if</u> the person can return to their previous state of decent functioning within a reasonable period of time. Normal grief is said to reasonably impair functioning for up to six months. That does not mean that feelings of sadness or loss are over at that point. But people can function. A person with persistent inability to resume daily functioning after a loss may easily come to psychiatric care.

Then there are other people who have an illness which they inherit, or a predisposition which may be inherited. A prototype of such a kind of illness is schizophrenia. Then in between those two, there are other illnesses which are partially genetic, which may have to do with early brain insult, and which may be partially learned (environmental) as well. A prototype of this type of illness is bipolar disorder. So the question, is mental illness heritable? is worth investigating at some length.

Then we come to discussing the phenomenon of transference whereby someone notes a similarity between a previous experience of theirs and their current situation and assumes that the current situation is just like the earlier one – which of course it is not, since the current situation involves different people than the earlier one, the patient is older than they were in the previous situation, etc. But this phenomenon of transference is responsible for much pain and suffering for the patient, so it, too, will be investigated at some length.

In Chapter 4 we talk about the types of mental illnesses that exist and in Chapter 5 we talk about choosing and changing providers. We also talk about the phenomenon of "split therapy", whereby the patient sees a physician rarely for their medications and sees a therapist more frequently for their psychotherapy.

In Chapter 6 we have a discussion of what a reasonable person can expect from psychotherapy (which is talk therapy), in Chapter 7 attitudes to medication, and in Chapter 8 what a reasonable person can expect from medication. More about medications follows in the next 4 chapters. In Chapter 13 we have a discussion of why the patient's history is so important, how to tell that story and the importance of diagnosis to the patient and to the provider.

Next in Chapter 14 we have some important decisions that the patient must make in life, and a discussion from the patient's perspective of suicidality. Chapter 15 concerns enlisting the help of providers with third parties such as an employer or school and some tips for the patient as to how to manage their providers (which is really about how to manage the time with the provider to get the maximum benefit from it). Chapter 16 concerns motivation towards psychiatric treatment, and how to make motivation more positive. Chapter 17 is a chapter about the effort that is necessary for a patient to invest in their care if they are to get the most out of it. Chapter 18 discusses controlling one's feelings and one's moods and also has a section about visiting the emergency room. Chapter 19 has a portion concerning getting "stuck" and about professionalism for patients (I will explain what I mean). Chapter 20 concerns responsibility in mental illness and Chapter 21 is about attitudes of providers; I would suggest this chapter is more for them. Chapter 22 is about how to make a geographic move (that is a move in which the patient has to change both their provider and their insurance plan) without running out of medications. Chapter 23 is to help families communicate better with their mentally ill family member. Chapter 24 has sections about treatment of mental illness and pregnancy and treatment before and after elective surgery and drug interactions involving psychotropics (psychiatric medications). Chapter 25 is titled 'A Bit of Philosophy – What Form Does Your Wealth Come In?' Some people have a lot of money but no time, while others have the reverse – a lot of time but little money. It is also about changing public attitudes and the importance given to psychotropic medications in non-psychiatric settings. Chapter 26 covers ending treatment, getting support, and how to feather your recovery nest. Chapter 27 is about hopes for the future of psychiatry and for the system. Chapter 28 is a summary and farewell chapter.

Thus, I hope to cover the whole gamut of questions from deciding whether something is a psychiatric issue or not to getting into treatment, choosing providers, managing time with those providers and ending treatment. I don't plan to pull punches either for patients or providers. My thesis in writing this book is that the people on the two sides of the desk need to work together better, and I hope might start some progress in this direction. Also, I believe that most patients, like most people, have almost limitless potential, of which at present we bring forth only a tiny fraction. We must learn to think, not of what is probable, but of what is possible, and stretch ourselves, patients and providers alike, to reach for our dreams until we hold them in our hands.

INTRODUCTION

My recovery story

My illness began quite suddenly when I was in the third or Major Clinical year of a prestigious medical school in New York City when I was 22. Looking back at it all now, I can see that the problem began at least four months earlier when I began to have difficulty sleeping on nights when I was not on call. I was living with my alcoholic and poly drug addicted mother. She got her drugs, as I found out years later, by being the patient of 4 or 5 doctors at the same time, all of whom gave her prescriptions for narcotics for her arthritis and a potentially addictive calmant for her nerves. She got reasonable doses from each doctor, who never suspected that there were several others providing her with similar prescriptions, and so she had a plentiful supply. Plus, she drank upwards of a fifth of whiskey per day which she ordered over the telephone from several local liquor stores. My sister later got our mother into many rehabs (including 9 in the last year of her life), but by then she was past helping. My sister was older than I but in the same class of medical school that I was (we thought we might make it through school if we were together so we could support each other). Unfortunately, my sister had a nervous breakdown over the 4th of July weekend that year. My mother became impossible to deal with when my sister fell ill, and I had the feeling that I would break into a thousand pieces under the stress. I lasted until the 26th of October.

That was the day I was first hospitalized. In one day I went from being a third year medical student to being a creature that in those days, over 40 years ago now, had almost no rights—a mental patient. And for the next ten years my life was hell. I would go to bed sane, and wake up bonkers. The medical school, in spite of having put me on a year's leave of absence and telling me that I could come back to school, did not let me come back a year (and one more hospitalization) later. So I went back to school at the Catholic University of Louvain in Belgium, and I finally graduated, not in 1974 (my original trajectory), but in 1981. By the time I reached the care there of Professor Guillemot who found me my sanity, I was on my fourth hospitalization; I was taken to his hospital after a very serious suicide attempt – I was found in hemorrhagic shock after I had cut through all the flexor tendons of my left thumb, though I left the nearby radial nerve intact. I remember thinking how beautiful and amazingly clever the human hand is, and I could not cut the nerve.

I had a hospitalization at that time that lasted nearly 8 months. I had several more over the next few years; they got shorter and shorter, until the last, about a year and a half before I graduated, was only for two weeks. I also had two more near-miss suicide attempts, both when I was already in the hospital for depression. A nurse left the pharmacy door open and I stole 30 barbiturate pills and took them late that night, and I did have a cardiac arrest once it was all absorbed; but having fallen in the hall I was taken to the local hospital, and staff were there to revive me when I arrested. I later went out on a pass by taking the bus into town and bought a serrated bread knife and returned to the mental hospital grounds and cut my own throat. I cut the jugular vein but missed the carotid artery by about a quarter of an inch, and then I walked back to my building soaked in blood. It seemed to me that a nice, calm, non-destructive part of me took over so that I was able to make it over bumpy ground, blood pouring from the cut in the jugular, without falling, and then I was taken to the regular hospital and stitched up.

The good Professor was very patient with me; between these various admissions to the psychiatric hospital I managed to hang on and get through school. Then I came back to the U.S. and did manage to get a pediatric residency program to accept me, only to discover after 6 months that I just could not manage the 100+ hours a week work schedule which was expected then, but which has been outlawed in New York State since. (The daughter of a well-placed staffer on <u>The New York Times</u> died because she was given two medications known to be incompatible, by two young doctors too exhausted to be able to think. The grieving father did sue the hospital but he did also push until a law was passed that no young doctor could be made to tolerate extraordinary sleep deprivation. But that was after my time.)

I will say that in December 1982, a year later, I was hospitalized for mania again, but this time I was given an anticonvulsant that was just beginning to be used as a mood stabilizer, called carbamazepine (brand name Tegretol®), which was added to my lithium. After two doses, I knew it would change my life, and so ended my decade of hell.

For the next fifteen years I was better, but still not very steady. In 1983, seeing a doctor whom I hardly knew, I told him truthfully I was not suicidal, but did not bother to contradict him when he said "I suppose to you life hardly seems worth living." So he called my sister in Rochester and told her that unless she came to New York City to pick me up and take me back with her, he felt he would have to hospitalize me again, which might spell the end of all my hopes. My sister, being the trooper she is, came and took me back to Rochester, where I was soon started on the Preventive Medicine Residency. So I got a Masters in Public Health, and also did six months in Rhode Island to make up for my broken internship.

The professors at the University of Rochester encouraged me to think of a Doctorate in Public Health. I was accepted into Johns Hopkins and Tulane University. Hopkins is a much larger school with many more course offerings, but having been in a big school before (the New York medical school) I was attracted to the idea of going to a smaller school where if I had difficulty they would be unlikely to just dump me. Plus, it seemed that Tulane had some connections in the field of worldwide public health, where I could use the fact that I was bilingual in French and spoke decent Spanish. Both of these languages have become rusty since then but at the time it seemed to my advantage to choose Tulane.

When I got to New Orleans my new psychiatrist suggested I work part time as a psychiatrist in one of the State mental health clinics. "That's a nice idea," I replied, "but I have no training in psychiatry!" I had left the New York school before reaching the psychiatry rotation, and though Louvain has two years of lectures, no patient experience is required. But, said my doctor, my lack of experience was not a problem in this instance. He thought I would be good 'doing psychiatry'. And the State system was in crisis. Some months before, the Louisiana Governor, anxious to resolve his fiscal crunch, had slated about half the State clinics for closure. A paranoid schizophrenic patient, faced with the projected closure of the clinic he had been attending without difficulty for 30 years, expressed his dismay by shooting 3 bystanders, killing two and severely wounding the third. A public outcry followed, and the order to keep the clinics open went out 24 hours before they were due to be closed. The doctors who worked in those clinics had found themselves other jobs in anticipation of the closures, but the clinics could not run without physicians, so the State was hiring physicians with licenses but not requiring any psychiatric training. I got a job there, and I continued working for the State until I completed my Tulane Doctorate in Public Health, almost three years.

When I had been working in the State system about 2 months, my supervisor, the Regional Director for the nine clinics in the New Orleans area, took me out to lunch and told me he had read all my workups and thought I had a gift for psychiatry. He said he would like to help me get psychiatry residency training. This made me very conflicted; on the one hand, two months of working without training in a place which was in an uproar had made me fall in love with psychiatry; but on the other hand, most of the psychiatrists whom I had met struck me as egotistical, arrogant bastards. Plus, my beloved Belgian Professor had told me I should never be a psychiatrist because I would identify with patients too much. After a year of soul searching, my love of the work won out. I accepted my supervisor's offer, and landed a residency in Philadelphia.

During my residency an unfortunate thing happened. The psychiatrist who ran the main inpatient ward, who had been diagnosed bipolar previously but who rejected the diagnosis and refused treatment, had a manic crisis and was taken to another facility in handcuffs for hospitalization at 3 AM. According to an attending who liked me, this made the leaders of the residency very uneasy. They thought about the fact that I had said I had bipolar illness and they would not like to be taken by surprise if I got sick, as they were by this attending. The fact that I had always been forthright about my illness, accepting treatment and complying with it religiously, seemed to escape their notice. The chief resident took up my cause, saying that one could not assume that because something happened to one patient with a given disorder, the same thing would happen to another. The hospital was also in an uproar with many people not wanting to do what they should (the place filed for bankruptcy two years after I left and the layoffs started when I was there, together with a general atmosphere of noncooperation and mistrust) so the faculty decided the only way to guarantee me extra supervision was to put me on probation. Now, probation is generally used as a sanction for people caught drinking or using drugs on the job, or behaving in some flagrantly unacceptable way towards patients (coming on to them, for instance). None of these reasons applied to me, and I never got an objectively justified explanation for the faculty's actions. I was on probation for 8 months, earned my way off, and for the last two years of my residency had no trouble.

But the effect was still there. Having been officially on probation early in my residency, I was unable, despite enthusiastic recommendations from several preceptors, to get a good permanent job in one place when my training was completed. So I worked a succession of temporary contracts all over the Eastern U.S. By some I was called the 'Mary Poppins' of the temporary contract world in psychiatry. This continued for 15 years. I heard what I call "The Speech" (it has 3 elements: #1, you have changed my life; #2, I will never be able to thank you enough, and #3, I will not forget you for as long as I live) about 200 times in those 15 years, and I got a total of 7 State licenses, all with full disclosure of my past as a patient. I am particularly proud of being granted the New York State license because I was the first physician in any specialty to have been honest about my diagnosis, and to have gotten a license to practice on that basis. Before I came, the New York Board of Medical Licensure had no record of being asked to license a physician with Bipolar disorder. From the numbers in surrounding states, it was estimated there were 2000 bipolar doctors practicing in New York State, but not a single one of them had ever admitted to having the mental illness, despite the fact that non-disclosure is "under penalty of perjury." I applied for the New York license, and then, receiving no reply, worked in other states (LA and PA) and got the New York license after11 YEARS of working elsewhere.

Then in 2009 I was diagnosed with a benign (non-invasive, non-metastasizing) brain tumor which was irradiated in 2010. The radiation did affect my brain function; it was about 7 or 8 months before I could say my Social Security Number or my most frequently used credit card number from memory accurately, and I have had an exceptional memory for digits my whole life. Also, while I am extremely grateful that the tumor is benign and will not kill me. a newcomer tissue inside the skull presses on the surrounding normal tissue which belongs there, and so may interfere with its functioning, and this tumor, pressing as it was on the part of the brain controlling balance, made me very unsteady on my feet. I was born with brain damage and cerebral palsy on my left side, and the tumor interfered with balance on the right.

At first I tried to keep going with my many moves, always going to wherever I had a work contract. But in 2011 I had a bad fall for no good reason (I did not trip over an obstacle or slip on a wet floor) and broke my right arm into 3 pieces, which required 8 pins to be put in to put my arm back together. Actually., in 2011 I fell a total of 19 times. So I obviously had to give up moving around so much.

So I came back to Rochester. It took me a while to get used to the idea that I wasn't going to look for another work contract as a psychiatrist. Although I could still listen to a story, make a diagnosis, and propose the treatment, I can no longer promise to walk down long corridors and not fall, and I did not succeed in finding an employer who would be willing to have call the receptionist, and say "Marie, this is Dr. Clark. I have finished with Robert, so could you please ask Martha to come to my office." Whereupon Marie would say, "Martha, the doctor is ready for you now, so please go to the fourth door on the left, and knock as you go in."

As for my mental illness, I am doing well. My last hospitalization was for 5 days shortly after 9/11/2001. I take my medication religiously, get my blood drawn every 6 months, and see the doctor about every 4 months. The clinic has a requirement that I be in therapy there, so I see the therapist once in 6-8 weeks. My mental illness is now no more burdensome than a somewhat elevated cholesterol or a low thyroid (for those conditions also I take medication, get my blood work done and see a doctor periodically).

A great deal of who you are is determined by how you see yourself. I will never forget receiving a welfare benefits card for New York, which arrived on the same day as a contract to work in Pennsylvania establishing a new inpatient psychiatry service for two months, for which I would receive $15,000 a month. So I was either a mentally ill person totally unable to earn a living, or someone who had a good earnings capability indeed. You can guess which path I took.

When I was in my twenties, I used to haunt the Self-Help sections of bookstores, thinking "Surely someone who has been through this already has written about how to find my way out of this illness!" (Nobody talked of recovery back then.) I vowed all those years ago that if I survived to tell the tale, I would write a book for those who follow. The last thing in my mind then was to become a psychiatrist, but it is the best qualification for writing this book. This is the book I sought over 40 years ago, but could not find, because it had not been written.

I was until recently trying to start a business as a life coach, (that is a person who helps reasonably healthy people find solutions and make changes in their lives that would make them happier.) Life coaching does not require a license, and clients could be anywhere, and they could contact me by email. My Author website is DrSWClark.com and my email is DRSWClark@gmail.com.

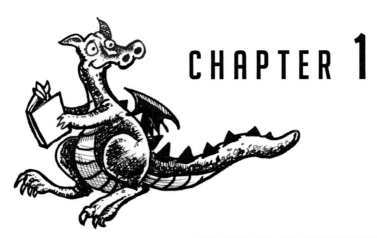

CHAPTER 1

WHAT IS A PSYCHIATRIC PROBLEM AND WHAT IS NOT

Psychiatric illness as now defined in the United States comprises almost all abnormalities of thought, feeling, mood, or behavior. For anybody who feels that psychiatrists make themselves into arbiters of what is abnormal thought without legitimate claim to do so, I will immediately give some examples of abnormal thought. Supposing your patient says to you, "I won the beauty contest, and the runner up was a lizard." Or supposing they maintain against all logic, as one patient of mine whom I will call Sandra did, that she was the mother of two sons, one of whom was currently the Pope and the other of whom was the President of the United States. The lack of an age difference between President Obama and herself did not deter her; she was his mother. In other words, she had a delusion. I think these two examples show quite well that these patients had a disorder of their thinking.

Now to get back to the main thread of my argument. An abnormality is variously defined as something that is far from the norm and/or something that results in trouble to the person who is behaving in that particular fashion. It covers learning disabilities and attention deficit disorders for youngsters (though we are increasingly finding that people who had

Attention Deficit Disorder as children do not necessarily 'grow out of it' as they reach adulthood – people are more or less able to adapt to it. Although over diagnosis occurs in children, increasingly, larger numbers of adults feel that they are better sticking to their stimulant medication now that the disorder has, as it were, come out of the closet and is something that is recognized. More adults seem to go on taking medication, if effective, who perhaps used to suffer in silence.)

Other mental illnesses are depression and other major mood disorders for adults and children, personality disorders in adults, disorders of aging and dementia for older adults, schizophrenia and other psychoses for children and adults, anxiety disorders in people of almost any age (these are actually the most numerous; the most common anxiety disorder is irrational anxiety when a person is asked to make a short presentation to their peers.) Also substance abuse, be it of a legal prescription substance or an illegal substance, and most recently, criminal behavior such as repeated killing or repeated sexual offenses. The repeated factor here is very important, because one sexual offense is unfortunate but is not usually enough to cause the individual to be registered as a sex offender. Being registered as a sex offender is reserved for people who are repeat offenders, who thus have established a pattern of sexual offenses.

We have here considerable spectra of pathology -- there is a wide variety of thoughts feelings and behavior which is considered abnormal, and which may become the focus of treatment.

I myself was hit with a bad case of manic depressive illness (Bipolar I is the newer nomenclature) when I was in my early twenties. My own feeling in those first few years was that I would go to bed sane and wake up bonkers. When the illness first struck, I was in the second half of my third year (which is called the major clinical year) in medical school in Columbia University in New York City. I was put on a year's leave of absence with the understanding that if I were better in a year I could come back to school, but when the time came around for me to re-enter school, I was told that my place had been given to the fiancée of a classmate so she could come in from Indiana and join her betrothed and they could live together in New York. It was explained to me that at that time (this being the early 70's) that 75% of the male medical school students who left school for any reason, returned, but only 2% of the females who left school ever came back, so they figured there was a 98% chance that I would never come back. Thus, they felt justified in giving away my place. After another year of struggling to find where I should go, I went to the Catholic University of Louvain in Belgium, which is world famous and which has been teaching medicine (with one short interruption during World War II) since 1425. Their reaction to my telling them that I had been a student at Columbia was to say "Why would you, as an American citizen, go to Bogota?" – in other words they thought I meant I had been to the country of Colombia, because they had never heard of Columbia University in New York City. I did graduate 6 ½ years later from the Catholic University of Louvain in Belgium.

People have a variety of reasons for having particular symptoms. They may have absorbed a negative view of life as young children and not even realized they were doing so. Or, they may have had some experiences in their teenage years or young adulthood which caused them to feel that they were fundamentally unlovable or could not succeed in life or were destined to have a particular form of difficulty. Patients need to learn that only if they will challenge these fundamental assumptions of their own inadequacy or unlovability can they succeed.

I will say from experience (both professional and personal) that the closer one gets to challenging these fundamental assumptions, the more painful the work can get, because much of one's own personality and approach to life was formed by the desire to avoid this pain in the first place. So if one is not willing to turn around and look at that pain and challenge the assumptions that underlie it, as most people, even the ones in therapy, may not be, they are not likely to get a good result of their treatment.

Being a psychiatric patient is a lot of work on the theoretical, philosophical level.

I once had a patient who was a self-possessed man who presented well; he was well-dressed and soft-spoken. On the initial visit he said he was depressed because he had been fired from his job two months before. I found out that he had been fired from his previous four jobs. I then went into a more detailed inquiry as to how these firings came about, and we discovered together that there was a pattern in his life.

He would take a job for which he was qualified, would initially do well. He would then undertake more than the description of his job entailed, would become increasingly annoyed with requests to do work that <u>was</u> originally in his job description, and finally would be so uncooperative that his boss would fire him.

It turned out that this man had an underlying assumption that "nobody is fair", which was based on his perception of his father's behavior. He would do more than he was asked to do, and then refuse to do the work he was originally asked to do, in order to provoke the firings, which would then substantiate his contention that a fair boss did not exist. When we were able to challenge that assumption, and when he was able to agree with me that some bosses may be stinkers, but it <u>was possible</u> for a boss to be fair-minded, he no longer needed to substantiate the idea that all bosses were unfair, and so he no longer needed to provoke his current boss to fire him. But the patient had to work a great deal, especially to challenge his underlying assumption that no-one is ever fair. It was very painful to change his whole view of the outside world. Because he was willing to do this, he was able to arrive at the possibility of having an employer who was decent and therefore his own work-site turbulence could settle down. I will add that he then met and married a very wonderful, stable woman who worked in the county library system, and that for as long as I knew them they were happy together. So being willing to challenge those underlying assumptions, painful as it may be, can certainly have a good payoff.

My point is that a person who comes to see a psychiatrist saying "I am depressed because I lost my job two months ago" and who will not look beyond that very simple explanation of their woes, will get out of the therapeutic situation what they bring to it -- a very simple solution to their problem which may or may not solve it on a deep level, probably not. This is because being depressed when one is out of work is a nearly universal condition; people need to solve problems on a more individual and personal level if they expect the solution to be long-lasting.

It is conventionally said that in psychosis (notably in schizophrenia) when the thought process is broken down and illogical, insight-oriented work is bound to fail. There have been a few notable exceptions to this, but certainly most therapists could not do insight-oriented work with most psychotic patients. One psychotic patient is not the same as another, and the general areas that are problems for one individual psychotic patient may be different from the areas that are problems for another, but certainly it is true that in most circumstances, schizophrenics and other psychotics will not be asked to do insight-oriented work. But this does not mean that they do not do work. What they work on is learning to discriminate between what is reality and what is a misperception brought on by their illness, so that they can at least some of the time join consensual reality. They may also work on things such as an adult work ethic that they did not learn as a young person because of the onset of illness. I would like to state that I do believe that there is immense creativity in many people with schizophrenia, and I do not advocate stamping out all their differences from us. But if they want to navigate daily life, they must cultivate some ability to process thought in the ordinary logic the rest of us use.

I have said that psychiatric illness these days is viewed as encompassing many different disorders of thought, feeling (emotion), mood, affect or behavior. 'Affect' is what is observable about a person's apparent mood state. Usually in psychiatry 'mood' means what the person <u>says</u> they feel. Affect is what we can observe. For instance, if somebody's old demented grandfather dies, they say they feel sad but we may not notice much reaction at all, especially if they haven't seen their relative for decades. Or, a person may smile and look very relieved if a family member had been in great pain before they died, but may say they feel sad. They feel sad because of their loss, but they feel relieved for the family member. But the relief may be more visible than the loss, so there is what we call incongruence between mood and affect. To say that mood and affect are congruent means that they match up. The person says they feel happy and they are smiling broadly. Or they say they feel sad and they look sad. That is the normal state of affairs, but, for a variety of reasons mood and affect may not match up, in which case we say they are incongruent.

In any case, psychiatry covers a very broad spectrum of illness. Psychiatric illness has to be distinguished from thoughts, feelings, moods, affects or behaviors which are less than ideal but which are not thought of as part of an illness. One of the most important factors in deciding whether to call something an illness or not is whether the person who exhibits these thoughts, feelings moods etc. is aware that they are a bit off track or not. If the person is aware, particularly if they are able to regain control of themselves, it is less likely to be illness. It is said, for example, that people who have a forgetfulness problem who are <u>aware</u> of it, are probably experiencing the minor forgetfulness that occurs as people age. But the people who are not aware that they're forgetting things – they are the ones that may very well be starting to be demented.

Then there is the question of the repetition of the poor thoughts or bad feelings or bad moods or difficulty thinking or bad behavior – that is, has this something been a one-time thing or is it frequently repeated? If a teenager gets drunk at a party one night, realizes their error, and resolves never to drink again or never to get drunk again, with good effect (meaning he never does get drunk again) then this is not a psychiatric disorder. However, if the teenager grows into an adult who frequently imbibes to excess, they are probably either an alcohol abuser or an alcohol dependent person, depending on how much of a negative effect this drinking to excess has had on their lives. Similarly, if a person overspends to the point where they are somewhat embarrassed, it may not be because of a psychiatric illness. But chances are if they overspend and cause themselves financial difficulty repeatedly, then even if they are not episodically manic (a situation where a person may overspend many times) they will probably benefit from some psychotherapy to determine why they engage in such destructive behavior over and over.

To benefit from psychotherapy, a patient must be willing to invest a considerable amount of time effort and money, and also be able and willing to cast a critical eye over their whole lives and what they have done well and what they have done not so well, with a view to coming up with a plan for how to do better in the future. No psychiatrist and no therapist can "make" someone better unless the patient is also willing to put in a lot of effort of their own. We do have medications these days that help people feel better, that make them calmer, that make them reason in a fairly logical fashion in this world (in other words, we do have medications which help with psychosis quite well), but no one will get better unless they put in effort to do so.

I'm going to put in something here about a small effort a patient can make which could pay them big dividends. This is, keeping an accurate medication history. A school notebook of one subject can be bought in dollar stores or in many grocery stores for about a buck, and this can be used to keep a log of medications.

This is what I would advise a person to do: make a list of all the medications they currently take starting each time with the name of the medicine, the number of milligrams per tablet, and the number of pills taken per dose, and when in the day those doses are taken; for example medication X, ten milligrams, three tablets every morning; or medication Y, 25 milligrams, one tablet morning and evening (twice a day). Then, if and when a doctor changes the dosage or changes the medication, or if a new medication is added or an existing one is discontinued, this is noted with the date in the log. For example, a person might write "1/21/13: medication X discontinued; medication Z started, five milligram tablets, two at bedtime." The patient should make every effort to note down why the change was made, for example, "medication X discontinued due to a rash on the trunk, or due to low white cell count appearing in the blood" or whatever is the reason. It is worth the patient's effort to ask why the doctor makes the change and to record it.

There is no necessity to record refills if the refills consist of more of the same medicine at the same milligram strength and the same daily dose. So it may be that a patient will continue for months or even years without entries in the log. Things like allergies should be noted carefully. If the person gets an upset stomach and vomits shortly after taking a given medicine that's not an allergy (that doesn't involve the immune system) but it is an intolerance; the way to note this is medication X discontinued due to patient's report of vomiting one hour after taking each dose. (Patients can obviously think that there are other things which could make them vomit, such as a true stomach problem, but these would not occur always with the same relationship to when the last dose of the medication was taken. In other words, if somebody is throwing up because they have gastroenteritis (an infection in the stomach) then the vomiting will occur when the infection is bad, not always one hour after they take the particular medication X.)

The reason I am advocating from the very first chapter of this book that a person keep a log of their medication history is two-fold. First of all, if a smart doctor has a record of the medications that a patient has taken for a given condition and the reaction to each medication, it is possible after several medication trials to be able to predict what other reactions might be like, and to use this most helpfully in making further medication choices. It is said that doctor number four is often so much smarter than his or her predecessors – just because he or she knows what happened when the patient took the medicines suggested by doctors one, two and three.

Secondly, if a new medication comes on the market which seems likely to benefit the patient, but being new, is under patent and is extremely expensive, the doctor can often make the insurance give assent to paying for the medication if the patient can substantiate having tried the older stuff and finding it unsatisfactory. But to do that, the patient needs to have the medication names, the milligram strength per pill, and the number taken per day for how long (in weeks or months) to show that a good trial of the older medicines has already been done. It is quite usual for insurance companies not to even consider paying for the newer, possibly improved, more expensive medication if they can't point to an adequate (a big enough dose for a long enough time) trial of at least three medicines which are available in generic form and which have proven unsatisfactory. After three unsatisfactory trials of a cheaper medicine, the patient becomes eligible for taking the newer more expensive compound.

It is a good idea also to record laboratory values and/or other diagnostic tests and surgical procedures by date in the log book. Diagnostic tests could be written in a different color of ink and surgical procedures perhaps with a red bracket around them. Anything which the doctor or doctors say about their reasons for choosing a particular procedure or a particular test should also be recorded.

To do as I have outlined would require perhaps five minutes when the patient gets home from the doctor's visit and what the doctor said and the change the doctor has made are fresh in the patient's mind. Since most of us, thank God, don't see a doctor every day or every week, this is not particularly burdensome. But the benefits to the patient who has a thorough history can be enormous. Imagine if you will how discouraging it is for a doctor who cares deeply about patients to hear that a patient has been a psychiatric patient for twenty years and has "been on everything" but does not know the names, dosages, how long they took the medicine, and does not even particularly remember why a medicine was discontinued. People say "I got a terrible allergy once, I nearly died" but they cannot tell the doctor which medication caused that allergy. A doctor may try by suggesting names of things it could have been, but if the patient doesn't know, it is very hard to find the history in a very thick chart, and it is hard to write to another town and get the medical records department to release information to the present doctor. So, if the patient has a list of their own pertinent records, this can be worth its weight in gold. If you will give your doctor the medication history outlined above, his or her present and future decisions in your case regarding medications can be immeasurably better and you will help yourself to a faster and smoother recovery.

I'll give you an example from my own history when I was first hospitalized after a manic break in 1972 which was not recognized as such and was thought of as an "acute schizophrenic episode" (a diagnosis which does not exist anymore). I was put on Thorazine[R], whose generic name is chlorpromazine. Since I struggled mightily every morning to get up, get washed, and get dressed in time for breakfast (which I thought of as normal, and therefore desirable, behavior) the doctor kept increasing the dose. A few days later I spoke to him and protested these dose increases. His reply was that he would continue to increase it up to three grams (3,000 milligrams) a day. I knew enough about the pharmacology of psychotropics to know that 3,000 milligrams or three grams is a potentially lethal dose of chlorpromazine. So I asked him, in some horror, would he actually risk killing me? To which he said yes, he wanted "a response to the medication". I found out from him that his idea of a response would be that I would not get up one morning – that I would spend the day in bed. So I did – resenting it all day.

During the time that I was trying desperately and with increasing difficulty to get up every morning before breakfast, I would get out of bed and hurry to the bathroom and as I got to the bathroom I would pass out because my blood pressure would drop suddenly and an insufficient circulation to my brain would cause me to lose consciousness. I would wake up with one foot against the commode, the other foot against the sink, and my head either up against the shower or against the door. I would feel my limbs to try and find out if the fall had broken something, and then manage to get up slowly and resume my washing.

This was all because I did not realize that when you take a medication which can cause orthostatic hypotension, which means a sudden drop in blood pressure; you may faint. A few times I asked the staff to measure my blood pressure after I had fallen, but it took them several minutes to get the blood pressure cuff which was kept at the other end of the hallway, and by that time my blood pressure was normal. So they never documented orthostatic hypotension in my case.

When I went to Belgium some years later, I noticed that one of my medications that I was given in the hospital after losing a sink full of blood when I cut my wrists was Largactyl[R]. I inquired, and found out that this was the French-language brand name for chlorpromazine.

On the morning after my admission, about a week after my suicide attempt (I spent the first few days in a hospital with my left arm in a cast after surgical tendon repair) I saw the director of the Clinique Regina Pacis, Doctor Guillemot, and I complained about a sensation of booming pain in the back of my head with each heartbeat, and told him that I was very sensitive to orthostatic hypotension. I also told him that I was experiencing a feeling that I was going to faint every time I bent down, for example to lace up my shoe, or to pick up a coin I had dropped.

Because I was able to tell him what dose of Thorazine[R] I had been on and what effect it had on me (including describing passing out every morning in front of my bathroom sink), he immediately discontinued the Largactyl[R] and put me on another anti-psychotic, which he then explained is used as a supplemental treatment to the mood stabilizer; he had put me on Lithium. He took me off the chlorpromazine because I could tell him that I had taken it before and what the result of taking it before had been. I was also able to discuss dosages. So even though I did not have a written record as I am advising my readers to have, I had the evidence that giving me chlorpromazine was not a good idea. This is much more effective than "I didn't like that stuff" because many people's initial reactions to taking psychotropics is not favorable and because I gave him the medical reason #1 (namely frequent drug-induced fainting spells) for discontinuing this drug. This shows the importance of putting down exactly why you did not like taking something. And if you complain of a known side effect of that particular medication, you are very likely to be listened to.

Many people come to psychiatric care saying they want to change the way somebody else behaves. Unfortunately, it is not possible to do therapy by proxy, generally speaking. If you come to a therapist saying you want to change how your mother behaves, the therapist will probably ask you why her behavior upsets you or in what ways you want to see change, and will set about showing you how you can react differently and establish a new pattern of response to your mother's behavior. This can oftentimes bring about change, but not unless you are willing to work on your own response. I have often said that you can change yourself and you can change how you interpret things, but if you're waiting for another person to change, it may be a long wait.

Many therapists conclude that some people don't really want to change; they want the right to complain about their present situation without any necessity of effort on their own part. Some people do seem to want to blame other people.

I will say a little here about being supportive to patients. We know as doctors and as therapists, that patients need some support in order to feel comfortable telling us the painful or embarrassing parts of their story; we must show that we understand the difficulty the patient is in, or the patient won't want to come back. But we must also sustain and cultivate whatever motivation the patient has to change. And being overly understanding/supportive of the situation as it is now, saying things like "Anybody would understand why you have difficulty" or "Of course you feel bad about (whatever)", does not sustain and empower the motivation to change. So a careful balance must be maintained, more toward support if the patient is having increasing difficulty in life, and more toward motivating change if the patient is in a relatively good place. As we will discuss in Chapter 11, motivation is a key element in encouraging the patient to change, so that their present difficulties are no longer so dominant, and therefore motivation must be sustained throughout the treatment.

So, to sum up; a pattern of thought, thinking, mood, attitude (by which I mean, something which might be more philosophical and less factual), or behavior can be considered a psychiatric illness when it is repeated, and when it causes difficulties with others, or with the law, or with the patient's internal idea of themselves, or effects their physical health. Most one-time poor decision making, if it is truly one-time, can be considered a learning experience which is not a psychiatric illness.

We have discussed a little why it is that therapists and doctors may not always be very supportive. It may be because they want to sustain what motivation the patient has, and perhaps increase it, so that they will change further in ways that are good for their emotional and mental and physical health, and good for their social and intellectual future. There are doctors, one has to admit, who do not empathize with their patients, and they also come across as not very supportive, which is a shame.

I'm going to finish with an example of how external circumstances can sometimes contribute greatly, even create, psychiatric illness. I knew a man once who had a mild stuttering disorder. This is speech pathology, but any speech pathology can create neurosis, and low self-esteem. Let's say the man's first name was Piper. He worked as an illustrator, and rarely spoke to more than one or two people at a time. He was a laid back kind of a person, very relaxed in his approach to life, and since he made his living by his drawing, and not by speaking, his mild stuttering did not really cause him any trouble. Also, he was fairly secure in his identity and knew who he was, so he had fairly good self-esteem. So, for him, there was little 'psychiatric fallout' from his speech problem.

Contrast that with someone I'll call Quincy, another man I knew who came from a very well-known prominent family that had had many achievers across the centuries, and for whom there is a very high expectation of achievement from birth onwards. Quincy also had a mild stuttering disorder, but for him the stuttering was a source of continual embarrassment and poor self-esteem and he often changed what he said to avoid the words that made him stutter, and therefore the stuttering had an impact on his personality which Piper's stuttering never had and never would. Quincy had developed neuroses because of his stuttering, because of his coming from a high-achieving high-pressure family and because pressuring Quincy made him stutter more. Quincy was a lecturer in engineering and he had to give his lectures without stuttering if at all possible, which caused him considerable anxiety. And he suffered from low self-esteem as I have noted.

You can understand that all these various factors made Quincy's mild stuttering much more difficult to live with than Piper's was. This should serve as an example of how external factors (meaning factors outside the patient and the patient's psyche) can condition the extent to which a given symptom impacts the patient's life. And so something which in one individual is not a psychiatric problem, for another individual certainly is one, and one for which treatment is very important.

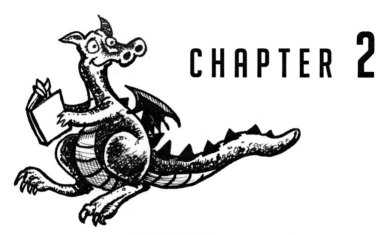

CHAPTER 2

IS MENTAL ILLNESS INHERITED?

This is a huge question, and this book will only skim along the top of some of the research on it. Nevertheless, it is important to address.

There are a few rare mental illness conditions that are unequivocally (and exclusively) genetic. Huntington's chorea is one example. The disease is named for the chorea, or twisting, undulating "dance" that occurs when the illness reaches moderate severity. It is one of a small number of illnesses in which a) every person who gets the disease has a particular identifiable genetic abnormality and b) every person who has the genetic abnormality eventually gets the illness. Unfortunately the disease manifests itself, often, in the forties or fifties, an age at which most people have already had children and grandchildren. Now, let us suppose that your father or grandfather has recently been diagnosed with Huntington's. (Women can get the illness too). You know the illness will progress with increasing motor and then some visceral (organ) difficulties, over decades, perhaps, until death – unless of course they die earlier of something else. There is really no effective treatment, other than to support people as much as we can.

Let us suppose that your grandfather is found to have one abnormal (Huntington's) gene and one normal gene. Yet he has the illness, because the abnormal gene is <u>dominant</u> – only one abnormal gene is necessary to have the illness; to be illness-free, a person must have <u>two</u> normal genes. Another way of saying this is to say there is no symptom-free, disease-free carrier of Huntington's.

Let us say further that to those who know how to do it, the test is very straightforward, and there is every reason to believe that two of your blood samples sent to two different labs would come up with the same result. So – would you want to find out if you inherited the abnormal gene, or not? If you're a child, it's likely that your parents will be deciding to test or not test you <u>for</u> you.

There is an argument for not testing. Obviously, you would not have the gene unless your parent who is the child of this grandfather inherited it from him. And even if your parent has it, you may or may not have inherited it in your turn.

Your insurance risk skyrockets as soon as it is known, if you do have Huntington's. And you would know your fate as far as developing this debilitating illness. But a lot of people might choose not to engage with you, from college admissions to employers, and a person might choose not to marry you. I realize it might be simpler to deceive a fiancé(e) than insurance, because the insurers can get hold of medical records.

The blood test can offer certainty, but would you want to know for sure?

One possibility is to find out the test results of your parent, who is a child of the afflicted grandparent. If he or she gets tested and you know that he or she does <u>not</u> have the gene, you won't get it, but if he or she <u>does</u> have the abnormal gene, you may or may not have inherited the abnormality from him or her. And, of course, if you don't know whether your parent, as the child of an afflicted individual, inherited the illness, you don't know where you stand at all. If your parent, child of your afflicted grandparent, survives to say, 75 without getting it, you probably have not inherited it, but by the time your parent is 75, you'd be over 40 yourself, and your children would have been born.

Now, you may wonder why Huntington's is being discussed in a book about mental illness. Huntington's patients may get very depressed, and/or irritable, and/or angry (after all, would you like to have inherited a gradually progressive brain disorder?) and sometimes they can be violent. Even when the genetics is simple, straightforward, and absolutely certain, the social problems that can be created are anything but.

There are other illnesses which are candidates for being genetic (heritable) afflictions, but for which the genetic basis is much less clear. Bipolar illness runs in some families though the majority of first time diagnosed patients may <u>not</u> have affected relatives. It is unclear how many patients have bipolar illness in the family because while in the 70's very few people were diagnosed as bipolar (it was underdiagnosed), today, 97% of the patients in a suburban clinic northwest of Philadelphia (mostly Medicaid and Medicare patients), who walked into my office in my first two weeks at that location told me they were "bipolar". In other words just about everybody in that public clinic <u>thinks</u> they are bipolar. Our estimates of the frequency of illness are perhaps 2% - 4% of the population. This is because many people think that any moodiness or unpredictability is bipolar disorder; it's more complex than that. Also, bipolar disorder is 'sexy' these days.

When I had my first manic break, I was misdiagnosed as schizophrenic. In those days, providers did not think of bipolar disorder very often. When they heard a manic patient speaking loudly and extremely rapidly and by the rapidity and complexity of what they were saying not seeming to make much sense, they tended to assume that the patient had taken a break from reality and was actually psychotic. It is true that when one is manic it does not seem possible to give a short, direct, to-the-point answer to any question. Everything seems connected with everything and the simplest inquiry elicits a very long story. But I have also seen when I have been an observer, that quite a few providers do not know how to listen fast, and so they say that what the patient is saying is nonsensical even though it does make quite a bit of sense if one can process auditory stimuli rapidly. People vary enormously in this ability as in others. I happen to be extremely unusual in that my auditory processing ability in English is matched by only one other person in ten thousand. I am quite limited visually, and other people have different groups of abilities and disabilities or weaknesses.

As I have said before, the official diagnosis when I announced to the doctor that I was leaving and walked out of the hospital was "acute schizophrenic episode", a diagnosis which no longer officially exists under that name. I should explain that I announced to the doctor I was leaving because when I was admitted people sat over me trying to get me to sign a document which began "I understand that under section so-and-so, so-and-so of the mental health laws of the State of New York...". I said several times, over perhaps forty minutes, that I understood nothing of the mental health laws of the State of New York and was far too tired to understand that document at that moment. So I never signed it. Since I had done nothing that would give anybody an excuse to hospitalize me against my will, they had no right to hold me there. I found this out by sneaking down to the telephones on the ground floor (there were no cell 'phones in those days) and calling the American Civil Liberties Union, who told me that I had the right to walk out at any time. I did not wish to be AWOL from a mental hospital (I wanted to get back to medical school in the future) and so I went back to the ward and told the doctor that he'd better write my discharge since he did not wish to have a court case over keeping me in the hospital.

The second go-round came almost a year later, before my second hospitalization. I noticed that there was a repeat of what had happened the first time, namely that I was unable to sleep. The first time, my mind had come unglued when I had had many weeks of sleepless nights. So I bought some over the counter Sominex^R (if you're old enough you may remember the jingle "Safe and restful sleep, sleep, sleep" on the TV ads) and when they didn't work at the recommended dose I took a much larger dose than I should have, quite forgetting the effect of an overdose of Sominex^R (which was, in those days, scopolamine, a cousin of atropine which is a major compound occurring in the brain). The result of an overdose of an atropinic is a very rapid heart rate, a rapid respiratory rate, difficulty focusing on near vision, urinary retention, and in large overdose difficulty standing.

When I was admitted to the hospital the second time I had all these signs and symptoms. But the intern admitting me did not think of a scopolamine overdose. That in itself is regrettable but forgivable. What is not forgivable is not to have asked a twenty-three year old patient who had been fully functional a week earlier if she had been taking anything. I was too befuddled to be able to realize that I should mention it without being asked, but if I had been asked, I would have said so. Since I bought a bottle of Sominex^R which cost only three or four dollars (I had some pocket money so I didn't have to ask permission to buy it), my mother never knew about it. For some reason, the doctor believed her and didn't even ask me. Not to ask a twenty-three year old patient about substance abuse is not easily forgivable. Added to which, the family doctor had seen me a few days before I was admitted and put me on haloperidol which not only potentiates spasticity but potentiates the incapacitating effect of an atropine or scopolamine overdose. My mother did find out about it, because I put the box top of the scopolamine with the date and the amount spent in the bin for tax receipts. (In those days over the counter medications were tax deductible) and she read in the Physician's Desk Reference that the haloperidol would have potentiated my acute scopolamine overdose.

Be that as it may, the doctor in the hospital concluded that I was having severe anxiety because my sister was preparing to go back to medical school and I must not feel up to going back. So he concluded that I had a conversion disorder, which was common in the nineteenth century when, for example, young men who did not want to go into combat would suddenly develop an inability to see or to walk which from the young man's point of view was totally genuine, but which was derived by converting his anxiety into an incapacity to do what he did not wish to do, such as walk forward into combat or see a target or pull a trigger. So my diagnosis in the second go-round was conversion disorder.

You may imagine that with this much misunderstanding to begin with, the doctor there and I did not fare well together. I found out what had gone on by becoming an emergency room volunteer after I was discharged and calling up my own chart, and in fear and trembling, sitting down and reading it for two hours. One of the things that hurt the most was this doctor taking the news when I was getting ready for discharge that I had actually found a temporary job as a secretary, and entering it into the chart with four exclamation points. I didn't see then and I don't see now why he should have found it so extraordinary that I could find employment as a secretary.

When I got over to Belgium, in August 1974, and did go back to medical school, I found out that in the beginning I could not study because I could not put a lot of very nasty family interactions behind me. When I sat trying to read a textbook, what happened in New York kept coming to the forefront of my mind and stopping me from studying.

Shana Wibberley Clark, M.D., Dr. P.H.

In the spring of 1975, I found a psychiatrist who was French-speaking and made an appointment to see him. The appointment was for three o'clock but I went at two o'clock, having mistaken the time. A Dutch-speaking psychiatrist came out and talked to me and I said "Okay, if the appointment is an hour from now, I'll go register for my spring exams". Whereupon he said "You're not going anywhere", hit me with what I believe is called a right uppercut to the jaw, and knocked me over backwards. I have never said that he cut my lip or knocked out teeth or something of that kind, but no man – actually I could say no human being – before or since, has ever punched me in the face. It saddens me to this day that the one person who did this was a physician.

The doctor then said he was going to take me to his hospital and I didn't know what would happen if I resisted. He'd already hit me – would he shoot me? Or rape me? – I didn't know. So I got in his car and was driven out to his hospital which is the Dutch-speaking mental hospital about twenty minutes outside of the town where the medical school was located.

At first my regimen of medications was accepted, as a matter of fact increased; I was put on a total of eight psychotropic medications. Then one day, two of this physician's former patients came to see me separately and each of them told me that he had sexually abused them and made them emotionally dependent on him, and that in their view I was going to be the next prey. So I did the only thing I could do, which was to play act a very brassy, loudmouthed, unattractive person, so that he would no longer wish to get me into bed. Two or three days later I found that all my medications had been cancelled and the good doctor was apparently persuaded that I had a personality disorder.

No doctor should ever cancel consequent doses of psychotropic medicines from one moment to the next. I have said to my patients that if they were on the fifth floor wishing to get to the first floor quickly, it might be true that the fastest way would be to fling themselves out of a window, but is that safe? Psychotropics should be tapered _slowly_ so that the brain can adjust to not having them. At first, when I was taken off all eight medications suddenly, I had a strong medication withdrawal reaction and became someone who was so nervous and anxious that I could not sit still for longer than perhaps twenty seconds. This same doctor just told me that I would have to learn how to calm myself down, and as the minutes and hours and days crept by, I did calm down, partly because the brain, which has made receptors for all the medications that you were feeding it, will resorb and eliminate these receptors when the medication stops. But immediately after stopping the medications, the brain makes the subject feel frantic because all those receptors are, as it were, screaming for the medications they had been used to.

In my own practice, unless a medication presented an immediate danger to a person, I would not stop it cold, but would taper gradually off. What one can then do is cross-taper, in other words start the new medication going slowly up while the old medication comes slowly down. If this is done right, there is little or no increase in side effects and the patient is protected from feeling either their symptoms or a medication withdrawal. In other words, it is possible to do this very slowly, though with all the practical limitations on the way psychiatry is practiced, including the brief amount of time the doctor is given each patient at each visit, and the separation of visits in time, it can be very difficult to do properly. Difficult, but not impossible.

To return to groups of different types of mental illness: some illnesses, like Huntington's chorea, are heritable as abnormal genes, and others are familial, though not heritable. That is, they occur in families which may have generations of affected individuals, but there is no single gene or "recipe" for the interaction of several genes which is responsible. These are some of the more behavioral illnesses, such as personality disorders. It is extremely difficult for a person who grows up in a family atmosphere in which their mother has a personality disorder to come out as a healthy adult. This is because the maladaptive coping of their parent will be their close example, and unless they also have known up close and personal someone else's better coping, they will think it is the only way to cope, and will get into emotional habits that are most maladaptive.

I will return to the question of some illnesses which are present in the genes shortly. Let me say that the vast majority of mental illness for which the question of heritability has been raised (because several cases may occur in generations of the family alive at the same time) are considered to be not genetically <u>determined</u> but genetically <u>influenced</u>. In other words there may be a certain predisposition such that if individual is brought up in a certain way they will manifest the disorder, but if the individual is brought up differently they may not.

Mental illnesses have been usually investigated by calculating the percentage of twin pairs which are concordant for the illness. These are pairs of identical twins (i.e., two people who are genetically identical) one of whom is reared in their family of origin and the other of whom is reared away. A twin pair is said to be concordant for the illness if both the one reared at home and the one reared away is free of illness, or if both the one reared at home and the one reared away come to have the mental illness in question. If there are significant portion of pairs that are <u>discordant</u> for the illness (one has it, the other doesn't) then environmental influence is larger than if there are very few discordant pairs.

In the unusual case of Huntington's, we know the mechanism of the illness. Normal DNA is made of a backbone of a particular sugar connected to variable base pairs, all wound like a spiral staircase. Below is a schematic of what it would look like unwound. S stands for "sugar" and B stands for "base". By "base" we mean the opposite of an acid.

	S	S	S	S	S	
NH3	B1	B2	B3	B3	B4	COOH
COOH	B2	B1	B4	B4	B3	NH3
	S	S	S	S	S	

Now, 4 bases make up the B1, B2, B3, and B4. Cytosine (C) and Guanine (G) are like the B1 and B2 above, always paired with each other. Similarly adenoine and thyronine (A) and (T) are like B3 and B4, always paired opposite each other. So if you put in C, G, A and T into the schematic above, you have

	S	S	S	S	S	
NH3	C	G	A	A	T	COOH
COOH	G	C	T	T	A	NH3
	S	S	S	S	S	

"COOH" is an acidic cluster, and NH3 is basic, and the two strands are paired up with acid and basic ends in opposite directions, as shown.

Now, the Huntington's gene gets "stuck" during cell division and causes a lot of repetitions of the same basic pairs. Let's say the bottom line reads, not "GCTTA" shown above, but "GCCCCCCCCCCCCCCCTTA, up to 100 C's. As replications continue through generations of individuals, the replication process gets more and more "stuck" and the number of repeats increases. And as the numbers of repeats increases, the manifestation of the Huntington's illness happens earlier and earlier in the life of those with the Huntington's gene. So a grandson or great grandson may get clinical illness in his early 40's while his great grandfather first began to show the disease in his 60's.

Huntington's Disease is the exception. Genetic predisposition which translates into illness in less than <u>half</u> those individuals strongly predisposed is the rule in mental illness.

Depression does seem to have some degree of heritability, but suicide, when it runs in families, is more often a learned phenomenon. This is something for parents to think about seriously. If a parent completes suicide, their child is several times more likely to complete suicide, eventually, at some time in the future, than someone else in the neighborhood. There are other people whose depression is as severe as the person who completed suicide, who do not complete suicide. It is thought that children "learn" that the way to solve your problems when life becomes intolerable is to complete suicide. Certainly, struggling with your problem, fighting it, getting professional help, sends a much better message to your children and grandchildren than completing suicide does. Seeing a parent or grandparent grapple with a problem, deal with it, and solve it is a powerful message for any youngster.

Schizophrenia is probably the most heavily genetically INFLUENCED one of the major illnesses. (Huntington's is very rare – I have treated 10,000 people and have only seen two cases, and heard about a third.) This is also studied by studying how many discordant pairs there are of genetically identical twins. If schizophrenia were entirely genetically determined, then both members of every pair would suffer the same fate. To the extent that there are learning features involved, if the twins are reared apart (so that they are not in exactly the same environment) then the proportion of discordant pairs (that is the pairs in which something happened to one twin did not happen to the other twin who was raised in a different household) is an index of how much nurturance and environment have a role to play. In schizophrenia, while genes are extremely important, they are by no means the only factor.

The same goes for bipolar disorder, which is a disorder in which the person has episodes of severe depression and also episodes of either full-blown mania or hypomania, a less severe form. Certainly there are family trees with many affected individuals, yet most patients in a doctor's practice do not have others in the family with the illness; they are sporadic cases. Mania is a state in which the person has too much energy, spends a lot of time trying to accomplish a number of tasks but tends not to finish anything, doesn't seem to feel a need for sleep because they wake up raring to go even if they have slept only two or three hours, and also may have grandiose notions and overspending, hypersexuality, and other "over the top" behaviors which can lead to trouble. Manics often talk loud and fast, and the person will often say that their thoughts are racing. Depression and full-blown mania together constitute Bipolar I. Depression combined with states of less dramatic mania called hypomania is called Bipolar II disorder.

Please note that people who are not bipolar will also sometimes say that their thoughts race. What they usually mean is that when they lie down at night their thoughts change subject fairly frequently. They may start out thinking about their son-in-law, then wonder why their daughter loves him so much, then ruminate about what life was like for themselves when they were younger and how things have changed, then think about something that happened recently in another part of the world to a young person the same age as their son and daughter-in-law, and how that was different, etc. etc. From a provider's point of view their thoughts are not really "racing" because the person who is thinking of all these things has no difficulty following the train of their own thought, whereas a person whose thought is genuinely racing is thinking so fast that they are lying down in New York and thinking of Shanghai, China and then saying to themselves "Why am I thinking of Shanghai? I don't know anybody there, I've never been there, I have no plans to go there – how did I get to that thought?" Bipolar disorder is sometimes thought of as part of a spectrum in which the severity, rapidity of "cycling" between a depressive episode and a manic episode, and so forth are variable, usually conceptualized as going from slow cycling of less than four cycles per year, to rapid cycling to ultra-rapid cycling to ultradian cycling, which means several cycles occur in one day. In some people's formulations borderline personality disorder, which is an Axis II disorder, is thought of as on the bipolar spectrum, because people with borderline personality disorder (BPD) can have marked mood swings in a matter of minutes to even as fast as a few seconds. But this is a minority view; generally, the mood swings of BPD are thought of as being not so much due to alterations in brain chemistry and membrane permeability (as in bipolar disorder), as due to an inability to have a sense of self which transcends the moment, a sense of "this is me" which underlies all their thinking.

A normal person has the sense that they are who they are, and if someone gives them some bad news, it doesn't get them at their core because they are still the same person they were a few minutes ago. A person without that strong sense of self can feel rocked by good news or bad news and fly to the extreme of elation or despair over minor things such as whether the weather will be good that afternoon or whether they were able to have their favorite food item for lunch. People with a truly intense borderline personality are not able to get through more than a few minutes at a time without a lurch to another mood state, whenever a good (welcome) or a bad (unwelcome) thought occurs to them.

The fact that many people with borderline personality do respond to Marsha Linehan's dialectical behavior therapy, which is a manual-driven therapy, (meaning that what to do next is specified in a manual, and so there is some uniformity of presentation made by different therapists/group leaders) suggests that borderline personality is indeed as we think it, a learned disorder, because the patient has not been able to develop a strong enough sense of self, such that Mary Jane is still Mary Jane whether or not she can accept life as it comes. Normally, moods go up or down with good or bad circumstances, but the change is relatively slight between a good day, a blah day, and a bad day.

It is certainly true that most bipolar patients may have someone else in the family who is bipolar, if not directly a sibling or a parent, then perhaps less directly as an uncle or a cousin. Certainly, there are gradations in the bipolar spectrum, and it makes sense that this might be genetically determined, though it isn't a simple matter of one gene. Interestingly, people with bipolar disorder may also have relatives with other ill nesses such as schizoaffective disorder (more about this later) or schizophrenia.

From the patient's point of view, bipolar disorder puts one in interesting company. Quite a few talented and justifiably famous people have come forward over the last twenty years and said that they are bipolar. Why should a patient not wish to associate themselves with such an interesting bunch?

No one should think that bipolar disorder is easy or fun, however. While being mildly souped up in hypomania can be agreeable briefly, full-blown mania can be total hell and certainly the depressive side of bipolar disorder (the depressive pole if you will) can be devastating.

I remember in early 1983, when I had been released from the hospital after another manic episode and my mother died when I was in the hospital at Christmas time in 1982, I was seeing a private practitioner in New York City. I had only seen him two or three times when we came to a crisis. The doctor asked me, with my medical career come apparently to a standstill, (I was neither working nor in school), if I was suicidal. I remember telling him truthfully that I was not suicidal at that point. A few minutes later he made a reference to the idea that 'life hardly seems worth living' and I said nothing. I didn't want to spend energy reassuring the doctor. I needed all my positivity for me, and I had already told him I was not suicidal. But he was waiting for me to contradict him, and when I did not, he told me he was going to hospitalize me unless he could get my sister to come down to New York City from Rochester New York and take me back with her to Rochester. I have thanked my sister many times in many ways because that is exactly what she did. Another hospitalization at that juncture would have finished all my hopes and I might never have done what I did manage to do which was to be not only a person with a medical degree, but with clinical training who was able to work with patients. Now, ten thousand patients later, I could not be more grateful to my sister.

The reason I put this paragraph in here now is that I would like to warn the reader against such manipulative ploys by doctors. If you don't speak up for yourself, they will try to put words in your mouth and then wait to see if you react. And if you don't react, they will conclude that what they just said is actually true. I do not support this kind of manipulative strategy myself, though I have become more sympathetic to the doctors since many times I had to assess a person's suicidality and all I had to go on might be if they said "No" when I asked them if they were suicidal. One does need more than one syllable. I would say to my reader, don't do as I did; tell the doctor your reasons for not being suicidal so he won't in desperation try to trap you in his own negative take on your life.

Now back to discussions of bipolar disorder.

From the physician's point of view, it has been difficult living with very rigid criteria. For example, if a person has <u>two</u> of the seven criteria listed for mania in bipolar disorder, but not the requisite <u>three</u>, what is the physician to do? Are they to be sticklers for the requirement for three out of seven? Or is two, if they are severe, sufficient? Similarly, what about the duration criteria? It has long been established that severe bipolar disorder (which occasions a person to be doing things which are very destructive to their own relationships, social reputation, employment status etc.) is called Bipolar I and that a milder form (milder on the manic side, not in the depressive side) is called Bipolar II. This is an illness which other people notice, but not enough to necessitate hospitalization, or to cause the patient to make a break with reality and to become psychotic. Some people have suggested that people who do not meet full symptom count be called "Bipolar III". Or that if they do not have the duration of four days of symptoms required for the diagnosis of Bipolar II, that this should be a different subset of bipolar.

Then there are those who think that a person who is rageful is automatically bipolar. That is not the case. People who fit the criteria for bipolar disorder, and who then exhibit ragefulness when they are in a disinhibited state are bipolar AND rageful, and should be diagnosed with bipolar and intermittent explosive disorder. But people who do not meet any of the bipolar disorder criteria listed previously, but exhibit only ragefulness when their wishes are contravened, should not be called bipolar. Bipolar illness is a matter of brain chemistry, which will be abnormal until the patient is treated or the episode blows over (in hours, days, weeks, or months); the ragefulness which stops when the person gets what they want and manifests again only when their wishes are contravened again, is clearly not the same thing. Real bipolar disorder depends on brain chemistry; ragefulness happens when a person is told "no."

This is something that many people in the family practice community have failed to appreciate. This is what causes many people who are not in the least bipolar to be called so. The question to the patient is, "Does your rage occur only when you are denied something that you wanted (which is not bipolar rage) or does it usually occur at periods when you have the grandiosity, the decreased need for sleep, the pressure to keep talking, the racing thoughts etc., -- i.e. when you are manic)?" In the latter case, it could be said that bipolar disorder disinhibits the individual so that his interior anger comes to the fore. But he still has bipolar disorder AND a different problem as well, namely severe anger. There are many bipolar disorder patients who do not become rageful when they are ill – they simply talk fast, overspend, say grandiose things, have a flight of ideas, gossip avidly, etc. etc. – but the content of their speech is not necessarily angry. Some angry people are bipolar and some are not, and some bipolar people have bipolar rages and others do not. As I said before, being angry only when life says 'no,' without ANY symptoms of mania, is not being bipolar. When we speak of ragefulness we are talking of property destruction and physical aggression (When a rageful person is told "We are fresh out of chocolate ice cream", he busts up the store and punches the person behind the counter – a reaction of anger out of any proportion to the stimulus, that he cannot have his preferred flavor of ice cream.

But I suggest that rebelling against rigid criteria, and going to another extreme, to the point where anybody who is a little bit pressured occasionally is considered manic, is counterproductive. We manufacture in these people a serious mental illness when they do not in fact have one. After all there are many people who by profession must show rather high-energy. Standup comics and used car salesmen speak at high pressure, as does anyone who for example is trying to call home in a few seconds before they board a train or subway. To call all that manic illness is not clinically useful. And if a normally high-energy person gets angry periodically, that alone does not make him bipolar, though he might benefit from anger management class.

Oddly enough we seem to have a better understanding with depression. All of us have dealt with feeling bummed out and blue when we didn't get the promotion or when the dog died or when something else that we are not happy with has occurred. It is possible that because the profession and the public alike all have experience of feeling blue, that we understand that there is a difference between a day or two of feeling rather down and a mental illness called clinical depression.

Now I'm going to get back to the main point of this chapter, namely, whether mental illness is heritable or not. You may understand from the above that differences in diagnostic criteria, differences in approach can very much influence who is considered to have an illness and who isn't. I think all of psychiatry has agreed that bipolar disorder does run in families, and that there must be a genetic component to it, but how much of it is genetic is very much open to question. I should also mention that today there is about 70-80% agreement between psychiatrists on diagnosing most people. This is as good as the diagnostic agreement between surgeons before they operate.

Schizophrenia also presents an interesting subject to study. Definitely, schizophrenia does run in families. Definitely it is partly genetic. Efforts have been made to tease this apart for example by testing twin pairs as previously described. The current estimates for schizophrenic has been as high as 60% in favor of the importance of genetics as a factor. Notice that this 60% means that 40% of the susceptibility to get schizophrenic is in no way dictated by genes. And there are other estimates of the importance of genetic endowment in schizophrenia which come out as considerably lower, leaving a greater role for the environment.

The interesting fact is that most cases of schizophrenia are sporadic. That is to say, most of the individuals who get schizophrenia are the only people in the family to have it. This may partially at least be accounted for by the idea that schizophrenia may be a final common pathway for many brain insults. (By 'insult', is meant injury.) That is to say that schizophrenia may be the end result of a number of different problems which have occurred in the individual's brain.

Let me try an analogy here. Suppose the car won't start. This could be viewed as the final common pathway for a lot of different problems. There might be no fuel in the tank. There might be malfunctioning spark plugs. There might be a problem with the transmission. All these things have as an end result (final common pathway) that the car won't start. In similar fashion, a great many brain problems coming from different causal factors might end up as the same result, that the individual having this particular set of causal factors will develop schizophrenia. The most interesting fact about all of it is that approximately one percent of all populations from places as diverse as New York City and Papua New Guinea develop schizophrenia. Now, in less "developed" societies there is far less negativity associated with being schizophrenic. In some so-called primitive societies, schizophrenics are thought of as gifted with a particular kind of insight which the rest of us lack. In our Western societies, it is more common to think of schizophrenics as people who cannot reliably think clearly, (they may hallucinate), who don't particularly want to wash, and have a curious lack of motivation to any organized activity. These people who as the result of a number of problems such as intrauterine toxicities, birth difficulties, lack of connection to their mother, poor nutrition, etc. etc. end up with schizophrenia can be said to have acquired it, which puts them in a somewhat different category, at least theoretically, from those who have inherited the illness.

The use of the words "genetic predisposition" occurs quite frequently in the literature. By this is meant that there may be a set of genes or different sets of genes that increase the statistical likelihood that a person will get a particular illness without one's being able to be certain that a single particular gene has caused the illness. In other words, in situations which we know are NOT as in Huntington's Chorea (as I discussed earlier in the chapter) where one gene causes the illness, everyone who has that gene gets the illness, and everyone who has the illness has that gene also, there may nonetheless be a certain increased probability of getting the illness with some constellations of genes.

To discuss genetic predisposition, I'd like the reader to consider anxiety for a moment. Let us suppose that the individual has several anxious people in their family. These people if they are employed are inclined to be very quiet and not assert themselves at all for fear of angering the boss. They may never have traveled or ventured into anything particular, again because they are anxious. They go always to the same place for vacation because that is comforting and the idea of adventuring into something unknown is very anxiety-provoking for them.

Consider a child who is born into this kind of household. Everything she hears is about safety, security, minding your own business, never getting involved in anything political or controversial of any kind etc. And she has daily examples in her entourage of people who are severely anxious and who have anxiety attacks and who perhaps take medication for anxiety. She doesn't know of anyone up close and personal who is daring or dashing or adventurous. One might expect that such a child would grow up with an avoidant anxious style even if she herself does not have an anxiety disorder. Then let us say she takes a safe job with an employer who is well known in the community, but that something external to that little community occurs such that she loses her job. Maybe the conglomerate which owns the company exports the job to China or whatever. The point here is that she is, in no way responsible for having lost her job. Now how is she going to react if not by anxiety, which is the only reaction she has seen thousands of times close to her?

Of course someone might grow up in that kind of environment and feel that they've had enough of these nervous anxious people and they want to strike out for the big city. This person would have to have a very strong sense of who they are; they could then develop a self which is more venturesome.

The above example illustrates how a worldview and behavioral characteristics can run in families, even without any genetic influence. Everybody in the family has always been anxious and retiring and many people born into such a family would not question this. So their worldviews that the world is a dangerous and scary place and the best thing to do is to venture to very little distance from home, become well-formed. This is perhaps more true of some anxious people because they may not go out and see the world even in their community. They may sequester themselves and always spend their weekends among the family, and never get to know anyone outside it very much.

But let's say that the family agrees a caregiver is overloaded, and the child is transferred to their non-anxious cousin's house at age 6. Does that six-year-old drop some anxious habits to fit in with their new home environment? Or not? Alternatively, perhaps the child has very calm next door neighbors, or a sensitive teacher who takes some time to help them, so that the child grows up knowing that he or she can choose to be much less anxious than the folks at home. That is the crucial variable – does the child see that other possibility as real, as something the child can imitate?

It doesn't take a lot of contact for this; it does take regular, reliable contact which may not be a lot of time (say once a week for a couple of hours). But the people who see the child regularly and reliably, even if not for a very long time, show a different view of the world. This is why Big Brother/Big Sister or mentoring programs can have a good impact which can be lasting.

Anxiety does run in families and there may be a genetic predisposition to it, but it is also a highly familial disorder ("We McDonalds have always been high strung" for example). I don't wish to be pessimistic here. Even a person with a strong genetic predisposition to develop a particular illness can get treated and fight it and win.

Schizophrenia and the psychoses are somewhat more difficult perhaps than other illnesses, but the face of schizophrenia has changed markedly over the last twenty years. This is one of the diseases for which researchers have been trying for decades to disentangle the question of what is the role of environment, and what is the pattern of inheritance, but this has eluded us so far. Schizophrenia is in fact a very complex illness and it may be that what we are seeing is a final common pathway, as I have said above.

Please remember that "crazy people" used to be chained to the stove, as for example the first Mrs. Rochester in *Jane Eyre* in the nineteenth century. Then we had the era of Thorazine^R shuffle and the zombification of people because they were given much too much medication in the 60's and 70's, and some still are in some out-of-the-way places. Now we have some fascinating cases of people who were schizophrenic years ago but are now motivated normal or almost normal individuals. It is very much to be hoped over the next twenty years schizophrenia will become far less daunting as a diagnosis than it is today.

Attention Deficit/Hyperactivity Disorder is also thought to be heritable at least to some degree, but there is so much confusion and misdiagnosis on both sides of the question (meaning people who do not have ADHD are told that they do, and people who do are not diagnosed) that at this point it is hard to say much that is meaningful about this. Also, some large numbers of the well-documented cases of ADHD (perhaps as many as half of these) will clear up and not persist past puberty, whereas the other half will persist into adulthood. The indications are that more cases persist than we used to think. At present we do not know exactly how to predict which child will be in which group.

Other disorders such as anxiety disorders and personality disorders are not considered to be heritable, although a person who has a mother with borderline personality disorder or in fact with any severe personality disorder may have something of a personality disorder themselves, because it is very difficult to be brought up by someone with such a disorder and yet turn out perfectly healthy as an adult. Crucial to this is whether there were other adults in the environment who did not have a psychiatric disorder, who were willing to care about the child, and show that caring by taking an interest. Severe psychopathology and a lifetime of suffering can be prevented by an aunt or uncle, a grandparent (stepfamilies and adoptive families can do nicely), a teacher, a neighbor, a <u>somebody</u> who cares, and who is willing to spend time with the child so that the child can see healthy reactions up close and personal.

Substance use disorders are considered in some degree to be heritable, although they will not manifest unless and until that individual takes the substance. I knew a psychiatrist, both of whose parents and all four of whose grandparents were alcoholics. He said that by any reckoning he would have bad genes for alcoholism himself. He had figured this out by the age of twelve, and he vowed he would never touch alcohol, which he had not when I met him in his forties, so he is not an alcoholic, does not have the disorder. He is unusually decided and determined to avoid the family curse, however.

A great deal about alcoholism is learned. Children who see parents not doing much of anything and not attending to what they should be doing will learn that the way to cope in life is not to cope. If, for example, they grow up on an Indian reservation where a large percentage of the adult population is alcoholic, they may become alcoholic because of the examples around them, and one cannot attribute all of this to a genetic disorder – or they may choose not to drink. I just gave you the example of someone who probably has strong genetic predisposition to alcoholism, but who does not drink, and so is not in fact an alcoholic.

The presence in anyone's life of one individual who copes with a difficult set of circumstances and deals with them not by becoming a substance abuser, but by doing what needs to be done, can be wonderful, because this one person can model healthy behavior for all who know them well.

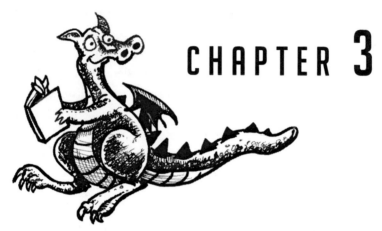

CHAPTER 3

THE PHENOMENON OF TRANSFERENCE

I am going to discuss here a phenomenon which occurs among all people. It is the cause of much suffering and so is placed early in the book. The phenomenon is called transference.

This is the phenomenon whereby we go from a definite past experience, abstract some but not all characteristics of that experience, graft the past onto the present by finding similarities of that experience to an aspect of our present life, and then assume that major parts of the present experience are going to be identical to what occurred in the past, which obviously is not true.

Everybody, I suppose, may have had the experience of feeling that someone they meet in the outside world is "just like Aunt Trudy" or "straight from the mold of grandfather" behaving as these people always do. There are also many situations whereby someone says that a person from another group (a different race, ethnicity, religious affiliation, age group, gender, sexual orientation, social class etc.), is behaving the way "they" always do. That is, we are assuming that because we know their race, ethnicity, religious affiliation, etc. that we know everything about them and that they will <u>always</u> behave in a way that fits our preconceived notions. Please notice that we would feel very insulted if someone else found out one characteristic about us and used that to predict our behavior;

but many people will predict the behavior of others based on one or two known characteristics, with no compunction about doing so.

Note that jumping from a past experience which is like the present in only one or two characteristics may be 'emotionally efficient' but is also quite dangerous. In other words, the assumption of sameness between the past and the present may be accurate, but most often it is not. You are not your grandfather, only Aunt Trudy was like Aunt Trudy and all generalizations can fall apart in the specifics.

Yet this is something we all do. We may recognize a few attributes as similar and we imagine that a whole group of other characteristics are similar also, rather than being willing to assess each situation and each person individually in the present timeframe.

This is also, as I mentioned, a source of a lot of suffering. People do not like to have it assumed that they are the reincarnations of others, and to the extent that the assumption is incorrect we are then building an incorrect perception of the world. Culture is replete with such phrases as "the fighting Irish" or "those tax-and-spend Democrats" or those "Republicans that always favor the wealthy." Sometimes it seems that we never allow anyone to be themselves – they are all considered more or less a carbon copy of someone else, or, if not the copy of an individual, more frequently the copy of some stereotype we have in our heads.

The unfortunate part of this is that circumstances which are in fact different are perceived as the same, and anticipations and beliefs are built up which might fit the old pattern, but not the more complex, real, current one.

I once had a patient who was employed to wash the floors of a grocery store. He worked on the back part of the store, and had nothing to do with washing the floors near the front, so he told me. An eighty-five year old woman slipped and broke her hip in the front of the store, an event with which my patient insisted he had had nothing to do. The supervisor took his anger out on my patient in front of the woman with the broken hip while they waited a few moments for the ambulance to come for her. The supervisor was apparently using my patient to make the customer realize he had taken the event seriously, so that the customer would not stop coming to this store and being a customer there. My patient was of course fired. Because he did not have a strong sense of self, or because perhaps he <u>was</u>

involved with making the floor wet where the customer slipped and he found this totally unacceptable to himself, he developed a severe obsessive compulsive disorder (which is an anxiety disorder). His obsession with checking that the floors around him are dry became so severe that when he met me, it took all the strength he had to sit for as much as three minutes inside his apartment when he was home, and not be checking for the nth time that the floor in front of his door was dry. He was deathly afraid that someone would come in with perhaps a little snow on their boots which might melt under their feet, leave the floor wet, and the next person would come in front of his door and slip.

Oddly enough, one day I (because I have very poor balance anyway) slipped in front of my own office door and dropped a big cup of coffee. I got it cleaned up and the floor was dry before the patient came. But no amount of my telling the patient that when there was liquid on the floor I simply got it dry, and there's an end to it, could make him imagine that he could do likewise. It is perhaps an extreme example of transference, because the patient is imagining that the circumstances from the case in which the customer <u>did</u> slip are going to be duplicated in later instances when the floor is wet. For example, the fact that the store customer was eighty-five years old and might have been somewhat unsteady on her feet anyway, which not everyone else is, was overlooked. The incident was seen as inevitably reproducing itself over and over in the patient's future.

I remember another patient who had an argument with his boss in a small room in the corporate headquarters, which was painted bright yellow. Shortly after, he left the firm for things having nothing to do with that conversation. But when he got to the job placement office he found the office at the labor exchange was also painted the same bright yellow. Because of the association of a bad outcome with the yellow color of the walls, he panicked and ran out of the room in the labor exchange office. It took a great deal of effort working with him to get him to remember the transferential circumstance (the point of similarity between past and present, in this case the bright yellow color of the walls) and to then explain to him why he suddenly panicked.

This is a good example of transference, because he had selected an unusual characteristic (that particular shade of yellow paint, while common in the 1950's, has fallen out of fashion since then) and he associated a disastrous outcome with this color, such that when he saw the color again, a disastrous outcome to him was inevitable, in his mind. When it became clear to him that he had reacted only to the color of the wall and not to the real situation he was in, he saw how he had let himself be distracted by a small detail which he magnified to something of much greater significance than it had in reality.

This is exactly why transference is such a destructive phenomenon. It makes a person assume, from a connection between a possibly trivial attribute of their current situation and a past situation, that the present situation is in all respects identical to the past one, and makes one blind, as it were, to what is different between present and past.

This is something all of us do all the time, and we all pay the price. It is also why therapists will spend a considerable amount of time and effort to get people to free themselves of these spurious connections. I would advise anyone who is thinking "my new boss is just like my Uncle Abner," as soon as they are aware of this, sit down and make a list of all the differences between the new boss and the Uncle Abner whom he may superficially resemble in some minor respect. Then perhaps one will be able to react to the new boss as a new person in one's life, although the more deep-set and unconscious the similarity is, the harder it will be to get rid of it. But if the reader gets the notion that getting rid of the spurious assumption of sameness would be a good idea then this chapter has served its purpose.

There is another situation which bears mentioning here. There are some women who are attracted to men who "live dangerously", as Bonnie was attracted to Clyde. These women may have had a series of romantic relationships in which the man was violent or nasty in some way. Yet they remain attracted to this at times violent kind of individual. These men are people, often, who cannot state definitely where they work, cannot mention a church or synagogue or mosque they attend, cannot mention any group to which they belong and have that same "dashing, dangerous" quality.

For these women, it is important that they see the similarity in how they have been attracted to their previous partners, and that they keep in their thoughts how disastrous previous romantic connections have been for them. Many women seem to need a lot of coaching to come around to the idea that their man is abusive. They tell themselves, for example, that they deserve to be beaten. The important thing for them is to see a system of transference. Their lives heretofore have been an endless repetition of the same story – attraction, domination, abuse, and separation. They need to wake up from the transferential myth that they learned that "dangerousness" means attractiveness. Until they are looking for a safe, reliable, non-violent person, they will keep meeting the dangerous types. One thing I say to start the process of shifting to a less dangerous attraction is "Suppose you go to a party where there are ten single men. Let's suppose that two of them treat their women very well, six are fair to middling as partners, and two are domineering, violent predators. Why do you always go home with one of the stinkers?" This may start my abused patients thinking about looking for someone who is not another abuser.

Transference, therefore, is the phenomenon by which we liken a present person or situation or circumstance, to something from our past. This assumed similarity is based on a superficial or at least imperfect comparison. We then assume that things will go forward as they did in the past, despite the fact that we are now in another location, the people in the scene are not the same people, and our circumstances are different if only because we live in a different time than we did before.

Transferential thinking is useful for routine tasks such as waiting for a bus, getting on it when it arrives and paying the fare – until we are in another country where people get on the bus and sit down and wait for the conductor. Making such assumptions does make a shortcut in the sense that it saves us having to reanalyze the situation, and if people are playing their parts rather than being individuals (if we are coming into a restaurant and the waitress is just 'a waitress' or we are in a doctor's office and the receptionist is 'the receptionist' rather than an individual, who will treat us as 'a customer' or 'a patient') then it may save some time to think transferentially. But as soon as we have to deal with individuals, such thinking gets in the way.

A great deal of psychiatry is in effect having to pick apart one's transferences, and see the sham assumptions that underlie them. Today in this moment is this moment; neither you nor anyone else, has ever faced this moment before, and you should make every effort to keep your mind open to whatever particular circumstance or happening it might bring to you.

I'm going to close the chapter with a brief mention of transference as particularly used in psychiatry. These days, transferential reactions would mean more to one's therapist than to one's psychiatrist, as psychiatric visits are so brief after the first visit. Transference used to refer to the collection of assumptions and emotional reactions which the patient projected onto the therapist. So it was a particular instance of the phenomenon of transference, namely the assumptions one had about one's therapist. Counter-transference is the particular assumption that a therapist may have about a patient (for example, the therapist may assume certain similarities between this patient and others with the same diagnosis, not all of which may be correct.). These terms have become more sloppily used lately to mean any reaction that the patient has to their therapist (transference), and any reaction that the therapist has to the patient without knowing the patient particularly well (counter-transference). But these are merely particular instances of the transference phenomenon.

CHAPTER 4

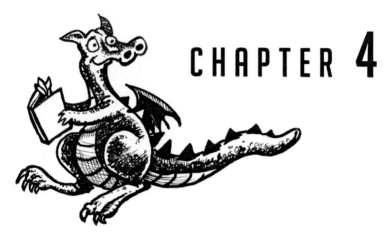

TYPES OF MENTAL ILLNESS

First, I think I should explain that for some time past psychiatric diagnoses are made on five axes. Axis I is most of what people would think of as psychiatric disorders as well as some other conditions that may be a focus of clinical attention although properly speaking they're not illnesses. Most of the diagnoses that members of the public will be familiar with, and some they are not, will be included on this axis. In Axis II are mental retardation (now called intellectual disability) and personality disorders, which I will get to presently. Axis III is concerned with physical illnesses, and they are important in psychiatry because just as psychiatric illnesses may influence physical well-being (for example, a person who is severely depressed may not eat, wash, or go about his daily affairs), a person with a physical illness may find it affects their state of mind; for example, people with serious heart disease can become quite depressed, and people who are treated for hepatitis C with interferon can also become quite depressed as a result of the interferon. Other equally serious illnesses do not necessarily connect to depression in the same way. Axis IV is concerned with the context; with psycho-social and environmental problems such as problems with the primary support group (that is either the family of origin for a child or young adult, or the spouse and children for an older adult), problems related to the social environment such as being the victim of entrenched racism, educational problems, occupational problems, housing problems, economic or money problems, problems with access to health care services (be these racial, or a matter of living deep in the country where certain health services are not readily available), problems related to interactions with the legal system and crime, and other kinds of problems. This is because it is recognized that the environment that a person lives in very much affects their state of mind. Axis V is concerned with the global assessment of functioning and results in a GAF score which is an overview of the ability to cope or the lack thereof of an individual. This isn't so much because of interest in a number, it's more a matter of a trend. If their GAF score is 60 which means they have moderate symptoms now, or moderate difficulty in social occupational or school function, what was it last year, and what may we work on to make it higher next year? One person may be doing much better than another even though they have the same diagnosis, because one person is much more resilient than another or is able to take difficult circumstances with more equanimity.

As to the Axis I conditions that are the focus of attention though not an illness, this covers things such as a partner relational problem in which the patient is not thought of as mentally ill, but having difficulty getting along with their partner, or a stage of life adjustment problem in which the person is having difficulty getting adjusted to a new stage of life, for example a young married person who has moved out of the parental home for the first time and is having difficulty, or an older person who is confronting the issues common to retirement, and having difficulty accepting what is happening. I would mention as far as Axis V is concerned that people are not necessarily very painstaking in how they apply the criteria of the GAF score. People are inclined to give patients who have been in a particular environment for over a year the same or a higher score than last year, without much regard as to how accurate this is. Psychiatrists pay a lot of attention, generally speaking, to the Axis I disorder, but may not be paying that much attention to Axis V.

Obviously something that is apparent during the pediatric age group used to be called mental retardation, now called intellectual disability, (the name change being mandated by federal law, (P.L.111-256). By that we mean a subnormal IQ level across the board, as well as adaptive functioning below that of age peers.

There are communication disorders, which subsumes old diagnostic terms such as stuttering, now called childhood-onset fluency disorder. For a schoolchild, a particular difficulty in a particular kind of mental task is known as a specific learning disorder. (Learning disorders were formerly called academic skills disorders). This category includes such things as reading disorder, mathematics disorder, and disorder of written expression. Plus, there are children who may even be gifted in mathematics but have little ability to generate a written statement in words or the reverse. There are also motor disorders.

Then there are a group of disorders called the pervasive developmental disorders in which severe and pervasive impairment in several areas of development occur together. The old term "pervasive developmental disorders" has given way to "autism spectrum disorders". The most widely known of these is autistic disorder, though it is by no means the only one. These children have significant difficulty understanding and reacting to social cues. Again, as my work has not been particularly in this area, I will refrain from saying more than that.

Also in disorders with onset in infancy or childhood is ADHD or Attention Deficit/Hyperactivity Disorder, which is both over- and under-diagnosed, depending on the situation. This is of several sub-types: a combined type in which attention deficit and hyperactivity are both present, the predominately inattentive type in which the patient is unable to focus their attention but they do <u>not</u> have motor over-excitation of running around and being very hyperactive, and those whose problem is primarily this motor hyperactivity/impulsivity. Children who exhibit inattention only without motor hyperactivity may not be diagnosed as early as children who do exhibit motor hyperactivity-impulsivity. The traditional ADHD has onset before age seven, but some purely inattentive cases may come to diagnosis much later because it may be thought that the child doesn't want to pay attention, (for instance the child may be thought to be daydreaming) rather than that the child is unable to focus. Last in this chapter are tic disorders, a tic being a type of involuntary movement or vocalization that occurs more frequently when the subject is under stress.

DSM-5 has put schizophrenia spectrum disorders next, and included schizotypal personality among these. Schizotypal personality is also listed among the Personality Disorders as a disorder characterized by acute discomfort with and reduced capacity for close relationships, as well as cognitive or perceptual distortions and eccentricities of behavior. It is listed among the schizophrenia spectrum disorders because it may be in evidence during the prodrome of schizophrenia, when psychotic symptoms are not yet fully developed. An example of a psychotic symptom is a delusion, which is a fixed belief not amenable to change in spite of conflicting evidence – such that others are conspiring to harm them (paranoia) or that others' communications are about them (delusions of reference), or that they themselves are a reincarnation of Jesus or are Satan (both grandiose delusions). A person who has been working in mental health but who is not known to staff where they are hospitalized may initially be thought to be delusional when they state that they have worked as a mental health professional – it has happened to me.

Hallucinations are another prominent symptom of psychosis, though not the only one, as severely disorganized speech and behavior are also. The most common form of hallucinations is auditory hallucinations, in which the subject hears voices that appear to come from outside his head but have no external source in consensual reality. Visual hallucinations are less common, (but note that in some cultures, it is considered normal for close family members of someone recently dead to be 'visited' by them shortly after their death), and gustatory and tactile hallucinations can occur also, though they are much less usual. The voices often say very nasty things to the people who hear them, and they can be terrifying if they say they are coming "to get" the subject. Nonetheless, some people can, over time, "make friends" with their voices which they say "keep them company". So some people do not want their voices to be silenced altogether.

These are the 'positive symptoms of schizophrenia', the things which schizophrenic people experience which people without the illness do not. Then there are the things which schizophrenic people are lacking which normals do have – such things as fluent, detailed speech and normal motivation. While our current medications do work well on positive symptoms provided they are taken consistently, we have yet to discover good treatment for the negative symptoms.

The next disorder I am going to mention is conduct disorder. This used to be placed in the beginning of the DSM because conduct disorder arises in minors, but conduct disorder is now placed with disruptive behavior disorders and impulse-control disorders. Conduct Disorder consists of repetitive and persistent pattern of behavior in which the basic rights of others or major age-appropriate societal norms or rules are violated. When these patients reach the age of eighteen they may or may not make criteria for the diagnosis of anti-social personality, which is characterized by persistent, major disregard for the rights of others. As you may guess, many people with anti-social personality are in prison. However, the usual statement is that about half the adolescents with conduct disorder grow out of it with maturity, and these people may make marvelous role models for other disturbed youth who come after them. The next category is oppositional defiant disorder, which is a recurrent pattern of negativistic, defiant, disobedient and hostile behavior towards authority figures that persists for at least six months. These are the youngsters who are defiant, who lose their temper, who argue with adults and do things which annoy other people, but they're not focused on ignoring the rights of other people, as the people with conduct disorder are. They don't steal other peoples' property, for example, but they throw a tantrum when asked to put away their own toys.

After the section on schizophrenia spectrum disorders in DSM-5 come sections on Bipolar Disorder, Depression, and Anxiety. Bipolar Disorder is thus placed between the psychotic disorders in the previous chapter and depressive disorders which follow because it is, in what is seen clinically, a bridge between the two. The word 'bipolar' literally means 'two poles' just as bicycle means 'two wheels'. There is an upper pole of either mania or a milder form called hypomania, and there is the lower pole which is depression. The depression in bipolar illness may seem to be like regular (unipolar) depression not associated with mania or hypomania, but is different biochemically, as many antidepressant medications may induce mania or hypomania in a bipolar patient. Before the term bipolar came into prominence, these patients were said to suffer from "Manic-depression". You can see the two poles in the name. So, bipolar disorder comprises two pathological (disease) states, the manic or hypomanic and the depressed. Some people may spend weeks, months, even years in a normal state in between these two extremes, especially if they take faithfully medication they can tolerate; for others the normal periods may be much fewer and shorter. It is said that people are more often depressed as they get older, perhaps because depressing things such as physical illness and the death of family and friends occur more often to older people and perhaps also because an older brain may be chemically more inclined to depression.

Depression comes in two basic categories: Major Depression, which represents a major decline in functioning, not only in terms of mood but also a number of other items, (see below)

There is also chronic depression, which may also be unpleasant to experience, but in which the subject is able to go to his or her job and perform at least minimally, can keep the house going by doing all the essentials, but feels very down and that everything is colorless or grey – the patient feels no enthusiasm, no anticipation, and no joy. The patient is getting through life, but looking forward to nothing. This chronic form of depression is called dysthymia. If a person is already dysthymic and hears some sad news such as the death of a close family member, they may have major depression as well as dysthymia, which in psychiatric 'slang' is called double depression.

There are nine criteria for major depression; five (or more) are sufficient for the diagnosis. Depressed mood (which is carefully defined so that it is a major impediment in the person's life, not a short period of feeling 'blue' after receipt of bad news) is only the first. Others are changes in weight (up or down) and changes in sleep (more or less). Agitation or slowing of movement is also included, as is having low energy, and certain feelings such as helplessness and worthlessness. The last two criteria are about difficulty thinking, and thoughts of death or of suicide, or a suicide attempt. Then there are other criteria, such as that the symptoms <u>do</u> cause clinically significant distress or impairment in important areas of functioning, that they are not due to other conditions, etc.

Those who have experienced the flip side of depression (except if it was induced by a medication or other treatment) are by definition bipolar patients. By the "flip side of depression" I mean generally speaking feeling too much energy, feeling perhaps too good, (although euphoria is not always part of mania, in fact there is a very disagreeable thing called dysphoric mania in which people have the energy of a manic episode, coupled with the thought content of a depressed episode. We used to say that people who were depressed were unlikely to hurt themselves, because just as they had very little energy to conduct their lives, so they had very little energy to kill themselves. But in a dysphoric mania people do have the energy to harm themselves and it is therefore a dangerous state.)

People with too much energy, little need for sleep, who desire and attempt to accomplish many things but have difficulty completing anything, and behavior which may be against their own interest (such as insulting the boss, screaming at the spouse, wild overspending on things they neither really want nor need, making sexual advances to inappropriate people, etc.) are experiencing, so to speak, the opposite of depression which is mania.

Then again we have a list of criteria to make sure that a manic episode is not confused with something else (such as a state induced by substance abuse), and there is a note that manic-like episodes that are clearly caused by antidepressant treatment (such as medication, electro-convulsive therapy or light therapy) should not count towards a diagnosis of Bipolar I disorder. This note is because some people who are naturally depressed but not bipolar can be artificially driven into mania by the treatment for the depression.

This is a description of Bipolar I disorder. Bipolar II patients may have just as serious a depression but the manic episodes are milder, since they do not involve doing things that are against the patient's own interests. Bipolar III disorder is a disorder which is similar to Bipolar I and Bipolar II, but the person does not meet full symptom count for the disorder. Also notice that there is a much milder condition called cyclothymia, in which a degree of mood fluctuations occur that is disconcerting to the patient.

Perhaps because I have worked all my life in public clinics where people often come to attention because a third party has noticed there is a problem, I have only seen one case of cyclothymia which was in a university professor who found his "upper pole" (that is, the manic side of his illness) very troubling. He was a calm, peaceful individual most of the time, and he found these episodes of increased energy distressing. But although he might have bought something he didn't intend to buy, he never spent the rent money on things that were unnecessary or ordered a custom built yacht, as did one of my other patients.

Before leaving the subject of manic depressive disorder, I want to have a little discussion of violence in mania. Mania is a disinhibiting symptom, which means that whatever limits the person normally puts on themselves to keep their behavior within acceptable bounds may not be operative in mania. If the person has violence inside them which is held in check most of the time when they are not manic, they may indeed be violent. But there are many manic patients who talk very rapidly and move very rapidly, but do not make any moves towards violence. This is because when they are disinhibited, when what is inside of them comes out, there is no violence. So mania can be associated with violence among those who are disposed towards violence or towards rage normally, but whose rage is normally held in check by their sense of what is socially appropriate, which may disappear in mania. But that does not mean the mania directly causes the violence, because there are many other manic patients who are not violent at all; rather, it is the rage that was already inside a person who through mania becomes disinhibited which causes the violence.

Now we pass to another category of disorders, the anxiety disorders. It is well known that the most common psychiatric symptom is severe anxiety when a person is going to be obliged to stand up in front of their colleagues or co-workers and make a presentation, even if only for a few minutes. Anxiety disorders are extremely common. There are many different types. People with generalized anxiety are "worry warts" who worry about at least four subjects at the same time and constantly rehearse the anxiety with "what ifs".

I had one patient who had a son who was a very good student. She worried about his finishing high school. Then she worried about his getting into college. He was admitted to Harvard, but she worried about his finishing his first year. He was on the dean's list, but she worried about his finishing his college program. She was never able to say to herself "Look, my son is brilliant, and he has always done well in school; therefore I have every reason to expect he will continue to do well." The son did finally graduate summa cum laude which means 'with the highest praise' and got a very nice job in his field. Thank goodness, the son did not adopt his mother's anxious stance when thinking of the challenges he faced. But it was nearly impossible to get his mother to realize that she didn't have to worry about him. His mother also worried about things like whether it would rain or not the day she had an appointment, whether she would get to her appointment on time, whether the new psychiatrist (me) would be understanding, etc. etc. The mother's inventiveness to come up with new subjects to worry about was quite striking.

Other types of anxiety disorders are phobias which are symptoms of severe anxiety when in a particular situation. Usually the motivation of the patient to get over the phobia is directly in proportion to the likelihood he has of being in the particular situation of which he is phobic in conducting his daily life. That is, if he is phobic of, say, elephants, he is not likely to encounter elephants in his daily life in the United States so he has little interest in getting over the phobia. But if he is phobic of bodies of water then he might have more of an interest in having his phobia treated.

Another type of anxiety disorder is post-traumatic stress disorder. This is actually a complex disorder which involves at least seven symptoms. Most people are aware that people with combat experience can have PTSD, and they may be aware that people who have been raped may have it. But many people are not aware that any situation in which they were threatened with death or severe bodily harm, or in which they were an eyewitness to someone else's being in danger of death or severe bodily harm, may get PTSD. Therefore, survivors of car crashes, air crashes, house burnings, etc. can also get PTSD. The key is being a participant or an eyewitness to death, near death, or the possibility of death (or loss of a limb).

Central to all these anxiety disorders is a repetition of impulses going round an anxiety circuit in the brain which reinforces and re-reinforces the anxiety. These situations can be tackled with medication and/or with talk therapy. Most psychiatrists prefer to have both used against the anxiety. It is interesting to note that the functional MRI's (that is to say a method of imaging which shows the present functioning of the brain when the image is taken) show exactly the same change whether a person gets better from medication or from talk therapy. Namely, the anxiety circuit I just mentioned becomes less active in both situations.

It is very important when treating a case of PTSD to point out that revisiting the place or the situation in which the PTSD took place in such a way that the anxiety disorder is not reinforced (for example, having the person get behind the wheel again if their PTSD is on the basis of a car crash) is extremely important. Obviously, they have to be calm enough while doing this to drive responsibly, so this is not the first thing that is done, but if the person can have a sense that what happened to them, although very upsetting, was certainly exceptional and not usual at all, then that contributes a great deal to their healing. Obviously this is different from combat-based PTSD.

Some people can benefit from revisiting traumatic periods in their lives mentally and imagining the outcome as different. I had a patient called Lianne who was a lady in her late forties who had been sexually abused by four members of her own family when she was a child. She benefited greatly from my use of something which is outside the realm of traditional psychiatry which is called the empty chair technique. It is a type of therapy in which the therapist invites the patient to visualize or imagine their abuser sitting in a chair which in reality is empty. Crucial to this type of therapy is to give the patient control. The patient may therefore say whatever they want to their abuser (about how hurt they feel, how angry they are, about how much what the abuser did has spoiled their lives etc.) and the patient is instructed that the abusing individual imagined to be present, is obliged to stay in the chair and listen to what the patient has to say for as long as the patient wants to talk. And furthermore, whenever the patient wants the abusing person to go away, all he or she has to do is click her fingers twice and the abuser will be gone. This does not take away the effect of the abuse, but at least for once the patient is able to imagine saying to their abuser exactly what they would like to say, and being in control of the situation rather than victimized.

For Lianne this made quite a change. She told me that another problem in her life was that she had split a forty hour a week job with another phlebotomist (that is a person in a laboratory who draws blood from patients when they come to have their blood tested) and she, Lianne, never got twenty hours – the other phlebotomist always got more than twenty, and she got less. Lianne was able, with my help, to set up a meeting with her supervisor's boss, who could order a change in the schedule. We rehearsed his interview with her so that she could learn to state what her problem was calmly, without rancor, and yet clearly. What her supervisor's boss needed to hear was that she was never given twenty hours a week, but always less, and so her splitting the job with another phlebotomist was not fairly done. She learned to walk in, say good morning, and say that she had been given a twenty hour a week job but she never got twenty hours, in a matter-of-fact voice, and she came back to me very excited one day and said that her supervisor's boss had picked up the phone and straightened out the problem then and there. Why I am mentioning this is that sometimes people will need rehearsal to alter the way in which they refer to some problematic situation.

Also critical in the treatment of PTSD is to teach the patient to pay attention to the present, to let the past be past, and to stop constantly revisiting traumatizing images over and over. If the patient has a loving spouse, she can help by pulling her husband back to the here and now, for example by giving him something to do which requires paying attention, such as a gardening task. All of us need to improve our connection with the present, with what is going on right now. Only in the ever-moving present do we have the capacity to influence what happens. Also, only in the present can we do things that might impact our future. Going over trauma constantly in one's mind serves no useful purpose, and can alienate people in one's present, and cause one to miss all manner of real opportunities, while rehearsing the trauma trains that anxiety circuit to be more and more demanding. People can get scared of going to unfamiliar places, so I would assign veterans to go with their spouse to a restaurant that was new to them, their choice which eatery they went to. They could choose to go at a time when it would not be crowded, but they had to order a meal, wait to be served, eat at a reasonable pace, pay for it, and only then did they have permission to leave. If they felt anxious, they were to take their attention away from their anxiety and try to engage in some gentle conversation with their spouse. I explained to them that just as they had to spend effort to stay alive on the battlefield, they had to fight to discipline their mind and get a grip on the present and the future. What is so sad is to see people who don't get a grip persuade themselves that life is not worth living, and some of them attempt or complete suicide. Incidentally, I treated over 2000 vets in 6 different VA's, and no patient of mine attempted or completed suicide on my watch.

Another anxiety disorder which needs to be mentioned which can be the result of a number of negative experiences is panic disorder. Essentially panic consists of 1) the presence of four out of thirteen possible physical symptoms of panic and 2) patients altering how they live their lives to avoid situations which they have known to generate a panic attack. One panic attack does not equate to immediate panic disorder, just as one episode of an experience of drunkenness does not equate to alcoholism. The person who has had the panic attack can only be said to have a panic <u>disorder</u> if they live in dread of the next panic attack and if they change their lives (for example, alter where they go or when they go, such as going to a 24 hour grocery store at night to avoid having to wait in the checkout line) to try and avoid the next panic attack.

One other anxiety disorder I am going to mention in some detail is obsessive-compulsive disorder or OCD. Obsessions, as the term is used in psychiatry, are intrusive and unwanted thoughts which come unbidden and which the subject would be only too happy to get rid of. The situation is very different from when we say, in English, that a young person who returns from a concert, say, and is constantly talking about the performer, mooning about her, and dreaming of when he may see her in person again, that he is 'obsessed' with her. The concertgoer is not having a profoundly unpleasant experience, and he can tear himself away from his daydream when he decides to. Nor is the situation similar to what we may say of a teacher who repeats an important point in several ways in an effort to see that her students learn it. We may say that she is 'obsessed' with this point, but she is only trying to do her job; she is not bothered by a most unwelcome thought which she would do almost anything to stop.

Compulsions are actions which the obsessive subject performs in an effort to counteract the intrusive thoughts. This may sound pretty farfetched until we remember phrases like "Step on a crack/break your mother's back." The idea of 'mother's broken back' is the unpleasant obsession; avoiding stepping on the cracks will mean this will not come to pass. Many people have mild compulsions: for example, that they must put the four cans of food they just bought in the cupboard in alphabetical order, though with so few cans there, it really isn't necessary; or, they cannot go to sleep until their bedroom slippers are placed at a precise 90-degree angle to the long axis of their bed; or that they can't start work until they have three new #2 pencils sharpened to perfection on their desk – even if they are going to be using a computer all day. Such mini-rituals may only become a problem if and when it is not possible to perform them as usual – for instance if the person is out of new pencils, and no-one else in the building has any. Can the person adjust or do they have a meltdown? Psychiatrists think the situation is serious when a person's work or personal life is affected, or when they are spending several hours each day pandering to their obsessions and compulsions. I'm not going to describe subtypes here.

The last disorder to discuss are the Adjustment Disorders. These are mild discumbobulations, often due to a change in circumstances. A young woman recently married moves across the country with her husband, and finds herself slightly disoriented and missing family, friends, and the familiarity of the surroundings she used to live in. Or, a high-pressure executive finds himself lost when he does get to the retirement he had been planning for a long time. Implied in the term 'adjustment disorder' is a) there is a recent change the person needs to adjust to and b) the adjustment will occur with time, with a possible return to their previous level of functioning.

Please note that one may encounter several anxiety disorders in one individual except that Adjustment Disorder is frequently seen alone.

Next in order after the anxiety disorders in DSM-5 come dissociative disorders (please note, it is not correct to say 'disassociative disorders' any more than it is correct to say 'preventative' medicine, the word is 'preventive'). The most commonly known among them is Dissociative Identity Disorder or DID. The Dissociative disorders are characterized by "a disruption of and/or discontinuity in the normal integration of consciousness, memory identity, emotion, perception, body representation, motor control, and behavior." DID used to be called Multiple Personality Disorder, but this is a misnomer, as I will try to show shortly.

To understand how DID occurs, let us imagine a little girl named Sandra whose family are very cruel. At the age of 4 Sandra is raped by an uncle. During the commission of this crime, Sandra's core self looks down from the ceiling (a dissociative phenomenon: when brutalized the victim imagines that they are not in their body, but are seeing it from afar). The recollection of this event is so painful that Sandra imagines that the rape was not done to her, it occurred to a make-believe friend Susan. (Make-believe friends are normal for a 4-year-old). When she is 5 and a half, Sandra is savagely beaten by an angry, drunken father. Sandra invents Amanda to carry the burden of this memory with its shame and guilt – Sandra feels responsible for angering her father. Shortly after this, Sandra invents George who takes over her voice and her body and becomes very aggressive when anyone is about to hurt her. These other 'people' who live inside Sandra usually do not grow older and bigger with her, and Sandra continues to be untroubled by traumatic memories or shame or guilt. Thus Sandra, who has no memory of these traumatic events, has a mild, untroubled "personality", whereas the others who represent trauma or protection can have all manner of drama in their "personalities", which may take over suddenly when there is a reminder of Sandra's tumultuous past.

It should be obvious from the above that the alters (Susan, George) do not have full, complex identities or personalities, but actually are torch bearers, representing the traumatic fragments of Sandra's experience. So Sandra does not have Multiple Personalities, but one identity which has become broken up – dissociated – into fragments. Interestingly, medical findings (including, for example, X Rays), may be very different according to which fragment (which alter) was in control when the X Ray was taken. Also, some fragments may "hang out" with each other and scheme with the others. A friend of mine who has DID says it's like having a 'committee' to answer to all the time.

There are other dissociative disorders, but since they are rare and the purpose of this chapter is to give the reader a sense of the complexity of psychiatry without being an exhaustive textbook, I will leave it at that.

Next comes a chapter which is new in DSM-5 which is called "Somatic Symptoms and Related Disorders." These are psychiatric conditions that exist in relation to a real, perceived, manufactured or feigned physical illness. There are several diagnoses having to do with excessive preoccupation with the (real) symptoms of illness, whether the medical cause has been pinpointed or not. There is also an "illness anxiety disorder" in which the individual is preoccupied with the idea of being ill, even though the symptoms are only mild in intensity. There is also what used to be called Conversion Disorder, in which a conflict (desire not to go into battle) is "converted" into blindness, the inability to walk or the inability to fire a gun, for example. The thing about Conversion Disorder is that these symptoms of incapacity are real to the individual since they are fabricated by the unconscious. There is a category for psychological factors affecting other illnesses. One example in this category is anxiety aggravating asthma. Then there are factitious disorders in which people do things in secret to make themselves sick or aggravate their illness (such as overdose on insulin or anticoagulants, or inject dirt to give themselves abscesses or make themselves septicemic, in other words they have a real an infection in their blood)). People who did something real to make themselves physically ill because they enjoy the sick role were said to have Factitious Disorder, whereas people who pretended to be ill without actually harming themselves physically (for the purpose of getting or continuing disability benefits, for instance – that is, for some secondary gain) were said to be malingerers. It used to be very hard to distinguish between these two groups unless one had irrefutable evidence that the person was harming themselves, and both Factitious Disorder and Malingering are based on deception. The word 'malingering' has disappeared from the index to DSM-5.

The next chapter is about Feeding and Eating Disorders. The first mentioned is Pica, which is eating non-food substances in a manner neither developmentally appropriate (small children will put almost anything in their mouths) nor part of the person's culture, for at least one month. Then there is Rumination Disorder, or regurgitating food which may be re-chewed, re-swallowed, or spit out. This may start in infancy, childhood, adolescence, or adulthood. Avoidant/Restrictive Food Intake Disorder is not because of an abnormal fear of weight gain, as Anorexia is. Bulimia consists of episodic consumption of much more food than would be considered normal (over a period, of, say, two hours); the bulimic individual does not have the feeling that they have control over this behavior. They may induce vomiting after an episode, to avoid the weight gain that would otherwise be associated with it, or do other things such as abuse laxatives or exercise excessively. Binge Eating Disorder is also characterized by episodic overeating, but without the ritualistic behavior after the episode to avoid weight gain. Next comes a chapter on Elimination Disorders, then a chapter on Sleep-Wake disorders which includes Breathing-Related Sleep Disorders like Obstructive Sleep Apnea, Central Sleep Apnea, and Sleep-Related Hypoventilation, followed by Circadian Rhythm Sleep Disorders, which are primarily disorders in which the natural sleep-wake rhythm does not correspond to the demands of the individual's environment. This occurs for instance when the individual changes shifts at work. Then there are the Parasomnias, in which various abnormal things occur during sleep, such as sleep walking. Restless Legs Syndrome is classed among the parasomnias. Then come Substance/Medication-induced sleep disorders.

Next come sexual dysfunctions, which include delayed and premature ejaculation, erectile disorder, and male hypoactive sexual disorder in men, and in women, female sexual interest/arousal disorder, (female) genito-pelvic pain/penetration disorder, and female orgasmic disorder. Substance/medication-Induced sexual dysfunction may occur in either gender.

Then there is a chapter on Gender Dysphoria, which means that the individual is unhappy considering him-or herself to be of the gender dictated by the anatomy he or she was born with. This category of disorders has become more complex than it once was; the interested reader is invited to get a copy of DSM-5 if he or she wants more detail.

Then there comes a new aggregation of diagnoses in a chapter entitled, "Disruptive, Impulse-Control, and Conduct Disorders." Conduct Disorder, a disorder of adolescence in which the young person has behavior (such as lying, stealing, destroying property, running away from home repeatedly and being cruel to small animals, for example) which decades ago would have earned them the name of 'juvenile delinquent', has been discussed previously. Oppositional Defiant Disorder (ODD) is milder illness in which children show a refusal to co-operate and may throw temper tantrums, but are not behaving nearly as aggressively as youngsters with Conduct Disorder. They are usually of elementary school age. In this chapter also is Intermittent Explosive Disorder in which people exhibit rage far in excess of the present provocation ("sorry, we are out of chocolate ice cream", "our offices close early today", or "this house has just been sold", for example). In response to one of these minor provocations, people with this illness become assaultive or destructive of property belonging to others or even to themselves. I remember one patient who came to me with a history of 4 arrests for assault in 6 months, but the reason he came to me was that he had just smashed his own new flat screen TV with a hammer. While people who are manic can become rageful when under the influence of the social disinhibition of mania, (another commonly seen socially disinhibiting situation is being drunk), this state of mind will not go away as long as their brain chemistry continues to be disturbed, whereas people with Intermittent Explosive Disorder exhibit rage for a short while when life tells them "no", without having the other symptoms mentioned above in the description of Manic-Depressive Disorder. Antisocial Personality Disorder is also mentioned in this chapter, as well as in the chapter on

Personality Disorders. The chapter ends with some specific impulse control disorders such as Pyromania (compulsive fire setting) and Kleptomania (compulsive shoplifting).

The next chapter concerns Substance-Related and Addictive Disorders. First are the disorders which come directly from using a substance, and then substance-induced disorders (intoxication and withdrawal). Substance/Medication-induced Mental Disorders are discussed in the chapter of the Mental Disorder they induce such as "Depressive Disorders" or Neurocognitive Disorders". Then each of 10 classes of abusable substances is discussed individually. Then Gambling Disorder is discussed at the end of the chapter.

The next chapter is concerned with Neurocognitive Disorders, which are disorders of the brain in which an acquired cognitive deficit is a prominent feature. (By an 'acquired deficit' we mean that this is not a developmental disability evident at birth or in early childhood.) The first to be discussed is delirium which is a disturbance in attention and awareness (as well as at least one other cognitive deficit) which may arise in a number of situations and which is often temporary, returning the patient to normal when the underlying cause is corrected. A very common example is the patient who is delirious after anesthesia for surgery; in fact it has been estimated that as many as 40% of hospitalized patients may experience delirium during their hospital stay. Other causes are such things as substance intoxication or withdrawal, medications, serious infections or some organ pathologies such as major liver disease.

Then there is another group of neurocognitive disorders, the dementias. Alzheimer's Disease is the most common of the dementias, but there are several others. These are not temporary; the average time between diagnosis and death for an Alzheimer's patient is 8 years. Other causes of neurocognitive deficits are traumatic brain injury, HIV infection, Huntington's Disease and Parkinson's Disease. This is not an exhaustive list; I am merely aiming to give the reader a flavor of the conditions that exist; this is by no means a textbook.

Next are the Personality Disorders, which, along with intellectual disability, are listed on Axis II. All personality disorders can be diagnosed as present as a 'trace' or as the full disorder. ('Trace' means that the person's behavior exhibits the flavor of this disorder, but the behavior is not as inflexible and maladaptive, causing functional impairment and subjective distress, as in the full-fledged disorder).

There are 10 different diagnoses in the Personality Disorders category at the moment. General diagnostic criteria for the Personality Disorders are enduring patterns of thinking, moods, interpersonal behavior, and impulse control that deviate markedly from cultural expectations. That is, unlike a person with a mood disorder who may "flip out" into odd behavior periodically, while having normal behavior and normal relatedness between episodes, an individual with a personality disorder has modes of interacting which do not fit in with what their culture considers 'normal'. And whereas these characteristics may be abnormal from time to time in a person subject to intermittent depressions, for instance. such abnormalities are always present in the person with a personality disorder.

The criteria go on to point out that the personality disorder is inflexible and of long standing, and not caused by another medical condition (i.e., a person is not considered to have a primary personality disorder if they have a history of significant head trauma, because changes in personality could they be attributed to the head trauma).

There are three Clusters of Personality Disorders. The three Cluster A disorders are characterized by exaggerated distrust and anxiety. People with Cluster B disorders tend to be overly dramatic and to act out. Cluster C personality disordered people tend to be anxious (and avoidant of what makes them anxious) and either avoidant of trying anything new in life, or clingy and dependent on others. The treatment of personality disorders can be undertaken with special techniques by people who have great patience with their clients. These are certainly the people most resistant to changing themselves, which is why the treatment of personality disorders is so demanding.

Those interested in more information on the personality disorders as a group, or who want to find out about individual disorders, should consult the Diagnostic and Statistical Manual of Mental Disorders. Fifth Edition, or DSM-5 for short, which is available in many public and medical libraries or which can be purchased from the American Psychiatric Association. Because the initials 'APA' designate the American Psychological Association, the website for psychiatrists is called psyche.org. But buying the book is expensive, so I will tell the reader that many private-sector medical centers, especially if they are part of a teaching hospital system (with doctors in training, called residents, who work there), will have libraries which these days are accessible to the public, and, if the hospital has a psychiatric service, they are very likely to have the latest DSM. State hospitals may or may not have good libraries. Usually one can call, speak to a librarian, and find out if they have the book and if a member of the public can read it (often, they will not let a non-professional check it out, as it is intended for use by the doctors).

Next come the paraphilias, disorders in which people find sexual satisfaction in something other than shared sexual activity with a consenting adult. There are quite a few of these, such as voyeurism (liking to watch other people engaged in sexual activity – being what used to be called in popular lingo a 'peeping Tom') exhibitionism (liking to exhibit sexual parts of the body, sometimes spoken of as being a 'flasher') and pedophilia, a desire to engage in sexual activity with children, which when acted upon is a crime. Recently, there has been a move in several states to give pedophiles and rapists – sex offenders – civil commitment (to a hospital, not a prison) after these people have served their prison terms. The offenders may enter prison for rape or child molestation at age, say, 20, and serve their sentence of 20 years or perhaps somewhat less if they get time off for good behavior. They are released from prison at around age 40. But if they go right back out on the street, they are likely (statistically speaking) to reoffend.

This particular civil commitment law says (at least for New York State) that they may be civilly committed if they have an 'anomaly' which predisposes them to repeat the offense. Of course they are committed to institutions which at least technically are psychiatric hospitals. But psychiatrists don't treat people with 'anomalies' but with psychiatric illnesses. The problem is that repeated rapes do not carry with them a psychiatric diagnosis – they are crimes, not illnesses. (Child molesters <u>are</u> considered ill because it is abnormal for an adult to be sexually attracted to children.) More problematical still is the fact that while the treatments we have do seem to reduce the likelihood of re-offense, they by no means eliminate the risk that an individual, once released into the community, will repeat past criminal behavior, and so many psychiatrists resent being turned into "jailers". Also the inmates, who thought they were going to go out into the world once they finished prison terms, are very angry to find themselves confined to another institution. I worked in one for 8 months, and I am very sorry to say that very little if any effort was made to stop the former inmates from raping each other, and the staff, many of whom had been maximum-security prison guards before becoming hospital staff, did not grasp the change in orientation/outlook that working in a hospital implies. So the place was much like a prison except that instead of being left in a cell all day, the inmates were required to attend classes designed to make them change their behavior.

After the chapter on paraphilias comes a chapter on other conditions that are the focus of clinical attention. These are such things as parent-child relational problems in which neither the parent nor the child is considered 'ill' but, say, the parent is something of a neatness freak and the child is not, or there is some other difference of outlook causing friction between them. There are other relationships in which differences of perspective may be painful, even though each party's viewpoint is within the normal range. The last chapter in the book concerns conditions which need further study to see if they should be made into diagnostic categories.

I hope that this chapter gives the reader some sense of the variety and complexity of psychiatric diagnosis. I will close this chapter by saying that it is my firm belief that the patient and the patient's immediate family that live with them have a right to know the diagnosis and to discuss the details of the diagnosis with the patient's doctor. There are sometimes difficulties because a competent adult patient will not allow the physician to talk with others in the house, but one can often get permission if it is pointed out to the patient that those living in the house would do better if they understood the patient. If the patient was diagnosed differently before coming to the care of the present provider, they are entirely within their rights to ask to discuss why the change in diagnosis and what it implies. What we need is more communication, and more effective communication, which is one of the reasons I wrote this book, and why I encourage patients and families to plan the use of their time with the doctor.

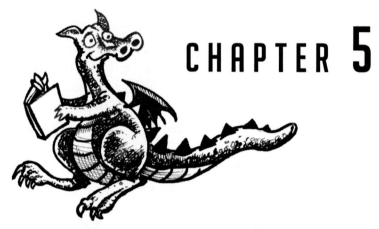

CHAPTER 5

CHOOSING AND CHANGING PROVIDERS; WHAT THERAPY IS ALL ABOUT

First, to get a referral to mental health care services, I would suggest speaking to your primary care doctor, or, if you have a friend or relative who uses psychiatric services and who is happy with their provider, get a referral from them. I would strongly suggest that your next step is to call the billing department of the hospital or clinic you have been referred to, or the office manager if your referral is to a private practitioner, to discuss whether or not that particular group or provider accepts your insurance. In mental health, there are some strange things that happen. For example there are insurances which cover physical illnesses treated at a hospital, which do not cover psychiatric services at that hospital – it is known as a "carve-out".

And, if you the individual are financially responsible for psychiatric services, you will be billed for the "charges." The charges are inflated so that when an insurance company pays an agreed-upon percentage, the providers still get a reasonable fee. Let's say the insurance company pays 60% of the charges. The original charge has to be large enough so that 60% of it will still allow the hospital to make a profit. But you as the individual consumer do not have an agreement for paying 60% of the bill, and so the hospital will require more than insurance (if you had insurance that covers this hospital) would actually pay, because you as an individual do not get the insurance 40% discount. I was caught when I paid the social worker's bill for an intake assessment; when I got the doctor's bill (over $800 for one visit) I negotiated with the hospital to pay what they would usually get from insurance, which was just over $550. And then after all that trouble to get to be that doctor's patient, she told me on my second visit to her that she had accepted to work at another psychiatric institution and referred me to a colleague who is very nice but who is much younger and so perforce less experienced.

I have two points in saying this. The first is, that it is wise to find out whether the insurance you have does business with the clinic or private practice you want to go to. The second is, you can never be sure that a given practitioner is going to stay put when you become their patient, so it is wise not to count on that too much. A short while after I to began to attend this clinic, I was able to change my insurance to one which does do business with them. I am glad that I found out that the other big insurance company with a lot of customers in Rochester did not do business with this particular clinic, else I might have chosen an insurance company which did not cover my psychiatric treatment. Since I had just paid over a thousand dollars out of my own pocket for the evaluation of me when I had my previous insurance, this would have been a costly mistake.

So my advice is to be referred to a particular clinic or individual, and then check whether your insurance covers the services of that clinic or that individual. Unfortunately, most of us regular folks are not in a position to choose a doctor who is a recognized leader in the field for our psychiatrist. These people generally have very little time for new patients, and while they may take referrals from a junior colleague, it is generally not the patient or the patient's family who chooses them. Also, I know from experience that being a patient of a famous doctor is not always easy, because the famous doctor feels at liberty to transfer the patient to an assistant as soon as the patient is doing reasonably well, so that the truly gifted psychiatrist can spend his or her time with people who are very much in need of his or her special expertise. This is not always pleasant for the patient. Since you as a patient or family member may therefore be negotiating with an average psychiatrist, there are a number of chapters in this book which are written to help you know how to do that. Most important is for you, the patient or family member, to focus on what you want to say, what you want to convey, and be able to get straight to your point without wasting time.

Now as to what therapy is about. The first thing to realize is that there is a continuum for the therapist between being one hundred percent supportive and one hundred percent challenging. Being supportive, empathizing, saying in effect "I understand your position; I can see how you got into the pickle you're in" supports the patient in how they are at that moment. By expressing empathy, the therapist is lending understanding to the suffering the patient is undergoing, without challenging the reasons for that suffering, the decision-making that led up to the suffering, or anything else about the patient. To be supportive means to support the status quo.

The problem with being supportive all the time as I have mentioned before is that continually supporting the status quo does not provide any motivation to change. And therapy is actually all about change. It is about changing a patient's outlook, changing how they see a particular situation, changing how they see their own history, their own present and their own future. Only if the patient is left somewhat uncomfortable are they motivated to change. In the beginning every therapist needs to be at least somewhat supportive, else the patient will not feel understood and will not return. Supportive expressions are used, such as "You're having a hard time, yes I can see you are, of course you feel bad, anybody would". The opposite end of the spectrum is absolutely challenging. Then the therapist would say things such as "Why do you think that?" "And therefore….?" "Is that really what you think or feel on that subject?"

Hopefully, the therapist will gain the trust of the patient and thus be more at liberty to cash in on some of that trust with challenging expressions when the therapist feels that he or she is close to the attitude or the perspective that most needs changing for this patient. Perhaps some of my readers are now thinking that they don't want to change, they just want to get over the death of someone close to them, losing their job, having a serious illness, or whatever it might be. But any one of life's milestones can be navigated with humor, increasing flexibility, increasing acceptance of life's adversity, or the reverse. Surely the marking events in one's life are most susceptible to changing a person, and we as therapists want them to change in a way that will make them more flexible and more open to life's possibilities after the experience than they were before.

Many patients do not actually engage in therapy until sometime after they have been seeing a therapist. By this I mean that they have perhaps enjoyed going to someone's office and having a professional listen silently while they talk about themselves. But do they really understand what their problem is, how they got there, why they stay there, and what they could do to get out of their difficulty or change how they see the situation? It is when they are considering these factors that we, the professionals, say they are "engaged" in therapy.

Many therapists conclude that some people don't really want to change; they want the right to complain about their present situation without any necessity of changing. Some people do indeed seem to want to blame other people for their hardships. One tactic to deal with this, is to ask them in what way they consider themselves an agent in their own life; in other words, what part of their lives have they made for themselves? If they continue to blame everyone else, then one might say that they don't seem to be an agent in their own lives, and that's possibly what their real problem is. People need to feel that they are able to bring about change in their own lives. Most often, people will profess that they <u>are</u> an agent in their own lives, but when they are shown that they keep blaming everyone else for everything that happens, it can be pointed out that saying they are an agent and then blaming others are not compatible positions. If this is pointed out gently, the person may make a bit of effort to take some responsibility for herself. That person is at one end of the spectrum; on the other end, there are some people who seem to think they are responsible for everything, people who don't seem to realize that there are some things (such as our ethnicity, the region we come from, the decisions of our parents) which are handed to us, for which we are not responsible.

The most fundamental choice that you can ever make is to continue on as you are, or to make a change. In order to make a change you need to see your own past as contributing in some way to your present dilemma. That is, you need to be able to critique the decision-making of your past. This is not to blame yourself, it is to look with the gaze of wisdom and see how your past reactions may have been not as helpful as they may have seemed at the time. For instance, if you have just split up from a spouse that you call a "stinking bastard" then how could you have failed years ago to have noticed that there was something about him or her which was not good? When could you have noticed something had you been paying attention, and had you had your eyes open? How can you protect yourself from making such a poor decision again, without feeling a need to barricade yourself against intimacy with anyone for fear that you might choose the wrong partner? Can you teach yourself to be a good judge of character, instead of falling for the next person who is good-looking and charming and attentive towards you, falling for that person and not noticing any signs that his or her character might not be stellar?

The therapist's job is to get you to look at your past with a kindly wisdom, learn from it so you would never repeat it, but at the same time approach your present and your future with more openness, more flexibility, more adaptability, and more of a sense of humor than you have ever had before. In order to make constructive change, you have to look back and see your life and see when you made important choices, and which choices there have been that you might have made differently – what the alternatives were, and why you chose the way you chose. Anyone who has been through soul-searching about alternatives knows that there were other ways of handling a given situation.

I would recommend that people with mental or emotional or job or relational difficulties see a psychiatrist for at least one session, to have a clear diagnosis so that some important aspect of their problem is not totally eclipsed. I have known a great many good therapists, but few indeed of these can include unusual diagnoses or unusual problems in what they look for and listen for. Oftentimes the practitioner gets habituated to seeing the population that they see, and they lose sight of the differences between what is usual for them and the people that are similar in some ways, but different in other important ways, from what they are used to seeing. A number of the clinics I have worked in insist that each new patient see the psychiatrist at least once, even if they do not wish medication, to make sure that the diagnosis is correct.

I have noted that in the 50's, 60's, and early 70's a number of large well-designed studies were done which showed conclusively that the <u>combination</u> of talk therapy and medication gave a much better result than either of these therapies alone. Yet over the last few decades we have turned away from this insight, with the result that one of the best-known algorithms (decision trees) for the treatment of major depression starts with the first decision being <u>either</u> talk therapy <u>or</u> medication. Those of us who are old enough to remember those earlier studies would say that both/and is the way to go. By choice, I have never worked anywhere where therapy was not available to all who wished it; to do otherwise in my mind is to mean that I would be stuck with less good outcomes than would be possible if I had the patients on combination therapy. And, I was trained to do therapy as some doctors these days are not.

Now as to particular characteristics of your provider. As to age, race, and gender, most clinics may try to accommodate someone if they express a pronounced preference for one race or gender. In some places, it seems to be assumed that a woman will have an easier time talking to another woman than to a man. Since I was sexually abused by my mother, but had a wonderful father, the reverse used to be true for me – in the beginning of my illness, I got along much better with male providers than with female. It is true that in some places there may be a shortage of providers of a particular race/gender combination, such black or latina women. This does not necessarily mean that the clinic is prejudiced against them; it just may be there aren't in that locality a large number of people who are qualified to be therapists who happen to be both black (or latina) and female.

Please do understand if something in your present life is making you uncomfortable, and uncomfortable enough to seek professional help and/or medication, then you need to find a new self which will be able to encompass the old self, and yet have more flexibility and be equal to the challenges which present themselves in your life now. This new self will be bigger and better, in some ways, than the old self. When I say bigger, I mean more vast in the way that the soul is vast, less limited by constraints of having been where and who we have been, and more able to accept difference in ourselves and other people, and not only accept it but work with it and even enjoy it. Oliver Wendell Holmes captured this well in his poem *The Chambered Nautilus*. The shell of the chambered nautilus is one we may hold to our ear to "hear the sea."

Now as to changing your providers: this section assumes that both you and the provider you are seeking to leave are going to be staying in the community so that the natural separation that might occur when your provider's program ends, when he or she moves on, when you get a promotion, when you decide not to come to the clinic for a while because you've got too many other concerns, doesn't come into play. First of all ask yourself, what is the real reason you are wishing for a change in providers? Is it because the provider is asking questions and making comments which get under your skin and annoy you, is it because the provider doesn't seem to be very sensitive to your need for support, and you need to be supported and emotionally sustained?

It happens fairly frequently that a good therapist will be very supportive in the beginning, but will be less supportive as time goes on. If your provider is making you feel uncomfortable, one good way to tackle the situation is to come right out and say what is making you unhappy. Something such as "Every time I mention my father, you seem to be dismissing what I say." Or "Last time you said that I was playing the sick role in my family. I never wanted or enjoyed or tolerated the sick role very well." An example that just happened can be very helpful. You may find that your provider either did not say exactly what you heard, did not mean what was said in the way you interpreted, or that he or she was trying to push you in a particular way because going in that direction seems to be your personal block.

Of course, there are certain behaviors which are not acceptable in any provider. Being consistently late is one (ideally one should never be late, but a five-minute lateness once in a long while, life being what it is, is, I think, excusable). Coming onto the patient, making any kind of snide or tongue-in-cheek or marking remarks to the patient, unloading his or her personal "stuff" (the therapist or doctor is supposed to be listening to you, not the other way around) or frequently falling asleep are some examples. When these occur, you should keep a record of it and then bring it up with the medical director of the clinic. I once had a provider who in one session took eleven telephone calls, absenting himself from the room in order to take the call (which was appropriate). What was not appropriate was having eleven interruptions in one hour, each of which took two or three minutes. Not only did that mean that my time with the provider was severely curtailed, it also meant that both he and I had great difficulty trying to remember where we were before the last interruption. I mentioned this to his superior and got a change in providers.

Don't forget it is you, the patient, who sets the agenda for each session. Don't do as I once did, shortly after I was raped by my boss, (having been a virgin until then), which was, walk into my therapist's office complaining of a dispute I had just had with the cab driver. The dispute with the cab driver took the whole session, even though I really needed to talk about the rape. I was just not convinced, and I remain unconvinced to this day, that my therapist would have been understanding about the rape. This was the fellow who had no regard for the values that led me to choose abstention from sexual activity as a young girl. I do not know what his reaction would have been, but I was very much afraid then that he would construe the matter that the man who raped me had in some perverse way done me a favor. I had told no one about the incident, and I desperately needed my doctor and therapist to at least take my part, at least in the period just after the rape, which I did not know that he would do with any degree of certainty. My point here in this book, is that whatever story you bring in to your therapist, the therapist will take whatever they are given, and go from there. So it is your responsibility to tell your story properly. Because I did not mention being raped, the negative effect of the rape stayed with me a very long time and did very much affect my experience with my doctor/therapist. I went through depersonalization (in which one does not feel real), derealization (in which nothing feels real) and could barely cope with daily life. If I had taken my story to my doctor, and if he had been able to empathize with and support me rather than saying something nasty, it would have done me a power of good.

After I was raped, several months later, I sought out some sexual experiences that, if not the pinnacle of love, were at least human and bearable, because I felt myself freezing and on my way to becoming like dry ice – so cold that it burns.

The irony of the situation is that if you find yourself not mentioning something over two or three sessions, I can almost guarantee to you that there, in what you are avoiding mentioning, is a major key to your difficulty. A good rule of thumb is to make yourself talk about whatever you would sooner avoid.

Say it! You can start with "I don't understand why, but over the last two or three sessions I am thinking about 'X'" – and then describe 'X'! The more you withhold, the more you barricade yourself against change, the more you will be stuck (and pained) by an entrenched status quo.

Change is scary, but refusing to change is very sad and can be quite harmful as time goes on. Don't hang onto your Peter Pan refusal-to-grow-up complex! As psychiatrists or other mental health professionals, we think one of the greatest marks of health is flexibility, adaptability, the ability to roll with the punches, accept the changes you cannot do anything about, and work on changing those things you need to change. There is an important balance in life between acceptance of what is, and willingness to change toward what you would like. Not to accept any change is foolish, and not to be open to changes that you could bring about or that come to you is to confine yourself to an unrewarding job, a loveless marriage, a depressive tradition (there are some families in which most of the adults are depressed at least to some degree) and an entrenched unhappiness. Be willing to change to claim your joy. If you are willing to change you, almost anything can be possible. You need flexibility, and the focus to keep your effort where it needs to be to bring about what you would like to happen. A little faith in the idea that most things in life do work out is good too, and if you have some religious faith you should hang onto it and pray for more – it is very precious.

There is a form of psychotherapy which was developed in the mid-twentieth century which is called cognitive behavioral therapy. It may be viewed either as something totally original, or as a very astute, clever repackaging of some psychodynamic concepts (by 'psychodynamic' I mean concepts derived from psychoanalysis) done in such a way that these can be generalized to almost any situation. This form of therapy explores hidden assumptions that people make as well as automatic negative thoughts. Hidden assumptions are generally negative assumptions about oneself or about people around one. For example, a young man many assume that the young lady of his dreams would never go out with him because he feels he is not attractive enough for such a gorgeous one as she. In this situation, the therapist invites the young man to engage in some personal research and ask the young girl out just to see if his assumption is confirmed. If it is, that may only mean that she declined for the particular occasion that he suggested. The possibility exists that she had a prior engagement for the evening when the young man was suggesting they go out. If on the other hand his suggestion for a date is accepted, then he can be shown that he made an incorrect assumption about himself and perhaps he is doing so in other situations as well. If she refuses him very rudely, then perhaps his perception of her as a heavenly, sweet girl, is incorrect. Similarly, if a woman thinks "No one will dance with me" if she goes to a dance, then she would be encouraged to go and find out if that assumption about herself is correct or not. As to automatic negative thoughts, these are the negative zingers that occur in the minds of people who have not learned to quiet them. For instance, if a person spills something and then his or her mind zings "You're so clumsy" or "Oh what a slob you are" – the mind is always critical unless the mind has been taught to be still – that zinger is an automatic negative thought, abbreviated ANT. Unfortunately people do not talk of automatic positive thoughts, but perhaps the purpose of repeating affirmations to oneself is to create them.

When I was fifteen my mind sent me automatic negative thoughts all day long. Every time I forgot something, did not say something perfectly, spilled something, dropped something or in general did not have the perfect reaction to whatever the situation called for, my mind would send me an automatic negative thought. So I began to combat these thoughts, since they were very destructive to my happiness and since I think picking on anyone, even oneself, is picking on a creature of God and is wrong. So I began to say to my thoughts "Get thee behind me, Satan". For the first month or so, nothing much seemed to happen. I kept getting negative thoughts and I kept sending them my defensive zinger right back, but they did not diminish. But slowly as time went on the force of the automatic negative thoughts decreased, and they were less frequent. By the end of a year of constant vigilance on my part, the only thing my mind would say to me when I spilt something or dropped something is that I should get the appropriate tools and pick it up.

It has been many many years since my self-talk was negative. Usually, I have no self-talk at all. And I enjoy the silence. Since this is something the reader could do for himself or herself without needing a therapist, I invite the reader to do it.

Shana Wibberley Clark, M.D., Dr. P.H.

Split Therapy

Almost everywhere these days, the talk therapy is done by one person and the medication is done by another. Unfortunately, communication between these two mental health professionals, is not always what one would want it to be. The person who does the medication does not know the patient nearly as well as the would had he or she also been doing the talk therapy as well as the medication therapy. But this division is here to stay, because the prescriber is generally paid a lot more than the talk therapist, and it is therefore possible for the prescriber to be a prescriber for hundreds of people, while the talk therapy is done by someone else who sees patients much more frequently, and who has a much smaller caseload. Most clinics insist that the patient be in therapy in the same clinic, so that, if necessary, the therapist can point out some events or some mood or psychosis in the patient's present which should be addressed by the prescriber. In the better clinics, some time is reserved for patients who are needing to see either their prescriber or their talk therapist more often than would normally be the case. So, if your talk therapist notices that your cousin's death seems to have a real effect on your mood and you seem to be getting more depressed, he or she may contact the prescriber to have him see you sooner than you otherwise would have, which would have been in two or four or even six months.

This system can work quite well if the therapists have an idea what medications can and cannot do, and if the prescriber is alert to the therapist who says the patient needs to see the prescriber sooner than would otherwise be the case. Unfortunately, some therapists take it upon themselves to try and dictate to a prescriber in what way the patient's regimen should be changed. I have no objection to being told that a particular patient needs more antidepressant effect, but I did not like it at all when talk therapists would tell me that the patient should be on, shall we say, Prozac^R. I occasionally would write a long note to the talk therapist as to why I do not think that was a good idea for this patient, but I was always willing to see the patient sooner than they normally would have and to keep in mind the therapist's alert that the patient needed more antidepressant effect in their medication. I think the best kind of communication from the therapist is to say "This patient is much more depressed than he was two months ago" or "This patient is very bothered by having hands that periodically shake" or "The patient is having a lot of diarrhea". What I used most especially to have a problem with is the therapist who would tell the patient "I'll tell Dr. Clark to put you on medication X" because that would give me an awful lot of explaining to do if medication X was not what I chose to use. To sum: up therapy is capable of changing your life as much as or even more than medication. It is your responsibility as a patient to bring up the important events in your life – the therapist cannot help you if you are not telling him or her what is going on. If you need to, write down for your therapist the important matters to bring up because trivia can easily overtake a session, unless you stop them from doing so. If you have a truly serious rift of values with the therapist, better get another therapist, but this is only for something truly serious. Also you may change if the therapist is not paying attention to you or is doing something definitely proscribed, such as coming on to you or being constantly interrupted with personal phone calls. In these situations, find a more attentive therapist.

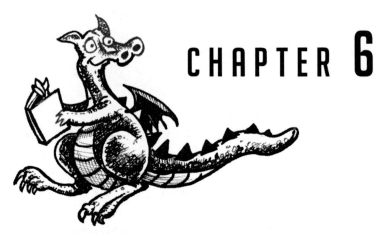

CHAPTER 6

WHAT A REASONABLE PERSON MAY EXPECT FROM PSYCHOTHERAPY (TALK THERAPY)

The job of a therapist is to offer support, particularly when you're distraught or anxious. But more than that, the job of a therapist is to coach you to handle your own episodes of being distraught. The therapist should get to know you very well and reflect you back to yourself so you get to know yourself well. Before you can work on eliminating your triggers (situations, statements, thoughts that worsen your symptoms), you have to get to know what your triggers are. Then, as you learn to be less and less stung when one of your triggers is activated, you get to have a much calmer interior. It may be that you still react slightly to something, but it can be your reaction which you have within yourself, and which you can choose to show to others, or not to show to them. And certainly the emotional force of your reactions should diminish progressively, as you see that reacting to a trigger is very largely a matter of choice.

Let's take a very simple example. Imagine a young man in his mid- to-late twenties. He comes from a fairly calm, and as far as we know sane family. No-one he is related to is known to have mental illness, nor is there anyone in the family who has a flamboyant personality with lots of sudden changes which might suggest undiagnosed mental illness. So far, the only major event in this young man's history is that he had a boating accident as a teenager, and he very nearly lost his life by drowning. So, he has developed a fear of the water so severe that he gets to white-knuckled anxiety at the very thought of crossing a bridge -- not particularly that he expects the bridge to collapse, but the mere thought of being close to the water is distressing to him.

Now let us suppose that he lives in a city which is on two opposite sides of a major river. He grew up on one side, went to school on that side, and has until recently been working on that same side. Just a short time ago, his boss suggested that he transfer his workplace to the other side of the river, where the company headquarters is situated. This transfer would be accompanied by a sizable promotion. It is planned a few months down the line.

The young man sits in your office (you happen to have an office on the same side of the river that he grew up on, where his house is, and where his whole life has been lived to the present). He becomes extremely fearful at the mention of the fact that if he takes this promotion he will have to cross the river twice a day -- once in the morning to go to work, and then in the evening to go home.

Some of the providers I know would give this young man short acting benzodiazepines to take every day, and leave it at that. I suggested a different approach. I pointed out that benzodiazepines actually dull cognition and would not serve him in his new position very well. I suggested a course of gradually increasing going near the water's edge, each time a little closer.

At first, the very idea that he was headed toward a large body of water was enough to make him have difficulty leaving the house. But as he became habituated to the idea, he was able to approach the water with more calm. After several months, he was able to take his four-year-old son to a little stream near the house and allow him to play with a toy sailboat there. The patient said he did not want to take his four-year-old to the big river, because he was afraid the boy would get out of control and suffer drowning. It was agreed he could delay taking his son there until the boy was seven or eight years old.

The man found out that there were a lot of other triggers that were somewhat connected to the big trigger about being near a body of water. He discovered that the sound of a whistling kettle made him nervous because after all the kettle contained water that was boiling. He never had been able, at least since the accident, (and he could not remember doing it before) to sink into a tub and luxuriate, enjoying being partly underwater. When he lost his great fear of the proximity of any water, he was able, for example, to wash his wife's back, and help her wash her hair when she was in the tub, which she appreciated very much.

Tackling his fear of water improved his life greatly. Fortunately for me, he was well able to admit at the outset that he was afraid of water, and willing to consider the idea that the best thing to do under the circumstances was to gradually overcome his fear. About six months after he was given benzodiazepines (by his general practitioner) to take twice a day, he came to see me and reported at that time that he used them very sparingly, reserving them, for example, for when he had to make a presentation to the president of the company. (When he shook with anxiety, the benefit of stopping his shaking outweighed the slowing of thinking.) Otherwise, he was going to work and going home every day without using them, which was much better for him.

This man had a phobia of bodies of water when we first met. Phobias are obvious to most people (though the person who has the phobia may be very obtuse) as limiting, and having a very negative effect on functioning. Therefore, it is intuitive to most people that getting rid of a phobia is important.

Most triggers leading to tangled sets of emotions under certain circumstances are a little harder to properly evaluate -- if it does not lead to a <u>simple</u> phobia, triggers can be harder to unravel.

Recently a friend of almost thirty years' standing who is an ordained minister talked to me about having a memorial service for someone she met when they were both patients at our local hospital, which has a psychiatric ward, as well as many wards for many other illnesses. My friend told me that this particular person, sometime after he got out of the psych ward, proposed marriage to her. She went on about this in some detail for quite a few minutes. I did not understand whether she was grieving a man who had proposed to her, or whether, now that he was safely dead and there was no possibility of accepting the proposal, she could review the entire phenomenon of what the proposal had meant to her and who he had been to her at the time, and the effect of her decision not to marry him on what transpired later. But it certainly was apparent to me that this was a very complex event, opening up the vistas of herself, her mother, her father's relationship to her when she was a young woman (this is always the prototype for later relationships, just as the mother/son relationship may have a great deal of influence on how a young man perceives women). This would have been a rich vein for a therapist. One of the reasons that most therapy has to be individual is that the personal connections that someone has made of a similarity between their boss, their teacher, their father, are individual.

For another instance, a soldier patient of mine talked about similarities between his mother who had wanted him to check various things daily on the home property when he was a teenager, and his tendency therefore to choose dependent women to marry who would look to him to be checking and arranging things.

Nobody is exempt; everybody makes these kinds of connections, but everybody makes their own individual ones, and if you are not aware of the connections which you have made, then you are fated to make them over and over and over even when they don't really fit, and that will cause problems. For example, my soldier patient was overseas for several years after his marriage, and he needed a wife who was strong enough to manage her daily life with the children, without him. He did not need a dependent woman who was forever in a crisis over minor upsets. It goes without saying that your boss or your teacher may not be at all like your father, just as the women you are courting may not be at all like your mother -- so these assumptions and connections can actually be quite erroneous and can lead you in the wrong direction (see Chapter Three on transference). And if you are understanding and reacting to people as if they were others that they are not, your perception of reality is skewed. Because of this skew you do not see other people as they are; you are reacting to and perceiving them in ways that are false, and so you are not truly in a "real" reality.

I will leave to your imagination what would happen to a young man with a water phobia if his symptoms were so severe or so entrenched and so much a part of how he lived his life, that he turned down the promotion or left the firm altogether on account of his symptoms.

The idea is that once you become aware of your assumptions and how incorrect they may be, you can change them and so change the reality you perceive, and because you are no longer doing a number of less-than-appropriate things because you think that people are people they are not, you will be better perceived by others. They will look at you as someone who has "his head on straight" and who "understands what's going on".

One more piece of advice to patients: if you notice that you have had any particular event in your life (which does not happen to everyone) happen to you more than once, I'd take a very careful look at that. For example if you have left a job or not shown up for a job more than once, if you have been fired more than once, if you have been passed over for what seemed to you an obvious promotion more than once; or, if you have been left, maltreated in some way, or divorced or abandoned by your significant other more than once. Look at it this way -- what is there about you (meaning, something about you that you could change -- remember that I have said before that if you are willing to change YOU there are endless possibilities, whereas if you wait for the rest of the world to change, it may be a long wait) -- what is there about you that has contributed to these events or has caused them, perhaps? Now, if your response is "Those stupid bosses are all the same. They want to work you to the bone, they don't pay you much of nothin', and they want you to turn up every day bright eyed and bushytailed, eager for more." I hate to say this, my friend, but there you are blaming the other guy. For in saying bosses are all the same, you DO NOT CHANGE you, and waiting for the other guy to change is not a winning proposition.

Now, what could be the cause of your dilemma? Is it that you get hungry and tired and needing to sleep indoors, and so you take a room somewhere and get a job which is of no interest to you, and then after a few days of doing this job which to you is boring, you get fed up and you don't show up for work anymore? Well now, that could be possibly remedied if you got some education and qualified for a job which you would find interesting. It would also help to counteract the sense of defeat you have when you work for many days in a row and don't have much to show for it. Or, could it be a matter that you don't persist in keeping "your eyes on the prize"? What I mean by that is maybe the work is not very rewarding in itself, but you don't think about what good you can do with your paycheck. Maybe, this time, when you get some money, instead of blowing it all on drugs and alcohol, you should get yourself a decent place to live in. Now, that's a scenario which would suggest that step one might be treatment for addiction to drugs and alcohol.

I have met people in all sorts of menial occupations such as janitor for a restroom in a railroad station or bus station where many of the customers are neither well-off nor well-educated and they may use a restroom very roughly -- not even caring that the waste the restroom is there to collect, lands in the right spot. So the janitors of these places really have thankless jobs. Yet I have met janitors who grin from ear to ear at the thought that although they are in a truly difficult place where it gets filthy very quickly, they leave the facility shining every day. One man even talked to me about leaving godliness behind him because he left the place very clean. I am only suggesting that it might be a good idea to look at seeing the work you do a little differently and reinterpreting what is going on so that you see that you have, as the janitors do, an absolutely vital role to play.

Once, in the seventies, the janitors in all of New York City hospitals went on strike. Within a day or two, used paper towels were piling up to overflowing, not to mention what was happening to the toilets. The senior administrative staff and some medical students (like me) were asked to volunteer to become janitors temporarily. Now, this gave me the chance to rub elbows with some very important people. We all had the job of cleaning toilets etc. because the strikers were not doing it. The problem is that in an environment like a hospital where there are many many very sick people, having massive filth, rot and infection can become disastrous.

Since we banded together, all grades of people from the top to the bottom of the hospital, to keep the place as close to free of infection as we could, the strikers had to come to the table and a settlement was reached fairly quickly. But this underscored for me, and it's a lesson I will never forget, that no one who is working to keep someplace clean is to be undervalued or ignored.

Let me tell a fable about three stonemasons who were working on one of the great medieval cathedrals built in Gothic style, which are now marvels to all who see them. The first stonemason looked sad and forlorn and a little bit sour as he said, "I work from dawn to dusk in a place which is very dusty, hot in summer and cold in winter, but that is how I earn money to feed my wife and children." Notice that he was thinking only of the effect of his work on his family. The second stonemason said, "Well, I have the interesting job of helping to erect a building which will keep out the rain and the snow and the cold for a long time to come. Sometimes, when I think that these buildings will last when I and all the people I know have gone to ashes and dust, it gives me the shivers, but it also gives me the courage to straighten up and go at the work with renewed vigor. I was chosen to be a foreman in this job, and I have the respect of everyone in town for the work I do, which makes the physical strain a lot easier to bear." Note that this man has a mix of self- and other-centered comments to make about his job, and he obviously has some pride in it. The third stonemason said, "I am building with my all-too-human hands an edifice for the glory of God which will endure for centuries to come. This is a place where the descendants of people I know will receive the sacraments for as far as I can imagine into the future. They will be confirmed here, will get married here, and their children and their children's children will be baptized here. This building will also be so beautiful that anyone who goes inside and even anyone passing by will be transported into the world of spirit and faith and I, humble stonemason that I am, have the great privilege to make all this possible. The good Lord has my profound gratitude. Glory be to God on high, the Father, the Son and the Holy Spirit!" This man does not even mention the difficulties of his job.

A Course in Miracles says that there is nothing in our lives that does not have whatever significance that we give to it. It may seem that someone else in the family or in our community has given this significance, but we assent to it. What I am getting at is that the meaning to you of everything you do is essentially yours to determine. Could it be that you have been undervaluing yourself, because of the mistaken notion other people have of how easy or inconsequential (unimportant) your job might be?

If you are unhappy with a particular circumstance, consider yourself on your way to a change in that circumstance. The one thing we cannot guarantee ourselves as time goes by is that everything will stay the same. This is why people who have a very good situation often get anxious, because how long can they make it stay that way? So they hire security, body guards, live in a gated community, and look for experts in 'wealth preservation.'

I met another janitor who was an expert cleaner who told me that he remained in janitorial jobs because "No-one hassles me, no-one pushes me to a better result or doing it faster – I have my assignment and I do the work in my allotted time, and there's an end to it." He said he felt freer as a janitor because it was a matter of saying "Yes, I have cleaned this room and this room and that room, and yes, I did clean the men's room and the ladies' room and so on." He was not tortured by trying to reach some theoretical wonderful that the actuality of good enough never seemed to touch. For him life was simple. Yes, he had already cleaned the men's room that day; or no, he would clean the men's room after lunch. The guys who are in the boardroom can make the performance this year better than last year, but there's always some perfection which they never seem to attain, so they never feel really satisfied. And then if they have a banner year this year, would next year be as good? None of these problems troubled him, and he was aware of this, and was a happy man.

Now, if you have a wife and several children at home and are really worried about meeting your obligations every month, then maybe the solution again would be getting some education so you can earn at a greater hourly rate.

I do realize there are people who have been disempowered and ridiculed and treated badly since they were born. The thing for them is to make sure they do not participate in that disempowerment and ridicule. In other words, when somebody says something disparaging, if you turn away saying, "Oh well, there's nothing I can do", then you are in essence consenting to that evaluation of yourself.

Please realize that I have had disability all my life, which has made it difficult for me to be accepted by other people in the economic stratum of my family, but also has made me keenly aware of other people who are not in that stratum and yet who are wonderful, worthwhile obvious child-of-God people. I remember very well when I was three years old and 'Shana the Shrimp' with the crossed eyes and stumbling gait, obviously a cripple, was never (according to most people) going to amount to anything -- meaning at that time that I didn't seem to be able to make it as a three-year-old. That is a very early experience which is still with me. I remember what it used to be like, and smile every day at how things are different now.

I really do look at people and see them. I don't see a man dressed as a waiter performing that role without also seeing the human being under the uniform -- the son, the brother, the husband, the father or grandfather, and the church member. I have to admit that when I encounter a young person of normal intelligence and normal physical health, I have difficulty understanding, at times, why he would throw away his noncripple status and get interested in drugs. I suspect that part of it is, he doesn't realize what a wonderful gift a normal intelligence as well as a normal physique is. So he does not feel gifted, he feels disempowered and neglected, and so trashes himself by using drugs.

I wonder if we could ever teach people to value themselves, so they can hold their head up even when other people say they are inferior? It's just too sad to see people accepting somebody else's take on them and using it to build limitations into themselves.

If you have been doing this, high time to stop. Remember you are a child of God, and your business is to get yourself drug free, trigger free, negativity free, and joyous.

Now let's take a person who has repeatedly broken up from significant others, been divorced more than once or something of that sort. Do you instigate the breakup or does the other party break away from you? More than that, look to the people you choose as partners. I once met a lady who had a succession of boyfriends who all seemed to live on the edge of danger. I made this comment to her and she accepted it. She said she found men who were living on the edge dashing and romantic. Then she changed her mind and said that's the way she felt about each of them in the beginning. As time went on in each relationship, however, she began to realize that these men each had their own obsession with risk-taking, and she as a person did not matter much to them.

Meanwhile that exciting danger was turning quickly into a life that for her that was plain old unsafe and this is why she split away from these boyfriends, but then when it came to meeting someone new, she was again attracted to the "outlaw" who was living dangerously, on the edge. This suggested that she might try people who were living an unusual individual life, possibly as an artist, but that had nothing to do with drugs or with flaunting the law. I said I could appreciate that she would not be interested in Mr. Conventional, but that didn't mean she had always to look for people who would very soon be providing unsafe surroundings. So she set about looking into why she found the "outlaw" aspect of these men attractive, and little by little she learned to be attracted to men whose rugged individualism manifested itself in one-man artist gallery showings rather than in having state troopers parked on the front lawn.

If you have had romantic partners who left you more than once, I would wonder what was there about them that made them susceptible to leaving their partners (in other words was there a character flaw in them) and how come you picked them out as romantic partners for yourself, or what you did in the relationship to make them want to leave. One patient I had was trying to "make other people better". They would change in her company, but then they would walk off into the sunset into a bright new life, leaving her behind as the "old" girlfriend; sometimes being someone's mentor can kill romance. In a certain way of looking at it, romance is more than likely to bloom if the parties feel themselves equally involved. This lady had to learn not to go home with the sort of fellow who needed employment or help. Unfortunately, a lot of people have the notion that they need to change their significant others. And the trouble is, the significant other often does not want to be changed, or at least not in the direction that their partner desires.

If you are a person who leaves your romantic partner and has done so more than once, would there be perhaps a point to improving your ability to communicate early enough in the relationship so that you don't get to the point where you think, "Oh, chuck it. There's no point in going on with this. I might as well walk out."

You obviously were attracted early in the relationship, else there would have been no relationship. At what point did your communication skills fail you, perhaps? Should you have a better set of communication tools at your disposal to avoid this happening more times, because this has already happened to you more than once, and nobody likes to get stuck over and over in the same play?

I'm going to close with a very funny conversation that I had one night when I was senior resident on call at Hahnemann University's psychiatric emergency room. A man in his early thirties telephoned, and asked me most earnestly, he was feeling dreadful, and if he came down to the emergency room to see me, would I hospitalize him? I replied that if he came down to the emergency room I would certainly see him and after getting some more details about his situation (I explained that the solution is always in the details) that if it was warranted we might consider hospitalizing him or whatever else was the best way to proceed.

He asked me again, saying in a very oblique way that he had had some thoughts about taking his life; and would I hospitalize him?

I commented that he had said that in a very oblique way and that I would want to know more about it, how it came about, how long he had been feeling this way, whether he had felt this way before and also what he had done before etc., prior to deciding on what course of action was best for him.

He again repeated his question, saying that he felt absolutely dreadful, would I hospitalize him? I said to him that I could not guarantee any particular outcome, if he wanted to be examined, what didn't he come down and see me?

He then changed his tactic and said if I hospitalized him tonight could I promise him he would be out of the hospital by next Tuesday? This was Saturday night. I told him that I could in no way guarantee that he'd be out of the hospital by Tuesday, especially if he were having definite thoughts of self-harm. Finally I said to him "Young man, what is really happening here? I have the distinct feeling that there are major things that you're not telling me."

He then said that his girlfriend had left him that afternoon, and that he figured if he could call her from the psych ward and say that she made him so miserable that he got himself hospitalized, that she might relent and return. I then asked him, "And what's so special about next Tuesday?" He said "Me and a bunch of the guys have tickets right next to the dugout for the Mets game in New York City, and I really wouldn't want to miss it."

Then I said, "Well, whatever your thoughts about harming yourself, you certainly do have a future orientation, for which I am very glad. We don't usually hospitalize a person in order to manipulate someone else into a particular reaction." I suggested he might call or write his girlfriend or send her some flowers or do something that wasn't destructive to convey that he missed her. I wished him an entertaining evening at the game, and hung up.

To sum up what a reasonable person can expect from psychotherapy: psychotherapy will help you become aware of your own repetitive patterns and your own non-acceptance of your life; it will also clarify for you where you may need to make some changes, such as get some education so that you can get a better job. It can also change your point of view about the kind of work you do, the person you live with, or anything else about your life where having a more positive attitude would be more fruitful in terms of bringing you closer to a future you desire. In short, psychotherapy can help you in any direction where you may need to change yourself so as to be able to become more the person you wish to be.

In sum, people have a variety of reasons for having particular symptoms. They may have absorbed a negative view of life as young children and not even realized they were doing so. Or, they may have had some experiences in their teenage years or young adulthood which caused them to feel they were fundamentally unlovable or could not succeed in life or were destined to have a particular form of difficulty. Patients need to learn that only if they will challenge these assumptions of their own inadequacies or unlovability can they succeed. I will say from experience, both professional and personal, that the closer one gets to challenging these fundamental assumptions, the more painful the work can get, because much of one's personality and approach to life was formed by the desire to get away from this pain in the first place. But if one is not willing to look around and challenge that pain and the assumptions which underlie it, as many people are not, one is not likely to get a very good result out of one's treatment. Being a psychiatric patient is a lot of work on the theoretical, philosophical level. It is also a lot of work on the personal level.

Many people do not challenge these assumptions and want to feel better and look for a new and better medication when the foundation of their psychological house is not well built. These are the people who get along feeling not so good to fairly well, but never get well enough to leave the clinic and conduct their lives without more and more therapy. I will say that it was my experience once to work in a well-run outpatient department which asked each of the patients every year or so what their main goal of therapy was. Many of them said that their main goal of therapy was to solve the problem they had come in with, and they were not interested in other issues that the therapist might see but that they might not see as an issue. So clinics are not apt to close out a case and decide that they are finished with a particular patient – unless the patient has a lot of no-shows.

SHANA WIBBERLEY CLARK, M.D., DR. P.H.

There is one situation in which the patient, in my view, should change therapists, or even change clinics. That is, when the therapist that the patient originally had does not seem to respect the patient's values. I remember when I was an inpatient and then an outpatient at Mt. Sinai Hospital in New York City in 1973 (which was only about eight years after oral contraceptives came on the market and so people were still working out how the availability of oral contraceptives should change their behavior).

I was someone who never had the desire to have a sexual relationship with a man unless I knew him and was in love with him. I have never been a person to treat sex casually as something to be engaged in on a whim or without a deep sense of commitment behind it. My therapist, on the other hand, seemed to be of the 'love them and leave them' philosophy, that sex should be enjoyed with anyone who was so inclined at the moment, without any idea that commitment at least of one's emotions should precede the actual sleeping together. He made a lot of fun of me because I did not share his easygoing value system. This caused me some pain at the time, and I felt he was undermining my sense of self rather than seeking to build up who I was. I did not seek to change doctors, but I grew to be less and less trustful of him and less and less willing to talk to him. This meant that when I was raped by my boss at the Congress of Racial Equality (CORE), I could not talk to my therapist about it. The therapist, on his end, grew to feel that I couldn't "say boo to a goose" which is what he said to me at our last meeting.

It is important to have a therapist whose theoretical outlook and whose values are not going to cause a block in trust and an inability to be honest with him. I did learn from this man; afterwards I fought when I needed to fight with my therapist so as to get him or her to understand what of my point of view was negotiable, and what was important to my sense of whom I was. Actually, when I went to the French faculty in Belgium, they were much more sympathetic to my old-fashioned sexual mores, and so it was not an issue. But I suggest that patients should talk to their therapist about what they consider really important, and if the therapist cannot agree, then change. I will say that in the United States, most therapists deal with many patients from many different cultures, and realize that the point of view with regard to such things as respect for one's elders, sexual mores etc. may be part of a patient's culture and the therapist has to be sensitive to the patient's values. Please realize that I'm not talking about one incident or one conversation here, I'm talking about the principle of what behavior is considered desirable and what is considered valuable. If there is a major misunderstanding between therapist and patient on this topic, then the patient has a good reason to change therapists. But if the patient changed therapists and finds that the next one has the same problem, then most of us would turn around and say that this is the patient's problem, and should be worked on in treatment. For a more comprehensive discussion of when to change a therapist, see Chapter Five.

If, after some time coming to a particular clinic, a patient has gotten much better because they have tackled their underlying assumptions and have rebuilt the foundations of how they see life, there is no doubt in anyone's mind that they are ready to leave the clinic. I would invite my readers to be this kind of patient. But in order to do that, the patient has to face the pain that made him construct the poorly laid foundation in the first place, and there are many people who are not willing to do that. For those that are, however, the rewards may be substantial.

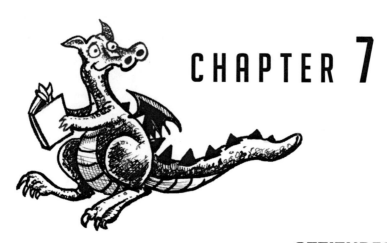

CHAPTER 7

ATTITUDES TO PSYCHOPHARMACOTHERAPY (MEDICATION)

The fact is, sixty percent of prescriptions written in the United States are not followed as they were intended to be. The patient may never fill the prescription at all, fill the prescription and take only a few doses and then stop, or fill the prescription but take consistently less than they are asked to take. (I'm just going to mention the problem of overdoses here, and of diversion, giving the medication to someone other than the person it was prescribed for.) This non-cooperation on the part of our patients is very distressing to providers; research has been done which shows that each provider thinks that he or she is an exception and that far less than sixty percent of his or her patients fail to respect the prescriber's recommendations as far as prescriptions are concerned. We think this is "the other prescriber's problem."

We don't often ask before writing a prescription what a patient's attitude to taking medication for their state of mind may be. Perhaps we should. Many people resent the idea of needing medication for their state of mind, and if the situation is that they do not absolutely require it but they might benefit from it, they still resent an implied dependence upon an exterior chemical to maintain their sanity.

If you as a patient have a preconceived objection to taking your medication, and you are seeing a psychiatrist or other prescriber in mental health, discuss it with the prescriber. I had a patient once whose grandmother had died not too long before I saw her. The grandmother died of peritonitis which ensued after her intestine ruptured, because her gut was riddled with cancer. She had been taking anti-depressants for some time before, since her primary care doctor thought that her state of mind might be helped by taking this medication. My patient had a confused idea that the medications had killed her grandmother, simply because of the temporal sequence that first she got cancer, then she got the medication, and then her gut perforated and she got peritonitis and died. My patient had an idea that somehow the medication had caused her gut to perforate. She had no understanding of the effect that cancer can have on the integrity of normal tissue. And she had a deep distrust of all psychiatric medications as a result of this. It took some effort on my part to detect this bias on my patient's part, and yet more effort to convince her that her grandmother had really died of peritonitis, which always follows if a person's gut is perforated for any reason, because the gut is full of disease-causing bacteria, and an inflammation of the entire lining of the abdomen is a redoubtable infection to be fighting. It took a while to convince her that cancer can make the gut wall so friable (a term meaning inclined to break apart) that it perforates.

There is another patient that I remember who had a different problem. She truly did not want any medication, and when I suggested one to her, instead of saying she wanted no meds, she mentioned a common side effect. I then suggested the medication that is commonly used to treat that side effect, and she grew even more incensed and mentioned yet another side effect, for which I mentioned yet a third medication. She was quite angry with me at this point, and so I asked her what she expected. Only then did she tell me that she expected to be referred to a therapist for some talk, and did not want any medication whatsoever. I did say to her that she could have saved both of us some wear and tear if she had said that at the beginning.

There is one caveat here. Physicians are positive people who are inclined to think that if a given medication were prescribed for a couple of months, that means the patients took it for two months. As physicians we know that about two thirds of our prescriptions are not followed, yet we are reluctant to acknowledge that the person in front of us may be one of those who did not follow the prescription. If a patient says, for example, that a given prescription made them feel "very sleepy", the patient should say how many doses they took before they gave up this medication for having an unacceptable side effect. It may then transpire that the medication was taken for only three or four doses, and that half the standard dose of this same medication may produce a very good effect.

The fact is, there is an enormous range that exists in patients' attitudes towards medication. I am going to try to point out the ways in which the attitudes that the patient has before coming to see a prescriber may be a help or a hindrance to his or her recovery. For example some patients do not want their mental health 'problems' called illnesses. Now, as a therapist (please remember that I come from the era before a person had a social worker or psychologist therapist and a doctor for the medication, and I was trained to do therapy AND medication together) I wouldn't mind what the patient wishes to call their symptoms. But, as a doctor, I treat illness; I don't treat a "health condition". I have sometimes compromised with patients on calling their illness their "problem", but health condition suggests something for which a doctor is not needed. For instance, in a "skin condition" in which skin is intact but it has dark spots or blotches (which occur in some people with age and can occur in young women as a result of pregnancy), the skin is intact and is still functioning as skin but the blotches or spots are unsightly and so the patient has the option of using various cover-up products, several of which are advertised on television. The problem is that the patient does not find these blotches, if seen uncovered, attractive – they are unsightly and cosmetically bothersome. But since the skin is not inflamed or infected or cut or showing tumor, the patient can consider that they are not "ill". Another type of health condition that I would consider a health condition rather than illness is a person who has perhaps a mildly spastic bladder with restriction in bladder capacity and yet whose professional work requires them to be in public view giving lectures for a couple of hours at a time. There are various approaches to this problem which I will not go into, but I am assuming that the bladder capacity restriction is not sufficient to give the patient a true "illness" – it's just that there's a mismatch between the patient's capacity and the capacity they need for the job.

There are the equivalent of health conditions in psychiatry. These are problems or sufferings that the patient has without having a diagnosable illness, but which become the focus of clinical attention because the patient is having a hard time. These are existential problems, problems of stage of life, or problems of communicating and getting along, when it is not obvious that the patient has a personality disorder or other disorder which is causing or aggravating the problem. But in my view, people with diagnosable illnesses should not be seeking to call them "health conditions." This starts a kind of collusion between the doctor and the patient about not calling a spade a spade which I don't think is healthy.

Let me hasten to add that I think complete mental health in all circumstances and at every moment of every day is extremely rare. Jesus was mentally healthy as were perhaps Zoroaster and, perhaps, in modern times, the Dalai Lama. I do not mean to put the Dalai Lama on a par with Jesus – after all Jesus had a message for the whole of humankind for all time, and I am not sure that the Dalai Lama would acquiesce to such a claim for himself. My point is, that only a very few people across the centuries have arrived at perfect mental health.

Now, it has been commented to me that patients have met psychiatrists who are not as healthy as some of the psychiatrist's patients. I am quite sure that it is true; the healthiest patients may seem healthier at a given moment in time than their psychiatrist. Please realize that in this conversation, all the patients' problems are spoken of freely, whereas the psychiatrist should be keeping his own difficulties to himself. I don't think it's a fair comparison to be juxtaposing a moment which for the patient is not difficult because he's not had any new or recent shocks in his life, to the morning after the psychiatrist has found out that his son has died overseas in a war, for example. I'm sure that examples could be found in which the patient is healthier over a period of years than a particular psychiatrist. My attitude is that most of the population does need therapy, though most of the population does not <u>need</u> medications, (though they might benefit from them) which are the subject of this chapter. But from their point of view, physicians treat illnesses which have symptoms.

Just as there are patients who don't want any medication, there are some patients who want a new medication for every little tiny change in their symptomatology. They are horrified if you suggest that they replace medication number one with medication number two, and very frightened of side effects if you increase the dose on medication number one to take care of apparently worsening symptoms. These people often come to a new doctor already on eight or ten psychotropic medications.

Please note that there is a thing called "polypharmacy" which is not good practice. It used to be thought that polypharmacy was the result of using any two medications for one symptom, but now that we have medications of the same broad class (both are called 'anti-depressants' or 'anti-psychotics' or 'anxiolytics' which means they are medications which break up or 'lyse' anxiety) – it used to be thought that giving two medicines of the same broad class to one person was a bad thing. But now we have medications that are in the same broad class that act by different mechanisms, so that it is sometimes possible to get two hits of therapeutic (desired) effect with two different sets of side effects, but each set of side effects is at half dose, so they never amount to anything for a particular patient. In other words, the desired effect can be cumulative while the side effects may not be. In that case it is perfectly logical to treat one symptom with two different medications.

On the other end of the spectrum are people who are very reluctant to take medication, and in one case that I can remember, the patient was absolutely horrified when I got out my prescription pad, and then she told me she didn't want any medicine at all. She had already seen a therapist and she was expecting to see me to check the diagnosis, but she had made up her mind she didn't want to be taking any medicine. Patients may figure, talk is easy, talk is cheap and a little 'counseling' is a good thing, but the idea that they should take medicine puts them in a category of not well people which is an offense to them. Well, you can stand on your pride and sense of offense that it should be suggested that you take medicine, but it has been proven conclusively many times over that the combination of talk therapy and medicine is the way to go for almost all psychiatric problems.

So you can see there all kinds of attitudes towards taking medication, from taking medicine for every little thing to refusing to take any medicine at all. I would recommend that you read the rest of the chapters on medications in this book, and that if you have any strong feelings about medications one way or the other, you should mention these to your providers. It is not fair to the prescriber if you have decided that you are going to allow the prescriber to write you a prescription which you have no intention of filling, for example. This will set up a dishonesty between you, and an antagonism because you feel you are not being listened to (though you haven't said anything to give the provider a chance to listen) and the provider will feel at the next visit that he gave you a good medicine and he doesn't understand why it had no effect. He may then choose other meds which are stronger, which might not be the best for you. So, go ahead and ask for more information or other sources, if you like. I would recommend being straightforward with your provider, who is, at least in theory, on your side. The provider wants you to get well, just as you do.

Be leery of accepting unquestioningly what somebody put on some site on the internet. The internet has, on some research sites, some of the cleverest psychiatry there is. It also has (on some disgruntled former customers' sites) things that are outright lies. And there are a lot of mediocre sites full of sweeping generalizations. The internet has no control or editing of sources. Somehow, some people, because they see something written down or on the internet, tend to think it is gospel, whereas whatever is said by their doctor or therapist is suspect, even if it is exactly the same thing. There are things on the internet which were written by close family members of a patient who suffered a bad outcome, whereby the family member tries to convince the world at large that this medication is "bad medicine", bad for everybody. Thank goodness, most people have one or two side effects from something, not every possible side effect, and there are a few bad side effects which are tolerated (i.e. the medicine responsible is not taken off the market by the system) because the medication has been so helpful to many many other people.

Question: supposing a medication relieves a difficult symptom for ten thousand people. Supposing this same medication is responsible for two deaths among those ten thousand. Should it be taken off the market? Or not? Sometimes these situations are decided by money. What that means is, the families of a very small number of people who suffer a severe adverse effect take the manufacturer of the medication to court and sue for many millions of dollars. If the amount that the people could win in a lawsuit is much more than the profit that the company could envisage from this medication, it will be taken off the market by the manufacturer's refusal to continue making it. Some of our best vaccines have at times been hard to find because major manufacturers stopped production because of lawsuits from a handful of parents who believe (rightly or wrongly) that their children were made autistic by the vaccination. Let us say one year, after being used on 10,000 children, we have five autistic children among the vaccinated instead of the usual two autistic kids per 10,000. Is that chance, or a real causal relationship, or is something else going on? For very unusual events, it's hard to say. But going from two lawsuits one year to five the next may decide the manufacturer to cancel production – and then thousands of people cannot be vaccinated.

For those people who have suffered a death in the family, the fact that it was an extremely rare side effect becomes irrelevant. They are facing a great sorrow, and for them, the thousands of people who have benefited from the same drug are not their concern. But if the thousands of people who have benefited from the same drug can be ignored, then there are many medications in existence which would not be there because of the few unusual people with severe adverse effects.

I don't pretend to have the ultimate answer to this – I don't believe there is an ultimate answer. One of the concerns is, is there another medication which does not have this adverse effect which can treat the thousands of patients who benefited from the medication that did cause these deaths? Or is there another way of treating the underlying condition which would avoid the question of this medication altogether? Sometimes medications which are particularly useful for a small number of people are kept on the market, and given sanction to be used only for those very small number of people specified to have particular unusual needs. These medications which satisfy a need that is in a very few are called "orphan drugs" – because no big citizen lobby has "adopted" them.

I think I should finish up the chapter with a few words on what I think the ideal attitude of a patient is. (Believe me, I will have something to say in Chapter 21 "Attitudes of Providers" about what I think a provider's attitude should be.) Basically, a patient should keep an open mind. Patients should come to consult the prescriber for the prescriber's expertise about what will help a patient on the way to recovery. Therefore, having an absolutely closed mind such that the patient refuses to take any medications whatsoever, in principle, without even hearing about what they might be, is unfortunate.

The patient should question the prescriber's choice straightforwardly but respectfully and be careful not to come across as a smartass. But if there is something the patient does not understand, the patient should certainly ask. Think about the fact that at any given point in time, 15-20% of the American public is taking psychotropic medication. This means that several people you know take medication, though many may get it from their family doctor (80% of prescriptions for psychotropics in the U.S. are written by people who are not mental health professionals). Yet these people are not 'zombies' nor are they shuffling along nor moving stiffly. You don't know, to look at them, that they take psychotropics. Think about this and realize that the medications we have now do not do what the old stuff used to do, so perhaps you should be more willing to give them a try.

On the other hand, if the prescriber does not want to give you a certain medication such as Xanax^R, the patient should realize the prescriber has experience and has reasons. The patient has every right to ask what those reasons may be, and to expect that the prescriber will tell the patient. If the patient has a close relative who has taken the medication the prescriber proposes and had a reaction, this should be shared by the patient, who might have the same reaction when they take the medication. They should ask again if the information given the first time is not sufficient. Some providers do not do much more than grunt at their patients, and they need to work to improve their 'bedside manner' with the patient. If they repeatedly fail to answer the patient's questions, this is certainly grounds for the patient to talk with the administrative director of the clinic and ask to change providers.

Perhaps it would be a good idea to understand what the provider thinks the right medicine might do for you, which is essentially the subject of the next chapter, Chapter 8, "What a Reasonable Person Can Expect from Medication".

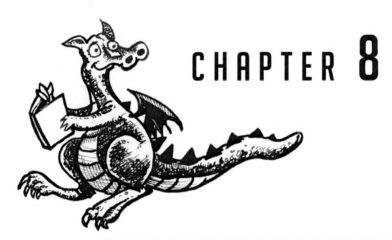

CHAPTER 8

WHAT A REASONABLE PERSON CAN EXPECT FROM MEDICATION

Medications in psychiatry are doubtless very important. The object of medication is to change your brain chemistry in such a way that you begin to feel some relief from your problem. Note here that it is extremely important to give a full description of your problem.

Let me emphasize here the importance of an accurate diagnosis. In the 1970's, it was extremely frequent to mistake bipolar disorder for schizophrenia. The diagnosis of bipolar disorder in the 1970's was quite rare, in fact there was a study done at Harvard in 1976 which found that most bipolar patients were not correctly diagnosed until their fourth hospitalization, as in my case. But let me tell you what a problem this creates for the patient. Antipsychotics are used beneficially in bipolar patients (in small doses), to help them stabilize. This is particularly true if they are inclined to go into a manic episode easily. A small dose of antipsychotics, taken at night or perhaps half in the morning and half at night, will help them keep their feet on the floor, so to speak.

But treating bipolar disorder exclusively with antipsychotics is a big problem. I can tell you from experience that it may quiet the manic patient in the sense that they are no longer running around or screaming, but it does not really normalize the thought process. What may happen is that the person is full of scream and running on the inside and unable to express that on the outside. Let me tell you, the suffering is considerable.

Such a big mistake in diagnosis has other consequences. The patient gets the idea that the doctor does not understand and does not know how to help them. They took me up to 1,800 milligrams of Thorazine^R per day when I was first hospitalized, and the doctor told me he would be willing to take me up to a potentially lethal dose of 3,000 milligrams per day. By the time I was discharged, the total daily dose was reduced to 900 milligrams per day. But I still could not think and could not really function as a thinking, feeling person.

So when I was discharged I stopped taking the medication altogether and went through a medication withdrawal which occurs if you go from 900 milligrams a day to zero milligrams a day in one jump. I did not know about tapering off doses at that time. Also, I refused to consider going to any psychiatrist or any therapist for follow-up treatment, which was also most unwise on my part. I was not really offered these because I forced the doctor in the hospital to discharge me because they had no right to keep me. I had not signed myself in voluntarily, and had done nothing to give them reason to hospitalize me involuntarily. They were, essentially, detaining me illegally. And when I forced my own discharge, I was not offered follow-up.

I can empathize with the doctor, who may have wished me to have a planned discharge with proper follow-up, but by the rules of the way the game is played, he was not allowed to do that. Actually I think this particular doctor was just glad to see me go because I had been contesting his every move. Not with threats, not with screaming, not with bad behavior, but with opposition which was all the more difficult for him because it was calm and well-reasoned.

At one point during that hospitalization the staff began to talk about me as if I were not taking all the medication, which up to that point was not true. But they gave me the idea of 'cheeking' the medication, that is parking it between my teeth and my cheek so as to be able to swallow in the large middle part of my mouth without swallowing this particular pill, and then going to the bathroom and spitting out the cheeked pill. This was a matter of survival for me because I could hardly hold my head up on 1,800 milligrams a day. I found out later that that is not (or was not in those days) an extraordinary dose for a schizophrenic, and that is why having a correct diagnosis is so very important.

I must say that when I got to be a psychiatric resident myself and I heard the old saw about how difficult it is to tell the difference between the bipolar patient and a schizophrenic, I kept a tally of the people I admitted under either diagnosis and found that I made a correct call 85% of the time. The reason is fairly simple.

A true schizophrenic may become agitated, may scream, may struggle, but does not try to relate to the other people around them. They may be standing in one corner of the room screaming bloody murder, but they're not screaming it to anyone in particular, and they're not particularly concerned whether anyone understands their point of view. The opposite is true of a bipolar (manic-depressive) patient. This patient, while talking very loudly and because of the rapidity of their speech and the way they may jump from subject to subject seeming to make little sense, is desperate to have their hearer understand. A bipolar patient will follow the provider around the room saying things like "Do you get it? Do you get it?" with a frantic desire to be understood. I don't quite comprehend why this is not generally noticed and written about – why it is still said that schizophrenia and bipolar disorder are hard to distinguish. I also think it makes a tremendous difference to both schizophrenics and bipolar patients if the providers speak with low volume and slowly. Unfortunately many providers jump immediately to high volume, high pitched rapid speech almost as if they were imitating the patient. It is a pity that the low and slow approach is not generally taught.

Let me just conclude that if a person is understood to be bipolar, a mood stabilizer is what should be given them with perhaps a small dose of antipsychotics, whereas a schizophrenic is not given the mood stabilizer, generally speaking. And having been through the experience of being misdiagnosed, a patient may have difficulty trusting other more savvy members of the profession later on.

Let's talk about what it is most important to say to your providers (or to have a family member say) when you first meet them. Let's say your problem is depression. It is extremely important, not only to talk about what "caused" the depression (the inciting event -- namely, you got fired, your significant other left you, the house burned down, or the fact that you have been dealing with a 'gray' mood most of your life). It is also extremely important to mention that others in the family have had a good appreciation of a certain medication, or conversely that others in the family have tried a certain medication and had a bad side effect. If your mother and your grandmother have both benefited from fluoxetine (Prozac^R), that would suggest that you might benefit from it too, because there is quite a lot of "brain chemistry" which may be inherited. If, on the other hand, three family members have all tried lamotrigene (Lamictal^R) and each of the three have had rashes, or blisters, then that would strongly suggest that lamotrigene is not the best choice for you.

What medication can do is to change the "background lighting" of your mental processes from dark gray to sunlight. Instead of thinking how bad things are, you begin to think that it's time to make a change; you begin to invest some energy in the idea that life will be much better once you have changed it. More importantly, you have the energy to think about a change in yourself, and you are no longer up to your neck in your symptoms and your suffering, so changing yourself and thus changing your life becomes a real possibility.

It is undeniable that changes in brain chemistry do produce changes in moods and feelings. But you would be ill-advised to count on the change in brain chemistry coming from the pill, and refuse to change your thought patterns. There are people in this world whose negative thought patterns can defeat even heroic combinations of medication.

A particular thought pattern, when it is new, is fairly easily changed. But 'rehearsing' the bad thoughts, as we call it, thinking the same bad thing over and over day in and day out, can make those thoughts habitual, and it is not easy to break a bad habit.

It is the same with self-esteem. I remember personally grappling hold of negative thoughts about myself every time they occurred and coming back with "Get thee behind me, Satan." At first I had this little snippet of conversation with myself many times an hour, in fact scores of times a day. As time went on, and I persisted in this direction, my thoughts served up less and less condemnatory self-criticism. I am a rather clumsy person; this is understandable if you comprehend that my balance is poor and that I do not perceive things visually as a normal person does. I made snide remarks to myself in the beginning every time I dropped things, I spilled things, I made a mess or I forgot something.

But at the end of a year, all that rose up in my mind when I made a mess was "Oh, you'll have to clean that up. I wonder where the broom is?" I also began to hear little voices in my head when I did not trip or spill something saying, "Hey, forty feet from the end of the cafeteria line to the table, and you made it! Good for you," rather than being critical of me. Change was very gradual, I remember after repeating the reply to "Oh what a screw-up you are" as "Get thee behind me, Satan" for three weeks, I didn't seem to have made much dent in the frequency of the negative remarks. But after a month or so, the negativity began to fade a little. Instead of "Oh, what a screwball you are!" it was "You are sometimes a bit of a screwball."

This is all talk, but I'm including it here in the section on medication because one of the things that shows your medication is working is that the negativity of your world view, of your appreciation of an afternoon, and of your self-talk will diminish in force as well as in frequency. Also, if you continue with very negative self-talk, no pill in the world will override it well.

Now a word about antipsychotic medication. We do now have a number of medications which can markedly diminish, even eliminate auditory hallucinations, and to a lesser extent visual ones. Gustatory and tactile hallucinations do exist in the literature, but I'm not sure that I have ever encountered people with them. For some people, it is hard to eliminate the hallucinations completely, but we can at least dial them down to a very soft volume, and some patients say the volume is soft enough so that they cannot hear the ugly things the voices say. Note there is a whole chapter of this book on Medications in Schizophrenia (Chapter 11).

This is an area where so-called polypharmacy is justifiable. I was once able to reduce the suffering of a man who was continuously completely irrational, and I gave him meds that helped him, I'm sure, to the point where, at a court hearing concerning his continuing commitment to the hospital, both the judge and the lawyer for the patient admitted they had never seen this man as good as he was that day in thirty years. The secret was that I had him on three different medications, each acting somewhat differently, which meant that he had a cumulative therapeutic effect without cumulative side effects, and, actually, he had hardly any side effects at all. However, just as I was leaving the hospital, the edict came down from the authorities that no patient could be given more than two antipsychotic drugs, which would inevitably mean that his symptoms would be back at least partially, compared to what they had been on three medications. This is because the cost of maintaining someone on three different antipsychotics would have been more expensive, prohibitively so in the eyes of authority.

It should be mentioned that after many years, some patients with psychosis do not want to have their voices eliminated altogether. As one patient said to me, "The voices are my company. I would be a very lonely person but for them."

A similar observation can be made about antidepressant polypharmacy. It makes no sense to combine Prozac^R with Paxil^R or Zoloft^R. They all have similar mechanisms of action. But, there are some nice results to be had by combining Prozac^R or Paxil^R or Zoloft^R with Welbutrin^R (bupropion) in some patients. Buproprion is known to lower the seizure threshold, so it is not usable in patients who have epilepsy or seizures. Bupropion also tends to make people somewhat anxious and edgy. But for patients who are sitting at home like a bump on a log, totally without energy, whose "get up and go got up and went" as a patient of mine once said to me, Welbutrin^R (bupropion) can be a very good idea. If on the other hand, the patient is depressed and wringing their hands, or pacing back and forth, (fairly anxious), then Welbutrin is not such a good idea.

Insurances do not look with favor on what <u>they</u> call polypharmacy. This is because insurances do not want to have to pay for two medications. Sometimes the case can be made for allowing two medications if one is a very expensive new medication (such that sticking to that one medication at a higher dose would actually be very expensive) and the other is a medication which has been around for years, and exists in unpatented, generic form. Also, if the patient has had an adequate trial (that means at least four to six weeks for antidepressants though less time for antipsychotics), then the insurance will pay for a combination that does work. The discouraging thing for doctors and patients is that the insurance may not pay for a particular expensive new medication unless at least three adequate trials have been made on old medications which are cheaper. And so the doctor is forced to try cheaper medications even if he or she is convinced that these are unlikely to work, unless the patient has a written record of having taken three cheap ones before.

What I usually do when I encounter someone on several medications of one class, if they are doing what they think of as relatively well (meaning that they are doing at their average or better of their functioning over the last ten years), if I think there is a significant possibility that they may get better yet, is ask them if they want any changes. If they say "Oh no, please don't change a thing, it was so hard to get to be doing this well; I don't want to rock the boat", I don't change anything. If they seem curious and open to the possibility that this is not the best regimen for them under the sun, then I may make a small change. If they say "I've been to six doctors and nobody knows what's good for me and I really am having a terrible time" then I may change their regimen substantially, keeping in mind that it is best to taper off most medications (decrease the dose slowly).

I do wish patients would come to me with an accurate medication history. As I said before, it would suffice to write down the names of medications when they were first prescribed by a doctor, whether it works, and then not write anything until the dose, the posology (that means, when the dose is taken, as, for example, 'two in the morning' or 'one in the morning and one at bedtime') changes. The reason for the change in posology should be stated in the patient's record. A note should be made also when the medication is discontinued, stating the reason for discontinuation, and specifying everything known about which side effects this particular patient experienced.

I wish that people would write this down, as I said in Chapter One, because if the patient comes to a doctor with a list of medications which were tried, how long they were tried at what dose, and what were the effects and the side effects, a doctor can conclude a great deal about a patient's brain chemistry. But if each doctor the patient sees is ignorant of their past history, each doctor will then start as if they were doctor number one (in other words, they will have to start at the beginning again).

Now a word about benzodiazepines. Benzodiazepines are a class of medication that is perhaps the best we have against anxiety. This class includes Valium[R], Librium[R], Klonopin[R], Xanax[R] and Restoril[R] as well as others. They are all potentially addictive, though Xanax[R] is considerably more so than the others. This is because Xanax^R has a very rapid onset, acts for three to four hours, and then has a very rapid offset. The rapid offset means that a person is experiencing a mini-Xanax^R withdrawal about four hours after they take the pill. This is a setup for wanting to take more for many people, a setup for addiction.

Even if the patient has no history of substance abuse (excessive use of alcohol, or any use of cocaine or heroin, or excessive use of prescription medications such as Percocet^R or oxycodone) benzodiazepines may represent a danger, especially Xanax^R. I have known clinic administrations decide that "we don't prescribe Xanax^R anymore here to anyone". I have worked in clinics that run the gamut from not prescribing any benzodiazepines at all, to prescribing 'benzos' to two-thirds of their patients.

'Benzos' are effective against anxiety, but they also diminish cognitive ability, and they may make susceptible people dizzy and more inclined to fall. The diminished cognitive ability is what I think some people dislike.

Now, I said 'diminished cognitive ability'. But if a person starts out so anxious they "can't think straight" then actually giving them a small amount of a 'benzo' can diminish their anxiety and their thinking can improve. It's all a matter of where you start from. There is one more thing that I should say about benzodiazepines. The reason they are addictive is that if a person takes a steady dose for a long time, they will build up a tolerance. What that means is that this same dose no longer has the effect it once did, and the patient will be wanting more. Many people start on the road to addiction when their doctor won't give them what they want, so they start buying more on the street, or they start visiting two doctors or something of the kind.

I once had a patient who took Doctor Clark's (my) prescriptions to CVS, Doctor Richardson's to Rite Aid, Doctor Edwards' to Eckerd's, and Doctor Foxe's to Faye's (please note, the first letter of the doctor's last name corresponds to the first letter of the name of the drug chain the prescription went to). People don't realize the danger of this in the beginning; they simply say, "This dose does not 'do it' for me anymore" and want an increase in dose. I warn everybody I put on benzodiazepines that if they lose the prescription, misplace it, leave the pills on the bus or whatever, I will not replace it before they should have their next prescription. I also say that I may be able to increase the dose slightly, but there will come a time, if they keep creeping up on the dosages, that I cannot go any higher.

So then I conclude by suggesting that they skip a dose once in a while. I invite them to choose the day on which they're going to skip a dose. For example, if a woman is going through a difficult divorce and has to meet with her husband and the lawyers about property divisions, and then has to go to court, I suggest she may want to take all doses of her medicine on those days. But if there is a day in between when nothing in particular is happening and she is going to be around the house all day, perhaps that's the day she can skip a dose of her medication. I remind people that people who become addicted to benzodiazepines may be just as much in need of substance abuse treatment (which is usually four weeks of inpatient treatment) as people who are addicted to alcohol or cocaine or heroin, and suggest again that they will not become addicted if they never become habituated to taking any given dose -- and the easiest way not to become habituated is to skip a dose every three to five doses so that they don't become "in the habit" of taking benzodiazepines daily and on time without fail. I point out that this is the only class of medication for which I say skip a dose; I do not encourage people who are on antidepressants or antipsychotics or mood stabilizers to skip a single dose.

I do not appreciate therapists who try to force the issue and try to make me change a prescription without even talking to the patient. I do not think it's a good idea to use a therapist as an intermediary between the doctor and the patient -- the doctor should see their patient and talk to that patient directly. Perhaps, rarely, both professionals can see the same patient together. I have sometimes made an extra appointment with a patient to see them sooner than I otherwise would have to discuss this issue, but no doctor should take anybody's word for it and simply give a prescription for a different dose. That breaks the doctor/patient relationship, and is most unwise.

I should add that when I first see a patient on antipsychotics for a psychotic disorder, I explore diminishing doses with them, because many are overmedicated. This may come about because they are given an "emergency" dose when they make a fuss sometime, and the "emergency" dose may have become part of their regular regimen.

Medications make it possible to change your old ways of thinking. Instead of feeling helpless continually, you find yourself wondering what you could plant in your garden. Go with the positive thought, get some seeds and plant your garden, or take the course, or get the job.

If on the other hand you cling to all you old ways of thinking, refuse to consider any positive developments in your life and refuse to focus perhaps on some details which you can change which make the bigger picture more bearable, if you devote all your thought energy and psychic energy to feeling bad, nothing is going to help you. Nothing will help you until you're willing to help yourself.

I have many patients who say to me at a certain point, "Doctor, you don't understand -- I have every right to feel terrible." I agree with them that they have the right to feel terrible. But then I say, do they really want to exercise that right? Would they not sooner feel a little less terrible?

Here too, whatever you use to engage yourself with a constructive outlook in life will be to your benefit. I have known some patients who felt much better after they started doing something positive in the community -- whether it is becoming a crossing guard for the school, walking dogs for the ASPCA, volunteering at the Lighthouse for the Blind, or whatever it might be.

I worked at a very large clinic once where the budget had been cut, and so the clerk whose job it was to take a folder and put in one sheet each of the many different forms used when a case is opened, had been terminated. One of my patients expressed interest in doing this, and so she came in for an hour or two a couple of times a week and put together new charts -- the folder and the copy of each blank page required to open a chart for a new case. She felt she was contributing something (which she certainly was) -- when the clerk had been fired, I was one of the physicians who was going slightly batty over trying to find all those pieces of paper and put them in order in the folders. She felt she was contributing something, the doctors found the papers they needed much more easily, and she volunteered at the clinic without ever coming into direct contact with distraught patients. She went on from this to become commercially employed as a clerk in an insurance claims office. Other people might have said that her job was very boring, but she enjoyed getting everything just right and keeping it all filed away just so. She enjoyed the triumph over chaos that this ability of hers represented.

I will talk in another chapter about how to negotiate with your providers when they choose what seems to be the wrong medicine for you. (chapter 12) But medication is a very important part of your treatment, and you should use it as fully as you are able.

Next I have to speak about something which occurs in psychiatry as it occurs in every other medical specialty, which is "me-tooism." Let us say a person has a diagnosis of major depression, and let us say he or she has chosen to have medication <u>and</u> talk therapy, which is by far much more likely to result in a positive outcome than either medication or talk therapy alone. In this respect, the algorithms (decision trees) which start out as either medication <u>or</u> therapy are basically flawed. Either one of those modalities can result in a positive outcome in perhaps thirty to fifty percent of cases. Together, there is a positive outcome in sixty to perhaps eighty-five percent of cases. There are unfortunately those unlucky fifteen percent of people we can't seem to help very much. But the amazing thing is that we can do a lot for eighty-five percent of the people that walk into our offices. But "me-too-ism" is a very dangerous. It is a situation in which a doctor goes along with diagnosis and treatment, in a patient who is not responding well, following what another doctor says without thinking for themselves – another doctor diagnosed this patient and started treatment and the new doctor just follows along. If the patient isn't doing well, the diagnosis and treatment need to be rethought. This is extremely difficult when time is very limited. Most insurances will pay for a diagnostic evaluation every year or two, however, and a diagnostic evaluation is usually given 45 minutes or an hour, so that can be used to find the time to rethink the diagnosis.

There are a handful of medications specifically used for substance abuse problems. One is Suboxon^R (for which the generic name is buprenorphine) which is used for the office-based treatment of opiate dependence. Its use should be restricted to only certain patients who are likely to comply with the treatment, and the prescriber has to have a special Drug Enforcement Administration license, which is generally the same number as their regular DEA license with the letter x before it indicating that they have had special instruction in the use of buprenorphine as well as that they have been determined by the DEA not to be in any difficulty regarding their prescribing of controlled substances.

As with any treatment for substance abuse, buprenorphine can work nicely if the patient is committed to it. Court committed patients are generally sent to inpatient substance abuse treatment facilities, but we do not have nearly enough of these and office-based treatment requires a lot less professional time. The thing is, only some of those people who can be prescribers are permitted to prescribe buprenorphine, and they must not have more than thirty patients total on buprenorphine to start out.

Here, beyond any other place in psychiatry, you should be candid and honest with your prescriber about what's going on. Of course, the substance abusing community (if one can call it that) is not known for being candid and honest about their illegal habits, and so there are various ways which I will not go into here about how they attempt to hoodwink their professionals when they do not wish to be abstinent. One of the scariest for those professionals is that the patient just doesn't show up – one wonders where one's patient is, and may be inclined to assume the worst.

There are other medications for substance abuse besides buprenorphine. One of the oldest, for alcoholics, is Antabuse^R (the generic name is disulfiram). This is a medication which is not recommended for those people who are first trying to gain their sobriety, but rather for those people who have been abstinent from alcohol for some considerable period of time and want a little extra reason to see to it that they stay that way. Antabuse^R will make the person who consumes alcohol while taking the medication extremely nauseated and may make them vomit. The idea is the person takes the medication and knows that if they then consume any alcohol they will be very sick. People who are just starting on their road of sobriety may very well consume the alcohol without consuming the Antabuse^R. It's only the people who really want extra help, an extra reason to stay off drinking alcohol, who will use Antabuse^R to good effect.

Other medications which may help a substance abuser by helping reducing cravings are Campral^R and Revia^R. These function to reduce the craving for the substance in question; some patients say they work very well and others say they have hardly any effect at all. But then, people's craving once they are abstinent may vary quite a bit.

Now something about personality disorders. It should be said that there is a hierarchy in treating psychiatric problems in terms of which comes first. Eating disorders are top priority to treat, especially anorexia because people with anorexia can literally die of starvation. Substance abuse problems would also be among the first to be treated, mood disorders (depression and bipolar disorder) and are in the middle, and personality disorders, being nonfatal as well as being the most difficult to treat, are approached last. People with personality disorders are given mood stabilizers in an effort to stabilize their moods, though if the underlying problem is borderline personality disorder, this may not be very effective. They are also given small amounts of antipsychotic medication, which is to say that antipsychotics are used as 'thought glue', rather than antipsychotics per se.

This is a time-honored use which does not have FDA (Food and Drug Administration approval because the cost of doing the research required to get FDA approval would be prohibitive. In this instance, the antipsychotic medications are intended to increase a person's ability to be in the present, and to improve their reality orientation, just as they are sometimes used in Post-Traumatic Stress Disorder (PTSD) or other severe anxiety disorders. This 'off-label (unapproved) use should not happen with the elderly, however. The purpose of using antipsychotics in this way is not to treat a psychosis, but to incline the patient's thinking to be more reality-based, and I have seen the addition of a small dose of antipsychotic do wonders for particular patients. I'm sure these medications are given to some people for whom they do little good, but a small dose does not do most young or middle-aged adults any harm, and when I encounter somebody with a history of a difficult personality disorder who is now on a small dose of antipsychotic and seems to be doing much better than they used to be, I leave them on it.

The lack of FDA approval does not mean that using a medication in a way for which it has not been officially approved is a bad thing to be doing. It may mean, as I said above, that the manufacturer has determined that the cost of doing the studies to prove that it should be officially permitted is too expensive. There may not be enough people who would use it in this way to make it worth the pharmaceutical company's while.

An off-label use is not necessarily a bad (harmful) use, however, particularly if among the professionals there are a number who use medications of a given class in a particular unapproved way. Certainly being a lone ranger and using medications off label in ways that other professionals do not, can be very risky, (in terms of liability) for the provider. Because if anything goes wrong, this will come to light; but using medications off-label in a way in which the majority of other prescribers also use them is not so regarded. Getting a use on label can be very difficult and very expensive for the manufacturer, as I indicated above.

It's not easy to tell whether a person's personality disorder is helped by any medication or not. Certainly, many of our patients would feel abandoned if they were refused medications, and there exist no specific medications for Axis II (personality disorders). These are indeed some of the most difficult problems to treat, and the relatively new group therapy for borderline personality (called dialectical behavior therapy or DBT) is a great help.

An exception to this idea that treating a number of conditions with a small amount of antipsychotics does not cause harm is the elderly population, specifically those who may be extremely forgetful or have dementia. The use of small quantities of antipsychotics, (and these would be very small doses since doses are smaller in the elderly than in the general population anyway) has been linked to an increase in overall mortality. That is to say that those who are taking small doses of antipsychotics tend to die sooner than those who are not taking small doses of antipsychotics. Here is an example of an important risk/benefit consideration. If the patient is quite wild and unmanageable, yelling, screaming, throwing things etc. then a very small dose of antipsychotic may help to make family visits possible. If the patient's behavior is less obstreperous, then the patient should not be given even small doses of antipsychotic because they may cause the patient to die sooner than he otherwise would have. Another consideration is, what is the older person's life expectancy without this medication. If the person is expected to die soon of their heart or liver or lung disease, then perhaps calm family visits are particularly important. At the very least, this should be discussed with the patient's family. There have been one or two families in my career who were so hung up on having their great-grandpa behave very well that I did not offer these antipsychotics because I felt the family would not give due consideration to the fact that the medication might shorten his life. But that of course is an individual situation, and it only happened once or twice in my career of treating over ten thousand people.

For other people, medications can stabilize moods, they can elevate moods, and they can decrease anxiety. But the medications still don't go out and get the patient a job, straighten up their relationship with their significant other, or plan their return to school. This is left to the patient, and this is where many patients do not succeed.

In short, the medication will not "make the patient better". The medication will make it possible for the patient to make him- or herself better. It is rather like stumbling around in the dark without medication, and then when you have taken the medication for a little while, the light comes on. Daylight by itself does not make you get a job or settle your differences with your significant other or anything else, but it makes it a lot easier for you to accomplish those things.

Therapists often provide what I call "staying power". This means that when it is possible for the patient to, say, apply for a job, the therapist can help by keeping the patient determined to get a job rather than giving up after one or two failures. Of course, I am probably talking about someone who was employed and had a good track record until they recently were upset by depression or anxiety or whatever. Most psychiatric patients never become competitively employed. I am convinced that it is because they don't have enough "staying power", and because there are some providers who do not have the imagination to see that they could get a job. It might not be a very fascinating job, but it would be a job, which for many patients would be a considerable advance in the world.

I think it would be a considerable help to state clearly what a doctor needs to know before he can prescribe medication. He or she needs to know what the patient has been on before (from another prescriber). It is very helpful to know the dosage. If the patient stopped taking this medication, why did he or she stop? Did she try the medication for at least as long as a month without skipping doses, or not? Is there anyone in the family who has a similar disease, who has taken this medication and had strong reactions? If the patient has been treated with these "wrong medications," what misled the doctor? This can be a very difficult question. Sometimes the way the history is presented can be very misleading. Sometimes, I will admit, doctors don't listen as well as they should. But the history that the patient has of taking medications for this problem – or for other problems – can be very important.

In the final analysis, a psychiatric patient is invited to make over who they are in the world. This can be painful, but it can also be very rewarding. Imagine someone who is always thinking of the negative, of the reasons they will not succeed, of the resentment of something someone else did or said, who is able to turn that around and become a very positive person. Such a person has done a lot of work, but the work pays off in that for the rest of their lives they are "walking on the sunny side of the street" – that is, they are seeing life from a positive can-do perspective. One does not often see this happen, because it takes courage and a great deal of work. But the person who has learned to emphasize that the glass is half full rather than half empty is happier for the rest of his life, and a wonderful example to everyone who knows him.

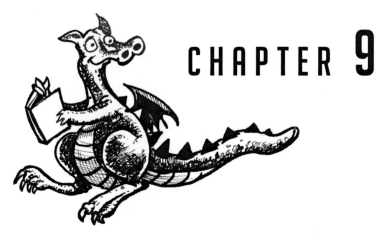

CHAPTER 9

HOW TO SAVE A BUCK (OR TWO)

The previous chapter was about what a reasonable person can expect from the right dose of an effective medication. This chapter is about how to save money. One of the most obvious things to do to save money is to pay the copay for your medication less often. Most insurances now do business with pharmaceutical supply houses for maintenance medication. For medications that you are planning to take indefinitely and for which you expect infrequent changes in dose, you can ask the doctor to write a prescription for a ninety day supply, and you will pay one copay for that ninety day supply instead of paying three copays, each one for a thirty day supply. This will cut your copays for those medications to one third. Note: this differential, one copay if you use a 90-day supply house versus three for a corner pharmacy does not work for all Part D plans that are used in the Medicare population. Some Medicare Advantage plans may still make prescription medicines quite expensive; in Medicare Supplement Plans, especially if you do use the 90 day supply house (which sell large volumes of medication and may get special prices from the pill manufacturer) you may pay nothing or next to nothing for your prescription medications, if they are commonly prescribed ones in generic form.

A maintenance medication, the kind of medication for which you may use the pharmaceutical supply house, can be most medications except antibiotics (for which you are given the exact number of doses for seven to ten days), or painkillers (analgesics) for things which we expect will heal so that a painkiller is not required for more than a short while, or cancer treatment drugs. Examples are painkillers for a sprained ankle, a broken toe. There are also some skin conditions which we expect will clear up after a few days to a few weeks of medication. For these short term medications, you use your local pharmacy and pay the copay for however many days' worth of medication we anticipate you will use. I am not going to go into cancer chemotherapy in any detail, it is a very complicated subject.

Nowadays, local pharmacies may also give a ninety day supply for three copays, but there are two disadvantages to using them. Refills are allowed only a few days before you run out. In winter, when you may get a cold or your car may be in the shop or whatever, not being allowed to get your meds until you are nearly out of them may be a bit risky. Ninety day supply houses, on the other hand, usually allow refills to be ordered on the 62nd day, which may be delivered a week later, still 3 weeks before you run out of your old supply. Furthermore, the pharmaceutical houses are at a distance, but they will send your medication to your home, which means you don't have to go and get it. For an elderly person who may not find moving around in wintertime so easy, home delivery is a distinct advantage.

There are a couple of disadvantages to using pharmaceutical supply houses. One of those is that they are set up to have members of the public talk, not to pharmacists or pharmacy assistants, but to customer service representatives. Should it happen, for example that your doctor increases your dose of medication X of which you take a 25 milligram pill twice a day to medication X 25 mg three times a day, the pharmaceutical supply house will not necessarily notice that your dose has been increased and that you will need a refill sooner. I would advise a patient to call the pharmacy a few days after the doctor has faxed the new prescription and point out that they are using up their supply faster and will need medication sooner than they otherwise would have. I personally used to write on the prescription for a patient of mine, "Note increase in dose, from 2 pills/day to 3 pills/day", and I ask my doctors to do the same. It is always a good idea to have the date on which your doctor faxed the new prescription.

The second inconvenience of using pharmaceutical supply houses, is it may take as much as seventeen or eighteen days for your medication to arrive. It may take three or four calendar days for the order to be filled, especially if it is called in on a Friday, and then you must budget two to three weeks for the order to arrive at your house. Some pharmaceutical supply houses will deliver an automatic message when they send the medication out. The message will give the order number, but not the name of the medication, so it is wise to have gotten the order number from them when you talked to them. They do have the option of your requesting for the medication to arrive in a few days, but this costs a surcharge frequently of the order of $15, and so you are not saving much money if you use this service. For that reason, you should have a method of regularly surveying all your medications to check if there are any that are three weeks away from needing a refill. If you get in the habit of doing this, you will be able to judge by looking at the bottle about how many pills there are left.

The pharmaceutical supply houses may list on the bottle the number of refills you have left, and they may say refills zero when you need a new prescription, or "call your doctor." The pharmaceutical supply houses may not remind you when you need to get a new prescription from your doctor. It can also be complicated if you see your doctor infrequently, because I firmly believe that it is in your interest to ask for the prescriptions when you're in front of the doctor. Some medical or psychiatric practices have efficient ways of asking the doctor to get prescriptions on a day that you're not being seen by the doctor, and some don't. Also, some practices will ask that the pharmacy fax them when you need a new prescription, and the supply houses may not be willing to do this. All practices which involve your speaking to someone who then writes a note to or speaks to the doctor are less certain of delivering the results you want because the intermediary and the doctor must both remember to do something that they're not in gear for. They are geared up to do their best to serve the patients they see that day.

But please notice that the solution of getting your prescriptions to a pharmaceutical supply house which will give you ninety days for, shall we say, $5 is actually cheaper than the offer made by a large national chain which sells many many different kinds of things besides prescriptions to fill some prescriptions of extremely common medications for $2. They mean a thirty day supply for $2, which would be a ninety day supply for $6, which is more by $1 than your usual copay for ninety days. Added to which, you never know how long this particular "special" of the national chain will continue.

I should mention that there are some medications which you consider to be maintenance but which may be controlled substances (narcotic painkillers, benzodiazepines such as Valium^R Ativan^R Klonopin^R Xanax^R and stimulants for attention deficit/hyperactivity disorder (ADHD)) which the provider may not by law give you as a ninety day supply. In some states, it is common to give two prescriptions, one of that day's date and one dated four weeks later, at one time. This is not illegal, so many clinics do do it.

But your doctor may not feel that he or she wants to give you access to that much controlled substance medication if you have ever been suicidal, or have been known to try and fill a prescription early, or if you have ever been known to give some pills from a controlled substance prescription to a person for which they were not prescribed. This is actually a crime and is considered quite a serious one, because you as a member of the public do not know what other incompatible medications the other party may be on, or what dangers these medications represent to them because they are not you. It also suggests that you may be buying some extra on the street to make up what you need to last the whole month if you give some away to someone, and yet have enough for yourself. So, that is the doctor's choice. There is the question of how much the patient trusts the doctor; there's also the question of how much the doctor trusts the patient to do what they're supposed to do and not be handing away or selling controlled substance pills.

Please realize further, if you do use a supply house for your maintenance medication, that you may have to remind your prescriber, when you do run out of refills, that you take a ninety day supply. If you take one pill a day, that's ninety pills. If you take two pills a day it will take one hundred and eighty pills to be enough for a ninety day supply; three pills a day is two hundred and seventy pills for ninety days; four pills a day is three hundred and sixty pills for ninety days, etc.

Personally, I recommend having the patient send in paper prescriptions with their new patient information when they have just moved or just switched insurances so that the patient is not counting on some overworked clerk to match up their new patient information with their doctor's prescriptions. If they're sent in the envelope together, there's a much better chance of things going through smoothly. I remember when I was first back in New York from Belgium and I allowed my doctor to fax in my prescriptions while I sent in my new patient prescription information. It took four weeks and I was down to my last pill when I finally got the prescriptions. And being down to your last pill causes an anxiety that I would not wish on anyone. Since I didn't have my New York State license yet, I couldn't just walk into a pharmacy and get myself a few pills. This is not regarded as good practice, and I would never do it except as a continuation for another doctor's prescription which the ninety day supply house has messed up. Of course it is not to be done at all for controlled substance prescriptions, and I never have. Because I don't like to live on the edge of running out of essential medications, I have learned to start asking perhaps five weeks before I will run out for my medication. In fact, I may fill the ninety supply house prescriptions after only sixty-two days periodically, so that I get a nice cushion of time before I will run out.

I should mention that your refill dates, although they start out in a particular location with a particular supply house and ninety days from the first fill, may tend to spread out if you change doses or if you change medications X and Y to some other in the same class that is similar but not exactly the same one. I currently take eleven different medications every day. I am tapering off one, which will take me down to ten, but nevertheless because of various things that have happened in terms of changing medications or changing doses, the refill times have spread out quite a bit. This can be annoying; it is a lot less efficient than being able to call the supply house and order all ten medications on the same day.

It is basically up to you to keep track of when you need refills or when you need a new prescription. Do not absolutely count on the supply house or on your local pharmacy to do this for you. If you have trouble remembering or figuring out such things, perhaps this is one of the things that a concerned family member or friend could help you with. It certainly is also is something appropriate to mention to your case manager, if you have one.

One of the great advantages of using the supply houses is that if you tell the pharmacy whenever you move, they are willing to send your medications, prescribed by a doctor in your home state, to whatever address you give them in the lower forty-eight states. Now, that does require that you will have an address. So if you were planning to be driving somewhere, perhaps it would be best to have a scheduled arrival at a hotel with a definite address at some point during your trip.

Usually, I don't count pills; I do it a lot less with years of experience than I used to. But sometimes I do. I count them in a slightly different way from the way other people might. I do not merely count the number of pills (say, one hundred) and then try to divide that total by the number I take every day (say four) and come up with the idea that I will run out of pills twenty-five days from now, and then look at a calendar try to figure out when twenty-five days from now would be. I have what I think is a more efficient way of doing things, and certainly less likely to result in error. I empty the bottle of pills that I have into a clean and dry saucer. I keep in mind that I take four of these pills a day (or two or three or whatever is the actual number that I take every twenty-four hours) so if today is 1/30/13 and it is early morning and I haven't taken any medication yet, I pick up four pills for the day and put them back in the bottle for January 30. I then pick up another four pills. If I have to I pick them up one at a time and say "January 31 one, January 31 two, January 31 three, January 31 four", and then I pick up more pills counting them with the date and with which pill it was until I have no more pills left in the saucer and that gives me the exact date that I'll run out of pills. You do have to be aware of how many days there are in the month you're talking about; for example there are thirty-one days in January but twenty-eight in February in a non-Leap Year, but I never plan to be within less than a week of running totally out of pills anyway. Instead of saying "January 31 one, January 31 two," you can say "January 31 morning, January 31 mid-day" or whatever you choose. I find this direct method of stating the date you will take the pill more likely to be accurate than counting the total number of pills dividing by the number per day and then looking at a calendar to see until what date your supply will last.

The last thing I want to speak to you about taking pills is to remember to check them before you see the doctor. If you are seeing your doctor every month and you get pills for three months, you are not likely to run into any difficulty. But if you get pills for three months and you are going to see the doctor next time four months away, then you will need two ninety day supplies or six months to make sure that you go past the next appointment date.

It is wise to have a card with all your medications on it in your wallet. This will help if you are ever in an emergency and the emergency personnel, who don't know you, will need to have the list of your medications. It takes a little time to update this list periodically and perhaps recopy it once in a while so that there are not lots of cross-outs and it is legible. Then when you go to your doctor's office you can get out your list and say them out loud. Some clinics are not very good at how they keep track of the medication someone is taking because there will be a notation of any new medication or any changes in dose, but many doctors don't bother to recopy the whole list at every visit. Personally I was rather compulsive about this, because as a locum tenens doctor, I never knew whether I would be there at the next visit or some other doctor, and I didn't wish by being a little lazy to create a misunderstanding.

I've given you some points about using ninety day supply houses. What about being able to get at least some of your medications for free? There are two sources of free medication; samples and programs for the indigent (which is a fancy name for 'poor'). We'll talk about samples first.

Samples

Samples are usually made by the manufacturer as a teaser when a drug is first available, in order to encourage prescribers to try it out on their patients who might benefit from it. It was fairly simple to handle samples years ago, because all the doctor was required to write was the patient's name, the date, the directions (such as "take one pill every morning" or "take two pills daily"). Since then, because the drug companies have realized that if a recall of a particular lot were required they would have no way of tracing their samples, the rules have changed and doctors are required to put on the label almost as much information as a pharmacist would.

Samples are usually given in boxes, and each box contains one bottle which contains four to seven pills. The doctor is not required to label every box but the amount that has to be written down has increased considerably and even such things as the patient's address may be a problem. I've had patients will say that their address is "396 East Main Street" and then say "Oh no, I suppose the front door is on Sycamore Street so I should say '396 Sycamore'". This is particularly true of a patient who may not be very stable and may be having to move a lot. And all that writing takes the one thing that a doctor doesn't have enough of, and that is time. So doctors in many clinics have not worked with the pharmacy to come up with a way of keeping track of the samples which is livable for them and satisfactory to the authorities. I remember a couple of meetings with the pharmacy of a hospital to get samples for the outpatient department. The prescribers were not always very diligent in recording the boxes they gave away, and it was extremely difficult to record everything required on one box. So giving away samples became burdensome to the doctors who worked there. Nonetheless, we did it.

More problematic for our patients was the fact that the supply of samples, gotten from pharmaceutical detail people, could be stopped at any time. If the drug had some innovative characteristics but did not sell well initially, the samples might be continued for quite some time (meaning a year or two). If on the other hand the drug was a "wild best seller" the company would not feel obliged to produce free medicine to get the prescribing professions more acquainted with it, and could stop the production of samples quite early. Personally, I promised my patients that I would give them samples for ninety days. This was enough time, if they paid attention, for them to apply for and get Medicaid. Now, Medicaid might very well refuse to pay for the newest, the latest brand name medication, but they probably would pay for what previously existed for that particular problem. Nonetheless, the patients might have a rude adjustment when they switched from the latest brand name to the old stuff, whatever that old stuff was. The problem was that I at one time in that clinic took all the new cases, most of whom were people who hadn't got their Medicaid yet, and I could not undertake to give one patient free medication indefinitely and therefore have to deprive other patients.

We as the physicians working in that clinic were obliged to spend a lot more time with the pharmacy detailers, so that they would be kind to us and give us many boxes of free meds. But I think the hardest thing for all of us was the amount of writing it took to be allowed to dispense free medication. And, the patient will have a considerable adjustment to make when either they get Medicaid and Medicaid refuses to pay for the new-fangled stuff, or they get commercial insurance and the insurance does the same thing. To give a patient samples is to put a nasty adjustment in their future, since new medications have to be on the market for many years before they go off patent and become available in generic form. Samples don't usually last that long.

Manufacturers' Programs for the Indigent

These are usually means tested, and the patient has to have proof of income. If the patient has no income (is living, for instance, with family) they may well be asked for a good reason why they cannot continue to do so and have their family pay for their meds. Different pharmaceutical companies have different thresholds below which they will supply free meds and some clinics have a nurse a large part of whose job it is to manage all the programs for the indigent.

From a doctor's point of view these programs are not satisfactory because there is no coordination of when the person gets a new supply of medicine in relation to when the person sees the prescriber. So if the prescriber wants to change the dose, that will go through only on the next time they get their prescriptions which may be eighty-nine days from now, if they got their supply yesterday. The pharmacy companies prefer to deliver the medication to the clinic, and this does oblige the patient to come to the clinic periodically, which is a good thing. One of the reasons why one individual may manage the indigent programs for the clinic is the difference in thresholds below which the indigent program would come into play, the differences between what money they will allow an adult for supporting children, etc. etc. There is little that is standard about this, which can make it quite confusing. If the threshold for losing eligibility is just above what the person has now, this is definitely a disincentive to getting a better job. But, the indigent programs do do a nice job of supplying medications for a lot of people. Pharmaceutical companies vary quite a bit in their willingness to have such programs, and I would ask the office manager of your clinic if they have such an individual to help people apply for the programs and to administer them from the patient's point of view. Usually, most of the physicians working in a clinic will know which medications have indigent programs funded by the manufacturers and which do not. It's worth asking. But if you are fortunate to have an income that is far above minimum wage, then the indigent programs would not apply to you.

There is one other possibility that I would like to mention in this chapter on saving money. That is, that patients sometimes decide to take half a dose per day, or to take a full dose every other day. I do have to tell you that this is very unwise, because you're courting disaster. Nobody, rich or poor, will do well with another hospital admission. If you're seriously thinking of doing this because of the cost of your medications, bring it up with your provider who may be able to come up with a better solution.

But you need to be a good friend to your brain, and giving the brain half of what it needs every day or a full dose of what it needs every other day or some other way of under dosing your medication is a rotten way to treat yourself.

I will conclude with what I consider a major failing of the psychiatric system. Patients are discharged from an acute ward with either a standard fifteen days' of medication or, if we're talking about a state hospital, then thirty days' of medication in New York State. Most of those discharges must be seen by an intake worker within seven days, but they may not get an appointment with an outpatient prescriber for, say, eighteen days. So if they have a fifteen day supply, they will run out of their medication three days before they see the doctor. And there's the rub.

Some patients are so fragile that they cannot go without their medication for three days without requiring readmission. I saw this so many times in so many hospitals when I was working around the country as a psychiatrist who would substitute (for someone who was out sick, or for a permanent employee who had not been found yet) that I took to telling the social worker that when and only when I had the date the patient would see their new prescriber would I write the prescriptions. If the date was eighteen days after discharge I would write a prescription for an eighteen day supply, so as not to create forced non-adherence because the patient wasn't given enough medication when they were discharged from the hospital. Then on the day they see their outpatient prescriber, they could at least get a prescription filled at a local pharmacy.

Shana Wibberley Clark, M.D., Dr. P.H.

This is a major failing of the system, because non-adherence is forced on people (and it is hard for them to believe in the importance of taking their medication if that is the case, and hard for them to believe that their prescriber cares). They are inclined to say "Oh, you're just part of the system and the system doesn't care". I hope some powerful people may read this and realize it is true and take steps to remedy the situation.

CHAPTER 10

THE SKINNY ON SIDE EFFECTS

I'm going to start by reviewing one of the commonest causes of miscommunication between doctor and patient. Let's suppose that you saw your doctor four weeks ago, at that time you were visibly and obviously depressed and he gave you a prescription for some medication. You filled the prescription and took a few doses, but after those few doses you had to stop because the medication made you unacceptably sleepy. Let us say you had one or two days when you were afraid you might fall asleep at the wheel and that you were actually seen putting your head down on your desk in mid-afternoon by your boss who let you know he'd seen it by giving you a dirty look. So, after three or four doses of your new medication, you stopped taking it. Let us say that you did notice it improved your mood or seemed to, and that you have no other complaint against it.

The feeling that your doctor tried to give you good medicine and was trying to help you, coupled with one or two minor incidents which made you feel your work is appreciated (when you're not falling asleep at your desk!) have helped you feel a little less depressed than you had been before the first time you saw your doctor.

Therefore, you come to your doctor's office and you look at him with a small somewhat rueful smile and say to him "Oh, doctor, that medicine you gave me last time made me SOO sleepy!" You don't tell your doctor what happened, that you stopped your medication after four doses.

Your doctor sees a young woman who is obviously not as badly depressed as she was four weeks earlier. He hears the patient complaining that the medication makes her sleepy, but here it is eleven o'clock in the morning and she is smiling and seems perfectly awake. He notices she's smiling with a somewhat hesitant smile which is not a full-hearted smile, but he reflects that she's only been on the medication for four weeks, and this particular medication may take a while for people to respond maximally to it. The doctor does not think to ask you directly if you are still taking the medication, nor do you think, knowing what you have been through in terms of your head on your desk and your fears while driving, (which you have not shared with the physician) that your doctor doesn't understand that you stopped taking the medication three and a half weeks ago.

So there you are, already not having the same conversation, because the doctor thinks that you are still taking the medication which perhaps has a sleepiness side effect for the first few days, and the side effect wears off after that, and you know that you stopped taking the medication after only a few doses.

Now, either one of you two could get the other to be having a conversation about how things are in reality if you would be truthful enough; on the patient's side, to admit "I took the medication for four doses but after being afraid to drive and being caught at work with my head on my desk at three p.m., I stopped taking it" or on the doctor's side by asking "Did you stop taking the medication because of the sleepiness?" But frequently, neither one states or asks point blank, so from then on they are having an unreal conversation. Note that the patient may correct the doctor when he gives her another prescription for this medication, and that may make him realize he has been living in an unreal assumption for a long time, or the patient may simply take the next prescription and leave, never to return.

Let's face it: doctors don't like a situation in which the patient does not take their prescription, every dose, when they're supposed to, until the doctor sees the patient again. Patients don't like to tell their doctor that they're not taking their medication. In the absence of absolute flat-footed candor, doctors tend to assume that the fact that at least sixty percent of the public does not take their medication as prescribed is the <u>other</u> doctor's problem, and to assume that this patient is taking it. And doctors will treat what they see; seeing is believing for any doctor.

I can understand a patient stopping her medication when her sleepiness is noted by her employer and she might get in trouble because of it. Faced with this situation myself as the patient, I have, on occasion, stopped a medication because I was obliged to, and then restarted it three days before I was due to see the doctor in order to appear very sleepy before the doctor, so that he or she would believe me and would prescribe a different medication which probably would not have this side effect. I was then able to confess that I had stopped taking the medication after four doses and had not had the benefit of the medication for most of the time between the previous visit and this one.

It's not that I am an enthusiastic advocate of stopping a medication and then restarting it so the doctor can see the side effect, but that is a viable strategy if the patient does not feel that the doctor will listen otherwise. Obviously, the patient will have to have someone else drive for those 3 days.

A strategy that's a very poor strategy for choosing a medication is to research the internet and come up with the patient's own idea of what they would like to take. The internet does not necessarily mention absolute and relative contraindications to using a medication. An absolute contraindication means that no-one with the given other condition should ever take this medication, usually because the risk of a dire event such as stroke or death is quite high. A relative contraindication means basically to use caution when giving this medication to a patient with the other medical condition. The doctor has to have a very good reason for using a particular medication if there is a relative contraindication for this patient about it. What I mean, for example, is that a patient may be depressed who also has diabetes or who also has an unsteady heart rhythm, or something of the sort. Since we have several subclasses of medication in every major class (in other words if the major class is antidepressants there are several subclasses which act differently, the same is true for antipsychotics, and the same though to a more limited extent for anxiolytics), so doctors generally want to stay away from prescribing medications with a known contraindication for some other medical condition that the patient has.

This is totally disregarded when patients try to come up with their own ideas for medications. I remember a patient who told me quite seriously that Aunt Mabel took medication X for a while and she did fine, and so they should be able to take medication X? The patient did not realize that Aunt Mabel did not have the heart disease that she did, and the medication that she mentioned would probably kill her by aggravating her heart disease, and so medication X had been dismissed as a possibility by me for that reason some time earlier.

If the patient really wants to mention another medication they should do it a little tentatively by saying "I've heard of medication Y. Is this something that I might have benefit from taking or not?" And if the doctor says no, they could certainly ask why, but ask why in a way that does not sound smartass.

The lists of side effects that pharmacies hand out are fine as far as they go, but they do not mention frequencies. They may mention horrendous possibilities such as, perhaps, stroke or even death, but they do not mention that stroke occurs in 1.5 per hundred thousand people who take the medicine, and death occurs in, for example, one per hundred thousand.

Your chances of being run over on the way to the store may be larger than one in a hundred thousand. The pharmaceutical company that supplies this information hopes to be protected from law suits if they list every side effect. Sometimes this works, sometimes it doesn't, but that is another discussion.

Of course, my heart goes out to anyone who dies of taking a medication and to their families. But such rare events are not predictable, any more than it s predictable that a person will be run over (and this has happened) while standing on the sidewalk waiting for the light to change – a car came up onto the sidewalk and killed them. Now, one may be inclined to accuse the driver of the car, but perhaps there was a malfunction in the car at just that moment (or perhaps the car driver had a heart attack) and mechanical malfunctions or bodily emergencies, like strange drug reactions, may not be one hundred percent predictable. Sometimes a person just has something bad happen for no reason we can fathom. Some people call this bad karma or bad luck – I prefer not to attribute agency to any particular occurrence, and just to say it was very sad that it happened.

Incidentally, a good source of information is a pharmacist because they have computer-generated lists of what goes with what and what does not go with what; it might be a good idea to run a new prescription by your pharmacist saying "Is this okay to take with all the other things I take?" and then ask him to call the doctor if a major problem looms. It's not always simple, because a computer-generated list of interactions will flag any two <u>chemicals</u> that interact, will not necessarily mention the mechanism or whether changing a dosage of one or the other might solve the problem.

To complicate matters further, the same side effects will affect different people differently. A gain in ten pounds, seen with indifference by a middle aged patient who will do almost anything to see their symptoms diminish, may be totally unacceptable to a young lady who is at ideal weight and proud of her curvaceous slenderness. Similarly, a student or CEO who count on being sharp-witted all the time may find even a mild degree of somnolence unacceptable, though they may not notice or mind a gain of a few pounds.

If you choose to restart the medication before you see the doctor, realize it's difficult to be navigating talking to a doctor when you're very sleepy, so it would be legitimate to go with a cup of coffee in your hand, but if the doctor sees you struggling to keep your eyelids open, struggling to stay awake, and you say "I brought this coffee this morning which I don't usually do, in an attempt to wake up to be able to see you" and "I can't take this medication because it makes me so sleepy", a doctor who sees somebody who is obviously fighting sleepiness will agree that that's unacceptable.

Sometimes, a person will incorrectly attribute a negative experience they had a few hours after taking a medicine to the medicine. Let me tell a short story to illustrate what I mean here. A patient of mine, whom I saw on a Friday and to whom I gave medication, made an extra appointment with me to come back the following week to tell me this story. He went to his pharmacy after I saw him and got the medication, and he took a pill at bedtime as instructed. He said he slept without difficulty, and got up the following day which was a Saturday, and went to lunch with a friend of his. They always lunched at a particular fast food restaurant, and they had double burgers as usual. This was perhaps at noon or one p.m. At around seven p.m. that night, the patient said he was "sick as a dog" and vomited several times.

Now, I know as a physician that if you take a medication at bedtime which is going to give you a severe side effect, it is unlikely to leave you feeling perfectly fine for about twenty hours and then suddenly give you a strong side effect. This is because medications reach their peak usually an hour or two after they are swallowed, and the peak level in your blood is associated with peak sensations of side effects.

My patient attributed his vomiting to his medication. So I asked him "How was your friend?" The patient replied that his friend was "sick as a dog" also.

"So," said I, "you took the medication almost a full day before you got sick, and your friend took no medication but he was equally unwell. Both of you consumed double burgers at the same time with mayonnaise on your salad and with your fries, and both of you got severe vomiting at the same time. But, if it was the medication that made you sick, how could your friend have gotten sick, because he didn't take any pills?"

Light dawned on my patient's face. "Oh my," he said, "I guess it couldn't have been the pill since my friend did not take any pills and got as sick as I did. Good gravy, Doctor Clark, you are a real detective! So do you think it was the burgers that made us ill?" I told my patient that I would guess it could have been the meat, or it could have been the mayonnaise because staphylococcal food poisoning sets in about six hours after the offending food is consumed. Through my head went a memory of an exercise I had done at the Tulane School of Public Health which was a real Centers for Disease Control case in which twenty individuals consumed different combinations of ten foodstuffs at a picnic. Some of the picnickers got sick, others did not. The question was to find out what the offending food was – in other words everybody who had the contaminated food should be sick, whereas no-one who had not had the contaminated food should have symptoms.

Then I explained to my patient why I had been skeptical about his attributing the vomiting in the evening of the next day to his medication. I told him I couldn't think of a medication which could be in the body for so many hours and cause no problems and then suddenly make a person very sick.

The patient smiled and said "I knew you didn't want to give me a medicine which would make me sick, and I'm very glad we figured it out."

Then I asked him if he would go back to taking his medicine, and he said he would, and he did. Let me say that the end of this story is very nice, because a man who had been hospitalized over twenty times in fifteen years saw his need for hospitalization decrease considerably. As a matter of fact, he was not hospitalized again for the remaining two years that I was in New Orleans. I discovered later that he told the story to many people saying, "I'll be darned, my doctor figured it out", and also, that he was kind enough to tell people that he had a "smart doc".

It's not a bad idea, if you are having what you consider an unacceptable side effect and the doctor keeps wanting to prescribe the same medicine, to ask your doctor why. What is his target? What is his end point? Why that medicine instead of another, similar one?

I tried, when I was working, not to have any preset limits that I placed on my patients because of their diagnosis. It seemed to make sense to me, since patients are individual people, to work with each patient to maximize their ability to function and if they could function extremely well, why that's wonderful. I retained the conviction that no one should be trashed. No one should be relegated to nonfunction by zero expectations from the doctor and other staff. Whether we have to start with teaching people how to get dressed, then that's where we have to start, but that is not where we end. I well remember before I was admitted the first time being very worried. I wondered if I could recall how to get dressed because my mind was going around the world about every six seconds; it was going so fast that I would put on one sock and forget to put on the other because I could not concentrate on what was in front of me. But I was ill, I was not stupid. Thank God several years later I encountered a psychiatrist whose attitude was "First we have to get you well, then we will see what you will do with your life."

The first thing you have to do when you have a significant side effect from any medication (assuming this is a problem or sensation you've never had before, and that it's onset is fairly abrupt within half an hour to three hours after you took your new medication for the first time) is to determine how serious it is. Do you need to go to the emergency room or to call your doctor's office right away? Think about how you would be if this side effect continued for some time. If you are mildly sleepy, and find yourself yawning in the morning but you're only yawning, not falling asleep suddenly, perhaps you can tolerate the side effect until you next see the doctor. Similarly if you are slightly dizzy but in no danger of falling, perhaps this can wait as a complaint until your next doctor's visit.

On the other hand, if you find yourself having to pull over while you're driving because you're feeling sleepy, then maybe you need to stop taking this medication. Or if you have already fallen, maybe you need help to get up, and perhaps you should not take this medication again.

I have written previously about assigning something as a medication side effect from taking a new medication vs. something that just happened shortly after you took your pill but which really had nothing to do with the pill. Sometimes these are hard to sort out, so <u>be sure to keep the facts straight about when you took the pill, when the side effect occurred, did it have its onset slowly or abruptly, is it something you have or have not felt before, etc.</u>

If you decide to stop taking the medicine as a result of experiencing this side effect, please notice whether the side effect goes away over time and whether it is gone by the time you should have taken the next dose of medicine. If you have felt something similar to it before, ask yourself whether you could tell the difference between the side effec you felt after you took the medicine vs. the feeling you may have without taking any medicine. For example, if the side effect is headache, is the distribution of the pain (that is, where the pain occurs in your head) different from your usual headaches? What about the time course of this headache? Have you ever felt a similar one before? What brought that on?

I'm laying stress on a lot of details here because often the key to what is going on inside of you is in those details, and if you don't notice them at the time, it's hard to bring it to mind later when you no longer feel it (in this case, headache).

Now as to management. I have previously told a side effect story, one about a man who was persuaded, having taken a new medicine at ten p.m., that the severely upset stomach he experienced at seven p.m. the next day (having had a fast food cheeseburger at noon) was caused by the medicine. In that case, since the friend who was with him who had also had a cheeseburger but who had not taken the medicine was also sick, the diagnosis was very straightforward as to what went on – they both had food poisoning from the fast food cheeseburgers.

I also had a patient who complained of trembling hands after taking a medication, but she did notice that the hand trembling wore off very quickly whereas the therapeutic effect of the medicine (the reason it was prescribed for her) did not wear off. Her side effect of the hand trembling was a "peak effect", something which is evident only when the level of medication in her blood is at its peak. She was able to rearrange her activities so as not to have to do delicate handwork when her hands trembled. In some cases, there may be a long-acting preparation of the medication which avoids this "peak effect" because the medicine is designed to have a lower steady blood level and not have a peak at all. I also had a patient who experienced the need to defecate about forty-five minutes after taking her medicine, who found that if she took it right after she woke up, (rather than after breakfast) the need to defecate would occur while she was still at home, when she was at liberty to do so, rather than on public transportation on the way to work.

I mention these ways of getting around the side effect here, because I think that far too often people abandon a medicine as intolerable when they could think of a way around the side effect if they gave it some thought. After all, your prescriber has spent some energy thinking of what medication would be best for the therapeutic effect for which you are being given it, and it may well be the best medication for the effect we desire. Therefore, such a medication should not be abandoned by the patient for a side effect which though inconvenient can be worked around if we put our heads together and think a bit. For example, I pointed out to this lady who had the urge to defecate forty-five minutes after taking her medication, that the instructions were to take it "in the morning" which is generally construed to be when you get up, but it doesn't specify exactly how long before you leave the house you should take it. If, as in her case, taking it after she rose in the morning rather than after breakfast would mean that her need to have a bowel movement could be dealt with before she left the house, then she was still complying with the instructions take it in the morning and this would make it tolerable for her.

Please don't forget, if you choose to give up taking a medication, to write down in your health record, which should ideally contain everything that was prescribed for you, and the reason you stopped taking a particular medication. This will help your doctor in choosing the next medication to tackle the therapeutic effect that the doctor wants for you, and that you presumably also desire because it was what your complaint was about.

I will close this section of the chapter about side effects with some information for Lithium takers which I have not seen anywhere. Not in textbooks, not in pharmacy handouts. Yet I have seen it affect many people. It concerns the fact that if you are from an area where the water you drink and cook in is very salty to an area where the tap water is very low in salt, you have a sudden drop in the sodium you are taking in every day, and for a short time at least your body may choose to conserve sodium at the expense of excreting more lithium in the urine, and your blood level of lithium may drop slightly. The drop is modest, but this can contribute to another episode of illness in a person who has recently moved and is trying to adjust to life in their new community. Obviously, if on the other hand you move from a place where tap water is low to a place of higher salinity, you will have a salt load which the body will need to get rid of by conserving Lithium, and you lithium level will go up slightly.

Part 2: How to Handle Forms

Now let us suppose you have an important form come to you, at least part of which must be filled out by your doctor. The first thing I do when I have such a form come to me is make three copies of the form, so that I have the original and two copies or three forms all told. One form I will put aside somewhere as my "accident insurance". This is to have in case I or someone else spills coffee or something else on their copy of the form and needs another copy of the form quickly. It means I won't have to go anywhere or call anyone or wait for the mail to get another copy of the form, if it is needed. A second copy I will fill out with my name, my address, my telephone number, my social security number, my date of birth. These are all things that I have by heart for me, but a doctor would have to go and look mine up because the doctor does not have, say, six hundred social security numbers of his patients memorized. Putting them on the form in the right place before I give the form to the doctor shows that I have done as much as I could to help myself and makes the doctor feel that I take the form seriously, so perhaps he or she should also. Also, I give the doctor a form for which he does not have to chase the chart – he can finish it quickly. Faced with a pile of forms for which he will have to hunt the charts, and one (mine) which can be filled out and completed in less than two minutes, he may as well do mine first. Further, the prescriber will realize I did everything I could to make things easier for him or her, and may want to reciprocate and make life easier for me by filling out <u>my</u> form first. Often, he fills it out while I am in the office.

I also fill out important dates. For example, I know the date I started seeing the doctor and the number of times I have seen him or her. Or, I know the date that I began taking medication or underwent surgery for a disabling condition. This is a matter of keeping records and being a conscientious patient. For those whose mental illness makes them not able to do such record keeping, they can either get a case manager (and many case managers go and pick up the patient to take them to a doctor's appointment so it's really worth having one if you can get one), or they may have a family member who might like to be helpful but who doesn't know how. Well, this is one thing a family member can do, help the patient keep records which I would advise would be on the patient's premises, put away carefully. It's not hard to understand, it does not get the family member in over their heads in the patient's incapacity – which the family member may or may not be able to handle – and does not embroil the family member in emotional controversies with the patient.

But <u>do not</u>, please do not fill in the diagnosis, the doctor's impression or prognosis (which means what is going to happen next – are you going to get better and when, are you not going to get better), professional opinions, the doctor's contact information, or his or her credentials. <u>This is the part that must be filled out by the doctor.</u> There are few things more annoying to a physician than to encounter a form in which the patient has written in the space where the form asks for the diagnosis something like "bad foot pain". That is not a diagnosis, any phrase with the word 'pain' in it is a symptom, and since the doctor cannot use any form of white-out or make erasures on the form, it will mean that your doctor has to start at least that page over again.

So I do fill out my own identifying information (name, age, date of birth, address, 'phone number social security number). If you cannot do this or feel that your handwriting is poor, at the very least put your name on the form. The doctor may have several patients who are going through whatever application or qualification process the form represents, and he or she may have no idea at the end of the day whose paper your paper may be if you don't even have your own name on it.

Whatever filling out you do you will have done on the form before you go to the doctor's office. Take the form to your doctor's office in a separate container (even if it's just a plastic bag from a store) which you put in your briefcase or bag or purse or whatever. Packed in a separate container you can get it out at the right moment without a lot of fishing around in your possessions which makes you look disorganized, and which loses precious time. Plus, there are some doctors who unkindly will not give a patient half a minute to find something, and who would just say "Well, I'll get to it next time" and stand up and usher you out of the office.

Do show this important paper to the doctor as soon as you say hello. If you have other things which must be discussed that day besides the form, say, "My form to apply for (whatever it is) has arrived," (as you get out the form) and then, before you hand the form over you say, "There is also a major problem with a medication you prescribed last time, which we need to discuss." Then, you hand over the form. If you hand over the form before telling your doctor you have another problem you have to discuss, he will be focusing on the form and may not hear you. I've been in this situation myself, it was wonderful how patients expected me to be able to fill out an important form while listening to them complain about a major side effect at the same time. You, the patient have been living for weeks or even months with the idea that you have two things you must discuss with your doctor: the form, and the side effect. But you need to give your doctor fifteen seconds to catch up with today's agenda.

I know there is still a great power differential between doctors and patients, but I don't think patients realize how much what they say sets the agenda. So, I would advise my patients to take the lead and set the agenda as soon as they have said hello to their doctor. My advice is, don't hand over the form until you have outlined your agenda for the day, but on the other hand hand over the form as soon as the agenda is spoken, so you're not doing what many patients do, which is go through all their time and then hand the form at the end. This gives the doctor a problem because he or she does not have a lot of time to do paperwork for patients apart from when the patient is there in the office.

So: first, set the agenda, then, hand over the paper for which you have filled out the patient's part in advance. And when you hand over the paper, if there is a particular deadline which you want to meet or a particular problem why it has to be done very soon, say so.

It is reasonable to expect the doctor to fill out the form then and there, if you filled out everything you possibly could except the part that he or she must do, and you have explained that you are under a time constraint with this form and you would appreciate it if he would fill it out right away. It is not reasonable to expect the doctor to be able to listen to you <u>and</u> fill out a form for you and return it to you then and there if you do not explain special circumstances.

My own personal limit was to say that no form stayed on my desk more than three business days. I am proud to be able to state without exception that I filled out everything I was ever asked to fill out within three work days. It is not reasonable to just show up in the doctor's office with a form when you do not have an appointment with the doctor and expect him or her to be able to fill it out without difficulty. I instructed my secretary to tell people who showed up with a form in that way to tell them to pick it up three business days later, late in the afternoon. I would then write on the top of the form the date they were going to pick it up.

Let me explain something. Taking care of you, deciding the right medications and helping you with any emergencies, is part of the doctor's job. However, filling out forms for you is also part of his job but it's part of his job that no doctor has any designated time for; his or her schedule is filled to the brim with other patients. We basically cope with forms it by gobbling half a sandwich at our desks instead of going on a lunch break, or coming in extra early someday to do it, or taking advantage of the patients who have appointments but who do not show up, to do someone else's forms. But doing paperwork is not on the schedule officially. Therefore, anything you can do to help your provider speed along through your paperwork is all to the good.

Next, I think it is extremely important that when anyone is sending forms filled out about you to some agency or other, you should have a copy of that form. Be willing to sign a release of information and have the form released to you yourself, the patient, so that you know exactly what was said about you.

Now as to mailing the form. If the form is one that the doctor's office fills out frequently for many different clients, then go ahead and let them mail out their copy, making sure you do have a copy with the doctor's signature and date for yourself as I indicated. If the form is one that few clients have asked for, then I would ask that the form be given back to you, particularly if there are other papers which you as the client must send in. It is easier to send the whole lot in one envelope, and then you don't have to imagine that someone in the agency or the organization to whom it will be sent has the ability to put the two halves of the application – yours and your doctor's – together in a file. If they are sent together, they are more likely to stay together.

More than that: if the doctor gives me back the form to send, I can make sure it is sent to the right address and it has the correct postage on it and it goes that day. If it is left to the doctor's office or the clinic to send out, it may well not be sent out for several days. I know one clinic which gives good care and is organized, but in which mail is sent out to the outside world only once a week. So if what they finished for you happened to be ready to go the day after, it would wait till the next week to get sent. This is a waste of time for you and no particular advantage to the doctor. So, if you can, I'd mail it out yourself.

Make sure before you leave the doctor's office that you go over the doctor's portion of the form. Doctors are people too, and it sometimes occurs that they can confuse one patient with another and fill out the form incorrectly. This is another reason why having brought a blank form (your 'accident insurance') to the doctor's office is not a bad idea.

Supplying the doctor with a stamped self-addressed envelope will make things go easier for you but it may still wait a week to actually get sent out. You can also take an index card and write 'your disability form has been sent, Doctor Smith' on one side and your address on the other, put postage for a postcard on it and ask the doctor to mail it when he mails the form out.

I remember when I was a patient I gave my doctor an application for a good program of supported housing which was filled out in front of me by the doctor, but then "lost" in his office for nearly 4 weeks (it had been put in the 'correspondence' section of my chart instead of being sent out). Unfortunately, by the time it was found, the deadline had passed and I never got my housing. Poor housing contributed to my needing a psychiatric admission shortly thereafter. This is why I have gone over every step – I don't want such a thing to happen to you.

CHAPTER 11

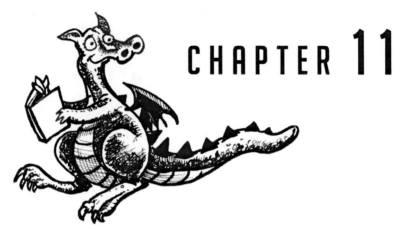

MEDICATIONS IN SCHIZOPHRENIA

People complain of being "medicine heads" when they take certain antipsychotics such as chlorpromazine (Thorazine[R]) or haloperidol (Haldol[R]). That to me means they may have needed the medicine they're on when they first came to attention because their disease may have been bad, but it suggests a reduction in dose might be very useful. Oddly enough, people who go home from the hospital may sometimes experience the need for more medication (because they are going from a safe, monitored environment to an environment with all the old stresses and strains) or they may need less because they are leaving the same monitored environment but there are other people newly arrived at the hospital who are screaming at night or carrying on during the day, and without this degree of upset around them, they don't need as much medication to tolerate being in their own house. Over the years I have met quite a few patients who are reluctant to tell me that they would like a dose reduction in one of their meds. They often can tell their therapist easily. Patients who were not willing to bring up the diminution in dose to me, but are willing to do so with their therapist, make me feel sad. Apparently, they may have seen doctors before me who would brush away any contributions from the patient. I hope that I listen for and ask about any possibilities that might help each patient, and I hope that it is not I who am so scary to the patient that they can't say "Doctor, could you just give me less medication X."

One of the things that disappoints me about many psychiatrists is how they prescribe not just the same medicine, but the same unchanging dose, for years. Biological systems do not go through years without change, and years of changeless prescription suggests that the doctor has not even been interested enough to inquire if a dose adjustment might be beneficial. If, for example, the patient has a history of trauma one winter, this patient might need more medication around the anniversary of the trauma and less in the spring and summer, to stay rational. Why see the patient if the provider is not contemplating a dose adjustment? Many psychiatrists willingly increase antipsychotic doses, but do not look for an opportunity to decrease them, even slightly. I think we should always prescribe the lowest dose that is effective, and I wish all my colleagues had this philosophy.

When I first encounter patients with primary psychotic disorders, I explore with them the possibility of decreasing doses, because many are overmedicated. In primary psychotic disorders, particularly, medication may be more important than even in depression or anxiety disorders. Unfortunately the exact mechanism whereby some people hear very destructive, negative voices talking to them is very poorly understood. But we do have a number of medications which can either diminish the volume or stop these voices altogether. We have quite a few choices, and it may take trying several to find the one that fits different patients. There is nothing I can say except to say to the patient that a little patience is well worth it here. I know it's hard to believe you can get better when you've tried a couple of medications which have not worked for you, but several trials are worth it because when you do hit upon the one or the set that works for you, the difference will be quite amazing. As I have said before, you can cut down the volume on the voices, usually, to the point where the patient is not able to distinguish exactly what it is the voices are saying. The voices become a sort of low background murmur to the patient's thoughts, which to most people is quite bearable.

This is a special chapter about medications in schizophrenia. Schizophrenic patients present a particular difficulty for us as prescribers, because they do need their medication and they are among the most difficult people to persuade to take it. We do have now some long-lasting preparations which can be administered by injection so that patients need, in the case of Haldol^R, only one visit for an injection every two, three, or four weeks, and in the case of Risperdal^R, one visit every two weeks. These preparations are recommended for those who A) are very difficult if impossible to persuade to take medications on their own and B) can be particularly violent or bothersome when they do <u>not</u> take their medication. Also, patients who have repeatedly been jailed for misdemeanors are considered candidates for depot medications.

On the other hand, there are many residents of state hospitals and others who have been overmedicated, and some of them have been overmedicated for years. This can occur in a state hospital because staff feel powerless when a patient has an outburst or an episode of misbehavior which is difficult to handle. Their immediate impulse is to request an increase the medication dosage, and they will pressure the doctor to do so, even without seeing the patient and without talking to the patient. I personally did occasionally increase doses, but never without talking to the patient, to get his or her side of the story.

Most people with schizophrenia (and please notice I do make an effort to say 'people with schizophrenia' rather than 'schizophrenics' because the former phrase emphasizes that people with schizophrenia are <u>people</u>, not a sort of embodiment of disease) are people to whom one can talk and use reason. Unfortunately, patients with schizophrenia are currently held in state hospitals often so doped up that they are, as people call them, like zombies. I once did a stint at a hospital in Wisconsin where the patients were so overmedicated that a number of them lost any connection to any part of themselves which could monitor their own behavior and decide what is reasonable. Therefore they hit out at staff members all the time. My major effort, (quite successful), while at this hospital was to decrease the number of staff injuries that occurred by <u>lowering</u> the medication dose of the patients. In the process, some of the patients 'woke up' and were able to begin to respond normally to their environment. These were patients who were given say, eleven milligrams of clonazepam (Klonopin^R) a day, in addition to heavy doses of two antipsychotics. They essentially were stripped of their cortical function (reasoned responses coming from the more civilized cortex) and all the mediating impulses which damp down our primitive animal reactions of hitting and fighting.

I am glad to say that things are not so bad in other places, but the tendency to overmedication of chronically ill people still exists. This is because with any incident or disruptive behavior on their part (which can include mouthing off at staff and is not always associated with physical risk) the doses they are given go up, and nobody ever takes it upon themselves later when the acute crisis is over to take those doses slowly down to the medication level they do need for maintenance of a reasonable outlook and behavior.

I do not think we are going to change the institutional culture of the chronic wards of state hospitals very quickly. Therefore I would invite every patient not to do the sorts of things that get them admitted into the state hospital system. Once you're in, it can be very difficult to get out. It has been my pleasure to successfully discharge a number of people from the chronic wards of state hospitals to mental health group homes in the community, and most of these people are still out there, or were out there for some time (months or years) before something happened that caused them to either create a danger or make someone nervous that they might create a danger, and they were readmitted to a state hospital.

It has been my experience that people with schizophrenia respond to straightforward direct analysis and criticism of their behavior much like other people do. It helps to put things tactfully; it also helps to put patients imaginatively in the staff's shoes, and say such things as "Well if you were a staff member and somebody yelled and called another patient names over and over, what would you do? Wouldn't you call the doctor and ask for extra medicine to calm this person down?" What is unfortunate is that in many state hospitals, staff do not try to calm the patient by talking to them, and staff may resent it, at least initially, when a doctor insists on talking to the patient rather than immediately ordering more drugs. In my experience, after a while, seeing the doctor talking to patients, staff may begin to think of people with schizophrenia as they think of other patients, namely as someone they can talk reason to, and the doctor benefits by getting less calls on the weekends for prescriptions after a dispute between patients, for instance.

By reasoning with patients, we help build in them the capacity to monitor their own behavior, and some ability to resist impulses to do things that a more balanced person would not choose to do.

By the way, schizophrenic patients are no more likely than other people are to do violent things. The difference may be that when a person with schizophrenia commits a crime of violence, it is perhaps more gory and spectacular than a crime of violence committed by a non-schizophrenic person. Therefore, it may be more memorable, and it may make the rest of the community very aware that patients with schizophrenia can certainly do very violent things. But statistically the numbers of incidents of serious violence committed by people with schizophrenia is not higher than the number of instances of violence of a group of non-schizophrenic individuals. So yes, they can be spectacularly violent, but they are no more likely to be violent than anyone else is.

Now, for outpatients with schizophrenia, it is very important, assuming that the diagnosis of schizophrenia is accurately posed in the first place (in the 60's and 70's many people, including patients with bipolar disorder, were diagnosed as schizophrenic) to get them started on a medication they can accept so that their experience of psychosis is brief and they can continue to live with normal people.

The trouble is that while many people with schizophrenia who recover from the first episode are willing to admit that something happened for the week or two they were in an acute hospital, once restored to themselves, they are not willing to believe they have an ongoing illness and that the psychosis will recur if they do not prevent it by continuing to take their medication. We have done such a good job for first episode of psychosis that the patient does not believe he or she has an ongoing problem.

They are discharged from the hospital quite well, and may even return to school or to their job, only to drift away from taking their medication because they don't believe they have an illness, and so to have a second episode. By this time, they may be thoroughly convinced that the doctors in the acute hospital were mistaken, and so may be quite resistant to taking their medication. These are the cases where things go badly.

When things go well, it is possible to explain to a recovering schizophrenic person that they do have an illness, that their illness is manageable and that their cognitive ability will not suffer as long as they keep the number of acute flare-ups of illness to a minimum. It is very helpful if their family, in this early stage of illness, can be invited to join the team of people that will help them and, for example, check up with them to be sure they are taking their medication if their behavior starts to seem a bit odd.

This is how we have today a number of schizophrenic people who are doing very well in full work, family and social roles and who do not look like the schizophrenics of previous times, who were much more likely to fall into a group with several acute episodes a few weeks or months apart each, and to begin to suffer the intellectual decline which several closely spaced acute exacerbations of schizophrenia do, to this day, bring on. The trick is to prevent the succession of a series of acute exacerbations by treating the schizophrenia properly from the beginning, and by having the patient understand that he or she has a treatable, if not curable, illness, and that he or she may well be taking medication for the rest of his or her life.

What I said in the last sentence is probably a hammer blow to many young people, but it is better if they face up to it early on than if they do not. If they do not face it, if they stop taking their medication, they very probably may have several re-hospitalizations in the first few years of illness, and begin heading towards a career as a chronic schizophrenic. The new outcome of steady effective treatment from the beginning is a real possibility; we as psychiatrists work as hard as we can to try and see to it that every new patient that is correctly diagnosed as schizophrenic choose this pathway, rather than the old, sad path of chronicity.

Of course there are a number of patients who complain of side effects, even though the side effects of the so-called atypical psychotics which are more modern than the older medicines (such as chlorpromazine, commercialized under the name of Thorazine^R and other names, and Haldol^R which is the most famous brand of haloperidol) – because the atypicals have less obvious side effects than the old stuff does. The new medicines are associated with weight gain, the metabolic syndrome, and the onset of Type II diabetes, which used to be seen only in older people hence the words 'maturity onset' diabetes. Some of the youthful complaining is because the patients, like many young people, imagine that they have a right to perfect health, without any need for medicines, and especially without the need for medicines which have side effects. For some, finding out that they have schizophrenia can be a rude shock.

But we, the adults, can shepherd them through their disbelief and dislike and rebellion against the idea that they do have a serious mental illness, and we can offer them a future which is so much brighter than the experience of their parents' and grandparents' generation. For these patients, a group experience in which their peers who have the same problem are able to agree about what a great shock it is but also to help them get through the initial negative reaction and take their medication so that they can get on to their bright future is, I think, essential.

Also, it is difficult for their families as well to hear that although schizophrenia is not curable, it is eminently treatable, and the real danger is letting the disease continue untreated. Not only do people then say and do things which are deleterious to their own future, they also (by skipping their medication) create a situation in their brain which is damaging to their intelligence.

This is what we in the profession must try and communicate, and this is the message we hope will be reinforced in the community, particularly if they meet some young people in a group who are a little further along than they are and who are doing very nicely.

I would like to offer some explanation as to why the more modern atypical antipsychotics are associated in many people with moderate to marked weight gain with all its attendant consequences (see above). A sensation of hunger is brought about by an empty stomach with acid secretions in it. Then the individual starts eating and the person will continue in eating mode until a small protein hormone secreted in the beginning of the intestine goes into the bloodstream and gets to the brain and in effect tells the brain "The stomach is now full; please stop eating". In other words, this hormone is required to get to the brain to turn off the eating behavior. In some way that is not yet clear, the atypical antipsychotics impair the secretion and functioning of this hormone, which does eventually get to the brain, but with some delay. People go on eating way past the end of their hunger, in fact they may continue to eat even when they are physically uncomfortable. This has been studied by asking people who are embarking with gusto on their fourth plate of food whether they are actually still hungry at that moment. The person will consider a moment and say "No" with a puzzled look on his or her face, and if it is pointed out to them that this is their fourth plate of food, they will stop eating without protest. Patients have told me that they will sit in front of the television set with a chocolate cake, intending to eat only one piece, and slowly consume the entire chocolate cake. Or, people may increase their snacking, and high-calorie junk food does not need to be increased by a great deal to result in weight gain over a week or a month.

Unfortunately, we do not have a complete understanding of why people who are taking certain medications tend to overeat. Some people may put on weight and we do not have very convincing evidence that they were overeating. Other people can take the same medicine and not gain any appreciable weight at all. That is something that we need to work on for the whole profession of medicine – we may know the effects, the side effects, the benefits and danger of the medicine in general, but we do not know very much about individual variations. This is probably as much of a reason as any why the practice of medicine is still largely one-on-one between an individual doctor and his or her individual patient. But I just wanted to get away from the idea that the medicine itself directly causes weight gain; obviously, in most cases, the weight gain can be largely due to even a modest change in eating habits.

I counseled my patients to first, drink three glasses of water before they sat down to eat; to fill a reasonable plate of food and consume it <u>slowly</u>; and to refrain, in any circumstances, from sitting in front of a television set or other distraction with a whole cake or gallon of ice cream, making it possible to eat the whole cake. I advise people to cut a piece of cake, put it on a plate, and take <u>that</u> in front of the television set. I also told people that the strange distortion of their hunger and eating patterns would continue about an hour or an hour and a half after they started eating. After the hour and a half was over, they would feel full if they had eaten normally, and very much overfull if they had markedly overeaten.

For the sake of consistency and completeness, I will reiterate here what I said in an earlier chapter, that today's schizophrenics can be separated into three groups. One third (roughly) will have only one psychotic break in their lifetime; another third will go on to have repeated breaks but with complete or nearly complete recuperation of function between them; and the final third will go along at a certain level of functioning for a while, have a psychotic break, (which is attended by a decline in function) and only partially recuperate their level of functioning after that psychotic break, so that after each break, the patient is descending step-wise down levels of functioning and declining in intelligence prematurely.

You can see how important it is now to have the correct diagnosis. I would say that if one has a patient who is loud, noisy, and not seeming to make very much sense in an emergency room, you should first think of substance abuse, but if you do not have a history for that, then think of bipolar disorder. The two most revealing questions for bipolar disorder are: "do you have bouts of waking up full of energy, raring to go after only perhaps two or three hours' sleep?" The second most important question is "Do you have times when you start many projects but fail to finish any?" These are questions that perhaps family members can answer if the patient cannot. Both of these questions should be answered "No" in the case of schizophrenia and at least one of them may be answered in the affirmative for bipolar disorder. Bipolar disorder is the only disorder in psychiatry so far as I know in which a person can wake up with so much energy that they run around the room even though they have slept only two hours.

I would caution someone who is doing well on medication not to presume they're going to be one of the lucky ones who will not have another disease episode and stop their meds. The cost to them and to society if they are wrong and recidivate with hospital admissions because of psychotic breaks is considerable. I have advised some students to wait till they get to the summer vacation and try tapering off their meds then. (I would also advise anybody not to stop their medication between one day and the next but to taper off.) An abrupt stop from full dose to zero is too hard on the brain, and someone who is capable of a healthy response to stopping their medication will not have a healthy response if they go from medium dose to nothing overnight. I have had one person who was able to stop his medication in the summer vacation between his sophomore year and junior year at college, and who suffered no ill effects. He did taper off slowly and he continued to do well throughout his college years. I have known one other person who had been taking antipsychotics for twenty-six years who managed, very gradually over years, to dial down the dose, and is now doing well completely off medication. So, it is possible. But I don't think anybody should have the chutzpah to imagine that they are going to be one of the very fortunate minority.

Tapering off your medication is only done, in my book, when the patient and his family have a close relationship with their doctor, they are not planning to move in the near future and start with new providers, and they are perfectly willing to stop the taper and stay on even a reduced dose of medication if symptoms rather like the prodrome – from the period when their disease was just starting (being a little bit off center in their reasoning, a little bit strange, a bit isolative) begin to reappear. I never consent to somebody stopping their medication if they're doing it just out of a feeling of being fed up with taking it. Meaning of course that people are free to do as they wish, but I register that I am not happy with what they are doing and they do not have my blessing. Sometimes, the same patient will come back to me saying sadly "Gee, Doc, I guess you were right, I should be taking medication."

I certainly would never advocate changing medications just as the final stress crunch of college or graduate school or starting a new job occurs. Pick your timing so that the stress on you is as low as possible, because it is quite possible that your brain has been accustomed to the medication and taking less will cause you upset. This is something which should be agreed carefully with your physician as well as with your therapist, and if possible also your college advisor and family doctor and any other knowledgeable person who is involved with the patient. It is not to be taken lightly, and will not do for most people; at most, it may apply to a third – two thirds have a chronic illness and need continued treatment.

Perhaps I should clarify what medications can do. They can silence or nearly silence hallucinations for the person with schizophrenia. Sometimes, people with schizophrenia feel that their "voices" are "company" and they don't want to be entirely rid of them, but medication can certainly quiet the voices to the point where they do not impede conversation with a living person.

How awful the experience of hallucinations is for the schizophrenic depends on what they are saying. If the voices say "You are no good, you will never do anything, you are scum" and things like that, it will be a very unpleasant experience for the person who is schizophrenic. But what is worse for them is a voice that is saying "We are coming to get you!" which is terrifying to be hearing. Sometimes a schizophrenic person hears that they are the devil or they are evil (which is unpleasant) or that they are Christ or that they have a special message for the world – which can be very pleasant for a person who has achieved very little that is real in their lives, because it makes up for their feeling of loss and of non-achievement when they hear that they are God. But my point is, that the medication can quiet whatever the patient hears, but it is still up to the patient to behave better and interact better with people and get themselves right. Schizophrenics very often can get to the point where they're not complaining of hallucinations anymore, but they have a curious lack of desire to do anything, including wash themselves or dress properly, let alone achieve anything that most of us would consider a good thing in this world. There are exceptions, of course, but medication as it is now is far from "the answer" to schizophrenia. We do have a few new additions to the treatment of schizophrenia (in terms of FDA-approved antipsychotic medications), but we still have to figure out what they each amount to in our tool box. Certainly, with the fact that about 1% of the human population, in all cultures all over the world, has schizophrenia, this will remain a very active area for research for some time to come.

CHAPTER 12

HOW TO TALK SO YOUR PROVIDER WILL LISTEN

If you have some preconceived notions based on your own experience or the experience of someone close to you with a medication which makes you particularly keen to take it or to avoid it, let your prescriber know.

I'm sure that a lot of the patients who say they have "been on everything" for some symptom and the medications have not worked, actually mean they have taken one or two doses of many different medications once. They don't realize that as far as the prescriber is concerned, there has to be an adequate dosage taken conscientiously for an adequate period of time, with little or no result, for us to say that a particular medication is not useful for that patient.

I say in more detail, in the chapter on "How to Manage Your Providers" (Chapter 15) that what you mention first when you see your provider is very important. Providers tend to think that if a side effect is a serious obstacle to you, you will mention it right away. We all notice that this is not true for every patient, because some patients seem to take five or ten minutes (during which time they say they are "fine") to realize they are in their doctor's office, and this may be the one place in their lives where it is expected that they mention in what ways they are <u>not</u> "fine". Such people may never get very far, particularly in clinics where the doctor is held to a very strict schedule of one patient every fifteen minutes or less. The doctor may witness a lot of instances of what we call 'the doorknob phenomenon', whereby the patient insists they are doing well and everything is fine and they have no particular problems, and then as they get up and turn the doorknob to leave, they say, "My mother died last night, my boyfriend has left me and I have lost my job," when their time is up and we can't respond. Such patients sometimes then feel justified in saying that they told us but we were indifferent, but this is really poor time management on the patient's part. If you want help for something, for heaven's sake mention it at the beginning of the encounter with your provider, not as an afterthought when you have your coat on and are reaching for the doorknob.

If you want to be taken seriously, be as specific as you can about a side effect and do not overstate the severity of it. Let's take three scenarios. In the first, a patient says "I feel dizzy sometimes since I've been taking that new medicine you gave me." They do mention a side effect which is dizziness, but all they say is "sometimes". Now let's take what a symptom exaggerator may say. A patient may come into your room and say "That stuff makes me incredibly dizzy!! My goodness, I nearly fell out of the car coming here! And yesterday I thought I was going to fall over backwards in the kitchen!" That the patient is exaggerating is quite clear because she mentions two instances of thinking something was going to happen which did not. Also, she has given no description of the dizziness phenomenon as she experiences it. Now let's take a third scenario: "Doctor, I feel dizzy and faint whenever I get up from bed, or after I bend over to pick up something such as a coin I dropped. The dizziness lasts only for a few seconds, but my scalp grows cold and I feel very faint. Yesterday, coming home on the train from Poughkeepsie, I felt particularly dizzy when I had to run up the steps outside the train, pick up the ticket which I had dropped at my feet, and dash onto the train in a great hurry."

This last patient is giving a good description of what brings on the dizziness and what it feels like. He mentions several real examples, each of which is associated with having dropped something, bending over to pick it up, and needing to rush in a micro-stressful situation.

What the patient above described quite well is orthostatic hypotension. What this means is that some medicines impair the normal mechanism by which it is possible for a person to go from lying down to sitting and from swinging the head down to pick up something, to straightening up, without having a sudden drop in blood pressure.

If you think about it, one of the ways in which the human body is amazing is that without any conscious effort on our part we can change positions quite rapidly and usually have no ill effect. By change positions I mean change in such a way that the heart, which is pumping sideways when we are lying down, suddenly starts to pump straight up to our heads against gravity when we sit or stand, with no ill effects that we feel. This is because of a mechanism which exists in the head which monitors our blood pressure and stimulates the heart to pump harder, and perhaps a little bit faster when we are sitting or standing – in other words, when the heart has to pump blood <u>up</u> to the head rather than merely on the same level, (the heart and the head are on the same level when we are lying down.) This mechanism is so clever that unless we are taking medication which interferes with it, we have no problem putting the head down to pick up something we have dropped (in which case the trajectory from the heart to the head is <u>with</u> gravity, and the heart has less work to do) than neutral (as when we are lying down) to pumping straight up against gravity when we sit up or stand.

Unfortunately, some medications interfere with this natural mechanism, and so we may bend down to pick up something we dropped and feel rather dizzy when we bring our head back up into the upright standing position again. If we are <u>not</u> careful we can actually faint because when the head arrives in the upright position and the heart has not been given a very rapid message to pump harder, it may for a beat or two not pump hard enough. If this happens, the brain is without an adequate blood supply for a few seconds. The brain's ultimate defense against this state of affairs is to make us faint, which corrects the situation because when we are on the ground the heart does not have to pump blood against gravity to get to the head.

Old-fashioned medications used to be much worse than recent ones are. We try to train our patients, if they must take a medication which impairs the natural mechanism, to come up slowly from having the head down, so as to give the slightly retarded mechanism of blood pressure correction a chance to get into gear.

When I was in medical school, there was one medication which was then still in use for blood pressure, which is no longer used. The generic name for it is guanethidine. I remember vividly a professor telling us most earnestly that patients on guanethidine must be told never to go into a telephone booth, the reason being that if a patient dropped a coin in the telephone booth and then bent over to pick it up and sat upright or stood quickly (which would cause the lack of circulation to the brain previously mentioned), the telephone booth was small enough that there was no room inside it for them, if they fainted, to sink to the ground. Therefore they could faint in a sitting up position, and the circulation to the brain would never be properly restored, and they might die because of their situational inability to lie down on the ground.

But I digress. Please notice that the third patient's attempts to describe the side effects he experienced included quite a bit of information about what brought on his dizziness. The one thing he did not say which is of interest for an episodic side effect is how soon after a medication is taken is the maximum side effect reached.

Medications which are swallowed are dissolved in the stomach or the small intestines, which may take up to an hour. Then they are absorbed, and the peak blood level is usually reached from one hour to three hours after the pill was taken. There are a number of side effects of a number of different medications which may occur if the peak level, reached within three hours of taking the pill, is too high for the patient's system. This is important to know because it may be that the for rest of the time (outside of the peak level) the medication will not cause the side effect in question (assuming that the medication is going to be in the patient's system for quite a few hours) An estimate of how long a medication will be in your system may be arrived at by how often you are asked to take the medication. If the medication is to be taken every six hours, then it obviously does not last very long in your system. If it is to be taken every twelve hours, that's a little longer, and if it is to be taken every twenty-four or forty-eight hours, that's longer yet. Good medications are sometimes put together with other compounds which delay their release into the body so that they last longer, and so that the peak level which comes with having the entire dose absorbed into the bloodstream at the same time is avoided.

What I'm getting at is, a patient may not tolerate the peak level, but they may like the effect after the peak is over with the particular medication. One easy way to decrease the peak blood level is to decrease the number of milligrams per dose. Another way is to increase the time interval between doses, since the level remaining from the last dose when the patient takes the next dose will be lower if the dosage interval is longer.

Note that most medications do not arrive at a steady state (that is, a state in which the addition to the blood level of a newly-taken dose equals the subtraction from the blood level by metabolism of the previous doses) until five half-lives. A half-life is the number of hours in which the dose has decreased to one half its previous concentration. Thus, if you take a medication at nine a.m. and you need to take it again at nine p.m. twelve hours later, then assuming the half-life is twelve hours, the concentration in your body from the nine a.m. dose at nine p.m. will be half what it was at say ten a.m. after the dose was absorbed. And for most medications, five half-lives (and you can usually translate that into five doses) is the time that it takes for a steady state to be set up in which the amount added to the blood level by taking the medication is equal to the amount subtracted by its metabolism. This is why some medications require the patient to have taken several doses in order to have any effect.

I feel I should say something about why psychiatric medications take a long time to have their effect. Patients may need to take some medicines three to four to six weeks faithfully before we see the therapeutic effect. This is because the cells in the brain need time to develop receptors on their surfaces which can lock onto the medication and take it into the cell. Also, there are a number of feedback loops which need to be navigated before the medication will have an effect. In other words after you swallow medication A, it gets into your bloodstream, then gets into the brain across what is called the blood-brain barrier (many things thank goodness do not get into your brain) where it needs to affect cell population B which will signal cell population C which will communicate to cell population D which will change certain things about the brain's metabolism, and then the effect of medication A may be in evidence. When television commercials say that a given medication increases neurotransmitters this is rather like saying medication A will increase D and not mentioning all the intervening steps.

We know not very much about how all this actually takes place. Most of us realize it's an extremely complex interlocking system, and to really make change takes time. This is also why people can sometimes skip a medication for a day or two and not feel any adverse effects. People with schizophrenia may stop taking their medication and not become acutely schizophrenic needing hospitalization for weeks to months, which makes it hard for them to understand that going off their medication a number of months earlier had the effect of the return of the acute illness most recently.

Now back to how to talk to your doctor about side effects. I once knew a patient who was a bookkeeper, who could do a lot of addition accurately in his head, and who was a whiz at adding a long column of figures if they were written down in front of him. He was the patient of one of my colleagues who prescribed a small amount of modern-day antipsychotics (not one of the old-fashioned ones with the horrible side effects) for his emotional instability. The patient reported to the doctor as he told me (when I saw him because his doctor was on vacation) that the medication worked well for the purpose for which it was given him. However he had told his regular doctor that he felt that his intellect was "befuddled". The doctor did not pick up on this word and ask him for more details, and he did not say that he could only add very slowly in his head or on paper; the befuddlement caused an unacceptable decline in his working acuity and productivity.

He had not told the other doctor that he was taking some Valium[R] which he got from a neighbor, which had never been prescribed for him. It was only with great difficulty that I convinced him that the "befuddlement" was most likely due to the long term effects of Valium[R], not to the Risperdal[R,] and that he should give up the Valium[R] rather than the Risperdal[R] if he wanted to come out right.

This patient made two errors. Number one, he took a medication which was not prescribed for him at all and of course did not tell any of his own prescribers that he was taking it; and number two he did not explain that the side effect he was complaining of was a loss of sharpness necessary for him to function on the job, and so to continue without a medication change would jeopardize his employment.

When these two items were cleared up, he was able with a great deal of effort to give up the Valium[R] and trust us to prescribe a non-befuddling medication for his anxiety, and to continue to take the Risperdal[R].

My point for this chapter is that the patient could have helped himself if he had brought out what he meant by 'befuddlement' when he first said it. As it was, his own doctor did not pay attention to his complaint which is the doctor's fault. He also could have helped himself had he admitted that he was taking Valium[R] prescribed for someone else, and allowed us to explain to him that Valium[R], Librium[R], Ativan[R], Klonopin[R], Xanax[R], Restoril[R] and others of the same chemical group have a side effect of causing loss of mental clarity. To sum up:

1. Always tell your doctor everything you are taking, including things not prescribed for you which you may have used to self-medicate before you came to see the doctor, or pills prescribed for friends or family members which you "borrowed".
2. If you experience a side effect, say in graphic terms what this means to you; "I get a little befuddled sometimes" is a lot less telling than "I can no longer add columns of figures with ease as I used to be able to do, and this is an important part of my work."
3. Mention when the side effect occurs in relation to when you take the pill. If you do not experience a side effect for many hours after you take a pill, it is difficult to ascribe that side effect to that particular medication.
4. If you experience a so-called 'side effect' shortly after you take a medication, do you have the same 'side effect' when you do not take this medication or when you have not taken it for a while? If so, that also would indicate that the 'side effect' in question is probably not due to that particular medication.
5. Be prepared to give a detailed account of exactly how you feel and what happens with the so-called side effect you are complaining of. For example, anxiety can induce certain physical sensations which people sometimes think are side effects of medication, when in fact they are part of the symptom that we are treating.

We have talked about getting your list out quickly, and the importance of what you mention first. Then there's the question of how you mention it. Saying "I got diarrhea an hour after I took the pill" while being good from the point of view of mentioning time course which I have stressed throughout this book, is too non-specific. If your prescriber writes prescriptions for this particular medication frequently, and if it frequently causes diarrhea, he hears that statement all day long, and may become inured to it.

The prescriber might try to say "How bad is the diarrhea?" What he wants to know here is not what the volume of your feces was or something like that, but rather how disruptive was this to your life. A good answer would be "I had to go to the bathroom six times in one hour, and I got several adverse comments from my work supervisor." Or, "That was the meeting at which we were handing out the prizes, and I had to interrupt so many times to use the restroom that the MC made a joke about it." Or, "I had to interrupt the dinner conversation many times, and I never could get to proposing to my girlfriend."

By the way, some doctors are still careful enough to say don't take your first dose of a new medication when you are going out into a social situation where you will be highly visible, and where such things as multiple sudden trips to the bathroom will be remarked upon. Try the first dose on a day when you are not working and nothing particular is happening, you're just puttering about the house and so several sudden interruptions (for bathroom visits for instance) will not be noticed by anyone else. Also, you can notice how clear your thinking is on this medication. There are quite a number of medications which say "do not drive a car or operate machinery until you are aware of how this medication affects you." They mean it.

But that is not all, because the fact is, a whole class of medications may be well-known for a particular side effect, but that does not tell us which person will get the most pronounced version of that side effect, nor does it say anything about the people to whom that side effect would be most obnoxious.

If I take myself as an example: it's difficult to give me a headache (so I am resistant to headaches as a side effect); and my innards seem to know how to arrange themselves so that even when I have very diarrheic stools, I don't have to interrupt myself a great deal for this, so that is not a problem for me; on the other hand, nausea is a symptom I tolerate very poorly, so even a little bit of nausea will have me feeling very uncomfortable – even if I am a long way from vomiting, still, I'm not a happy camper. Now, I have met other patients who tolerate nausea very well but diarrhea very poorly, or have some other ranking of preferences as far as side effects go.

If you have a particular side effect that you have experienced and that you do not tolerate well, or conversely a particular side effect which even when you have it does not seem to bother you much, please tell your prescriber that. Some side effects may be pronounced when you start the medication, but may wear off as time goes on and your body gets used to the medication. We have gotten to the point as prescribers where we choose what we prescribe in a broad class (by broad class, remember I mean 'antidepressant' 'antipsychotic' or 'anxiolytic' or 'mood stabilizer,'– we choose within a broad class the medication which we think has side effects that the patient will tolerate well or may not even notice.

So now you know what you're going to mention first, and you know you are going to mention the most objective reason why you have difficulty tolerating this side effect. By 'objective' I mean as shown by someone else's reaction – the adverse comment of your work supervisor – or by some outside measure of your behavior, such as interrupting yourself six times in an hour. This also gives a target in that if you only had to interrupt yourself once an hour, perhaps that would be acceptable. I have known prescribers, when a medication is ideal from other points of view, (for example from the point of view of its effectiveness for the psychiatric symptom), give the patient medication to take which treats diarrhea at the same time as they take their particular psychotropic medication. If the patient will tolerate it, this sometimes works quite nicely. Sometimes the best way to make this tolerable for the patient is to tell the patient "You seem to be particularly sensitive to the tendency of this medication to cause this particular side effect, so what we're going to try to do is to treat the side effect so that you can continue to take this medication."

Allow me to mention in passing that there is nothing wrong with preparing your visit with your doctor in terms of knowing the description of the side effect that you want to give. Practice not so much that you drive yourself crazy and the delivery is wooden, but a little bit so that you don't leave out some major aspect of it, because you may be intimidated by the presence of your doctor. That is also a good idea because then you are not spending several minutes trying to find the right words to describe the problem, and wasting that scarcest of all resources, time.

Next, let me point out something. Suppose the doctor says that he wants to see you back in a month, and gives you a prescription for a thirty day supply of your medication with no refill. This is not a very good idea for you, because the scheduler may be unable to give you an appointment less than thirty-five or forty days away, and you only have a thirty day supply of your medication. Provided that your medication is not a controlled substance, I would ask the doctor for one refill, giving the above as a reason. In other words because he does not know what the schedulers can do for you, if you have a refill at least you don't run out of your medications and have what I call forced non-adherence because you run out in the last few days before your doctor's visit. I do not think most psychiatrists are very resistant to refills of non-controlled substances. They would far sooner give somebody extra refills than see them readmitted to the hospital because they ran out of meds.

In truth, however, if you ever find that you have seven pills left and you don't see your doctor for another twelve days, there is nothing to prevent you from calling the doctor's office and getting a refill called in to your pharmacy. What I am trying to say is that it is your business to see to it that you don't run out of refills. Doctors do try, but a doctor may have hundreds of patients and you only have one, and if you're soon to run out of your medication, for heaven's sake pick up the phone and tell the doctor's office what's going on.

Here's what I do, as someone who still is a patient. If the doctor wants to try me on a new medication that I have never tried before, I will have the doctor call in the prescription to my local pharmacy, a thirty day supply without refills. I will pick it up that day or the next day and take it for a few doses or a few days to see if I have any particular problem with it. If I have a really significant problem with it, then I would call back my doctor and say I cannot take this medication and can I either have the old medication or we'll try another idea. The medication I just got will have been used for three or four days so I'm wasting perhaps a twenty-six or twenty-seven day supply. It wastes a lot less if you only had thirty days to begin with, than if you had ninety days and had to waste an eighty-six day supply. Then, as the doctor calls in a thirty day supply of my new medication to my local pharmacy, I ask her to write out on paper prescriptions for my ninety day supply house which, if the new medication is okay, I mail to the ninety day supply house on about day ten or eleven after I got the prescription. It takes about a week for them to arrive at the ninety day supply house so they'd arrive at about day seventeen and that is fairly close to day twenty-three of my thirty day supply which is the day that I can have a new prescription. I now have a ninety day supply house which will hang onto my prescription until the day that they are allowed to fill it if that is not too far away. If I were still dealing with what used to be the ninety day supply house that I had to use dictated by my old insurance, I would hold onto the prescription for the new medication longer and send it later.

I once had the rather odd experience of sending in a prescription which arrived at the ninety day supply house two days before it was allowed to be filled, and it was sent back to me which took another week, and it took a second week for me to turn around and send it back to the pharmacy, and I nearly ran out of my medication, but not quite.

You also have to realize that mistakes can be made. Your prescriber may agree to a ninety day supply and then forget about that and write a thirty day supply when it actually comes to writing the prescription. This is probably because most of the world still goes to their local pharmacy and gets a thirty day supply, and the doctor is not thinking about the cost savings to you represented by getting ninety days' of medication for one co-pay instead of thirty days' of medication.

You should check all your prescriptions before you leave the doctor's office. If you need to have your medication list and the number of pills you're given for each medication to check, do that. If the doctor ushers you out into the waiting room when you still haven't checked the medication prescription, do that before you leave since if you walk up to the receptionist desk and say that your doctor has made an error in your prescription, the prescriber cannot very well let you go leave without correcting the error. Calling back later after you have left the office is much more difficult.

And it is not only prescribers who make errors. I remember years ago going to a big medical center and being handed, not my psychotropics for Shana Clark, but digitalis (a heart medicine that I do not need and do not take) for an eighty-odd year old woman named Ms. Sarah Clark.

And then very recently my local pharmacy doubled the dose of my lithium (which would be very dangerous had I not noticed). The prescription I had previously from my doctor was lithium 150 milligram capsules, take one in the morning and four at bedtime. Please note that I used to take 300 milligram tablets one in the morning and two at bedtime but the morning dose was reduced when I added a decades-old medication for high blood pressure, amlodipine. Amlodipine competes with lithium for a site on an enzyme for metabolism. Most lithium (perhaps 80-85%) is excreted directly through the kidneys but the 15-20% that is not so excreted is metabolized in the liver and there is this competition between amlodipine and lithium. Amlodipine binds more easily to the site, and so the lithium loses out (so to speak) and therefore the metabolism of lithium is slowed down in the presence of amlodipine. So, any given dose of lithium will result in a higher blood level in the presence of amlodipine because of the fact that it takes longer to metabolize the lithium. Therefore, if you want to keep your blood level constant, you may have to lower the total dose of lithium.

So my dose was lowered to 150 milligrams in the morning and still the same 600 milligrams at night. I had asked my doctor to make it all 150 milligram capsules so that I would take one in the morning and four at night, because I have been through the problem of having two dosage strengths of the same medication and the people who talk to customers in ninety day supply houses never look beyond the name of the medication to the dosage strength, so if you need to renew one and not the other, you may not be talking about the same thing. So having two dosage strengths of the same medicine is not a good idea.

Before the amlodipine, my old prescription at the local pharmacy (which I used because I was waiting for my insurance to change, and that would mean I would have a new ninety day supply house, since different insurance companies work with different ones) was lithium 300 milligrams one in the morning and two at night. After I got the 150 milligram one in the morning and four at night from the ninety day supply house, I went to the local pharmacy, which did not read the prescription correctly and made it lithium 300 milligrams one in the morning and four at night; they didn't notice the change in dosage strength from 300mg. to 150mg.

Now this is not too terrible because the supply of five doses per day of 150mg. when I only need to take one will last me a long time and I can take two times 300mg equals 600mg. at night instead of four times 150mg. equals 600mg. at night. My point is that most patients don't read the whole prescription and an unwary patient might have been in a coma from the error of the local pharmacy. I checked with my doctor and she had not written an improper prescription; it was pharmacy error.

So I say to you again: read the prescription when you leave the doctor's office and read the prescription when you leave the pharmacy. I must say in favor of ninety day supply houses that in the fifteen years that I've used several different ones (because I've had 3 different insurances and different insurances make contracts with different companies), I have never seen an error such as the above made by a ninety day supply house. I think they really do have a good quality checking system.

I have never seen a prescription which was actually one thing that was labeled as something else. So before you leave the pharmacy, open the paper bag with bottles of pills in it, and check the pills, check what it says, check the total quantity; try to be responsible as a patient.

By the way there has been for many years now a huge drive to prevent medication errors led by a Federal commission. Every doctor has to go through training every time they renew their license. I presume pharmacists do too, so everything possible is being done to correct the problem – but you, as the consumer, are the last quality control checker. If you don't want problems, learn to check your meds.

If I'm giving the impression that checking your medications, and what you say to your provider should be very planful, so that you say exactly what you mean in the least amount of time possible, and so that you check the work of other people as it affects your health, then I have done my job.

When I was in my 20's, it did not occur to me that the schedulers had given me an appointment 2 weeks beyond the 8 weeks the doctor wrote on my paper. I didn't notice when I was running out of my medication, and ran out 10 days before my appointment, but didn't want to bother to say so, and I was back in the hospital before I could get to see my outpatient doctor. Again, I'm trying to warn my readers so they won't make all the mistakes I made in the early part of my illness. I will finish by saying that I personally, as a patient, once had <u>six</u> items I wanted my prescriber to get done in one ten minute visit. As soon as I had said hello I said "I have six items for you." I even drafted the letter I wanted him to write, so that he could write it immediately without having to think very hard about what he wanted to say. Since I did everything to help him accomplish the tasks in as short a time as possible, he did not fail to pay attention to all six items, and all six were accomplished in only twelve minutes. I would rate that as a highly successful interview.

And I say that with sorrow for what has happened to psychiatry – it's very hard to learn to talk fast. One of the good points of having a family member with you, is that they can help you keep on track about the main things to be said. A family member would also be very good to check your list of what medications you take against the items written out as prescriptions for you, and the labels of the pill bottles once you get them.

CHAPTER 13

HOW TO TELL YOUR STORY

You may read this title and think that on the face of it, it is preposterous. How absurd – how can I possibly pretend to tell someone how they should tell their own story? Doesn't the person who lived it know their own story a thousand times better than anyone else ever will, even if that other person stayed up all night listening sometime?

Yes, they do know their own story better. But that, in a way, is part of the problem. When they say "Mother" they have a mental image of what she looks or looked like, an olfactory memory of what she smells or smelled like, an appreciation of the sound of her voice, the way she keeps or did keep her house, the way she would smile when sitting on the porch, the way she looked sitting at the Thanksgiving table, and so forth and so on. Now, the hearer who hears this story for the first time knows nothing of this. So it behooves the talker (patient or family member) to choose what they want to say. What is it about their mother that is essential for the provider to understand at this moment?

Note that the picture becomes all the more complex when we are talking about something like "Mother," who has an archetype. There is an age old set of imagery attached to that word which makes it unique in our lexicon. There is also our cultural icon, which is different according to the culture we come from. In China, they don't eat apple pie, so "Mom and apple pie" is not part of their picture of mother. Then too, there is the reality of a particular person's mother, and what she was like. For those, like me, who had poly-addicted and episodically highly abusive mothers, it can be hard to get the provider to detach from his or her own notions of what Mother must have been like. So strong is their conviction that she really did care or she tried that it can be very hard to convince them if I say, for example, that she abused me at times and did try to kill me a number of times during my teenage years. If I said that boldly, although it was true, the provider might think I was becoming psychotic or irrational, especially if I had a known history of mental illness and he had spoken to my mother, who was always charming to outsiders. Therefore, I had to face my own reality basically alone. Only after I was absolutely certain how my story should be told, was it possible for me to tell it.

I still recall very clearly the numbers of times after my father died that my mother would come upstairs to the room where I slept alone (because my sister slept in my mother's room almost every night until she died in order to be there to help her get to the bathroom or navigate around the apartment, since my mother was often drunk and would often fall over in the middle of the night unless she had someone to guide her). So, I was left in my bedroom upstairs and I would wake up to see my mother standing over the bed with a carving knife in her right hand pointing downward.

The first thing to do was to roll off the bed so as to not be directly under the point of the blade. The next necessity was to get the knife out of my mother's hand. How many times as a preadolescent and adolescent did I do hand to hand combat with my mother at night just to stay alive! Please note that my mother was often so drunk that it would not have mattered whether she intended to stab me or not – she could have fallen forward with the knife in her hand and I might have been under it. I remember very well that people in school at the end of Friday afternoon would say "Okay, Shana, see you on Monday," and I would privately think that I would see them on Monday if I were still above ground on Monday. I also remember when I got to college and I had just turned sixteen that a bunch of my classmates were talking and one of them said "My mother would kill me if she found out about my making out in the car with my boyfriend." I felt a swell of sympathy when she said 'my mother would kill me if…'. I just managed to dash down the hall and make it into the women's room to cry my tears by myself when it dawned on me that when <u>she</u> said 'my mother will kill me' she did not mean her mother would make her dead – she meant that her mother would express a moderate to severe degree of displeasure. And as I dashed down the hall to go and sob privately, a college official happened by and told me how proud my mother must be of me, to which I replied "Yes, ma'am" and ran all the harder to the bathroom. Both my sister and I longed for some praise from our mother.

I remember also once when I was in college that my mother took a carving knife and was chasing my sister 'round the dining room table. It seemed to me that my sister was losing, so I picked up the 'phone and dialed 911 and pulled myself together and said in a very level-toned factual manner that my mother was chasing my sister with a carving knife in her hand and we needed the police forthwith. I gave my name and my address in a similar level tone and put the 'phone down.

But the police did not come. It then dawned on me that the police would not believe it if they heard a teenager being so cold and factual, because the police had no notion of what our life had been like. I had to learn at a very early age to deal with the hard facts of the matter and not let my emotions cloud my coping. So I called up 911 again and this time deliberately allowed myself to give vent to all the hysteria I felt. The police were there in less than two minutes. They explained that all they could do was calm down the disturbance, since my mother had not actually done anything – she had just threatened. But they were very understanding about why I called when they saw the situation.

Decades later, about twelve years after the onset of my mental illness, when I would have been in my middle thirties, I discovered that I could 'put on a strong editor' and tell my story when I was manic simply by keeping silent when I reached the irrelevant portions. This had the effect of making what I said come out slowly, with long pauses. I explained to various providers that I was 'putting on an editor', but they did not seem familiar with the phenomenon. I have since encountered people who have suffered from mania who have learned to do the same thing, and have had the great pleasure of telling other providers that not everyone who was a manic patient wishes to be obnoxious and hard to understand, and that some of us can learn to edit out the irrelevant or illogical parts of what we say.

I will say that in my experience of this, type of editing, that it is extremely exhausting and I don't know that I could keep it up for more than perhaps a ten minute conversation. I would like to hear from my readers, patients or providers alike, whether they have encountered this in others, because I have never seen it in a book. But then, it is only relatively recently that the profession has caught on to the idea that a severely manic person may be slowed down in their motor aspect, because their mind is going so fast that it is not possible to execute any of their ideas. It is interesting to think that I may have developed this editing skill because of the violence and the chaos I had to deal with at home when I was a youngster, and my ability to grasp and do what is needed in a crisis and not get caught up in all the emotion and emotionalism of crisis, stems from that experience with my mother.

"Mother" may not be relevant at all if what the patient wants is a medication adjustment. In this instance, the history of the patient in terms of their triumphs and their defeats told in parallel with a history of what medications they were taking would be most helpful. A story that starts "I want to have my medication changed because......" is what is needed here. And, as I have said before in this text, a prescription history, including an honest accounting of when the patient took the medication as prescribed, when they took it in some other fashion, and when they did not take medication at all, is what is required.

Now back to telling a story. There are basically two ways to do this. One is to headline, the other is to punchline. In headlining a story, you tell the main point of the story first, and then fill in the details. This works best when you need to catch somebody's attention and when you don't have any credibility problems. For instance, someone who comes home and cries out excitedly, "I got the job!" is headlining. They give the end result first, and then they will tell interested listeners all about the letter or the interview process or the encounter that got them hired, or how they heard the news.

In the punchline method of storytelling, you do not let on what the end result is at the beginning. Rather, you make the person in imagination follow through with you every step of the way until they reach the startling finish. This works best with people whose attention is not difficult to get, but who might be rather skeptical of the outcome if you blurted it out at first. And the thing is, if you say an outcome that your listener does not believe, they may spend the next few minutes fighting the truth of this outcome, and not listen to you at all.

Let's pretend that the job applicant mentioned above lives in a rooming house with strangers who don't know the applicant very well. So the applicant comes back to the rooming house and says "Well, I never thought it would take so long! When I got there, I had to sit in a waiting room with twenty other job applicants, and we were each seen by four different people one after another. With waiting time between each interview, this took about five hours. But, you won't believe it! It's amazing, I know, but I got the job!" That is the punchline approach. The talker may add in descriptions of the four interviews, who interviewed them, what the talker said and what was well-received. This will help to convince the listener that what the talker is saying is genuine.

There are considerations about the choice between headlining and punchlining in psychiatry also. Because emergency rooms are busy and people may not pick up on things, I would encourage a family member who goes with a patient to headline "My (boyfriend or husband or son) Jack has been complaining of suicidal thoughts for two weeks, escalating over the last three days and becoming very focused this evening" before we get into a long list of Jack's recent stressors. Punchlining is not a good technique in this situation; if you punchline, the provider may have gone by the time you say that Jack is suicidal.

Telling a story with a careful eye for the timeline of the symptoms and the taking of medications is a good idea. I have listened to many stories when the family got off onto a tangent concerning something totally different – the family was offered a trip to Japan, the boiler burst, someone stove in the side of the car when it was parked in a parking lot, which is more about a stressor to the family member speaking than about the patient. Please also try to keep family disputes out of it – you are coming to the ER for medical help for a family member. Try to stay on topic. Keep in mind that the provider needs to know, when did the symptoms appear, when did they get worse, when was medication prescribed, and above all why is the patient and the family in the emergency room. More especially why is he in the emergency room now – not yesterday, not last week, and not next week; what happened to make the family to decide he needs to see a provider (and possibly be hospitalized) now, this evening, today.

Shana Wibberley Clark, M.D., Dr. P.H.

Don't forget that you have come to the emergency room concerning an emergency. Most urban emergency rooms these days are full of people who have acute health problems but which are probably not life-threatening emergencies, and a much smaller number of people who have been shot, are having a heart attack, bleeding internally, or something of that kind. But the vast majority of people in an urban emergency room today are people who have sprained ankles, cuts on the fingers, coughs, colds, or maybe a broken wrist or arm; something that needs to be attended to as soon as possible, for sure, but something from which they will not die. Nevertheless, you are in the emergency room to be seen. There are some places in the US today which have what is called "urgent care" which is for the broken arm, the broken wrist, the nonlethal cut etc. which is urgent but which is not an emergency. These have done good service in being much faster for the patient (you don't have to wait hours while the staff is concerned with the person who got shot or the person who is bleeding or some other emergency which *is* life-threatening) and urgent care services are possibly nearer the patient's house than the big medical center, so they do good service. If you have this kind of service near you, please do use it.

If, on the other hand you are going to the emergency room for a true emergency, please do *not*, out of a wish not to bother anyone, hide what is going on. I sometimes think that our medical personnel have been taught 'cultural sensitivity' to certain cultures where people dramatize and seem to exaggerate their symptoms. I know for a fact that they do not know how to assess people who have spent a lifetime working on being unobtrusive, unobnoxious, self-effacing etc. The stiff upper lip (which comes from the fact that when a child is about to cry their upper lip trembles, and so it is a call to be stoic) is part of British culture which did not translate to this continent. My sister was having her first child and since our mother was dead, a friend was with her. When she began to experience the pain of giving birth, she said to the friend, "I wonder if it would be possible to begin a discussion of analgesia". The friend said "Tedda, just scream! Just let it out! That'll make them come running". My sister did as she suggested and they did come running and gave her some pain medication.

With that in mind, don't please be like another acquaintance of mine who went to the emergency room when she was having pains through her chest and into her back (a classic picture for heart attack in a woman) and every time the nurse came to say "How are you doing?" she answered "Oh, I'll manage. I'll manage." She never said the pain was terrible or that she couldn't cope or demanded to be seen. She died of her heart attack before she was ever seen by a doctor. Don't do that.

Something needs to be said about how things may appear to a third party (such as a provider or the police) which may cause them to come to a conclusion which may not be what the family expects. First of all, I will say that the emergency room personnel will make a decision: to admit or not to admit. If they decide that the situation is not grave enough to admit, they may tell the family to call back during the day to the outpatient department and make an appointment. Families are often upset at leaving the emergency room without an appointment. But the emergency room is run twenty-four seven on a completely different schedule than the outpatient department, and the emergency room does not have any given provider's schedule – when he or she is working at that institution, when he or she has a pre-existing appointment with another patient, and when he or she has an open appointment time. So, that is why the emergency room says to the family "Call tomorrow and make an appointment for your son (or daughter.)"

If the family is uncomfortable with going home with the patient and coping with the situation until they can get to an appointment, then they should say why. I have known situations in which the family says that Grandpa is not thinking clearly. Yet they do not mention any danger or any particular fear about what Grandpa will do in this state. It is only when the emergency room says, this being on a Friday night, "Call the outpatient department at this number on Monday and make an appointment for Grandpa," that the family comes out with the fact that Grandpa has wandered away three times in the last forty-eight hours and they are uncertain what they would do or how they would find him if he did wander off yet again. Sometimes, one says to the family "Well, those of you who are in your right mind should be very careful to lock the doors every time you come in or out so that Grandpa will not have a possibility of leaving." Sometimes a family can take such an instruction, and other times they cannot. Sometimes one has to say, "Putting Grandpa in the hospital is not a substitute for you guys' locking your doors."

On the other hand, sometimes families come in and give a very good story for the idea that Grandpa is dangerous, and then are horrified at the prospect of having him hospitalized. I'm not saying that we as providers expect families to be very logical. It is a good idea if they come in knowing what they would like to have happen, and why.

Let me give a story about someone who presented themselves in a manner that was very misleading to the police. The story concerns Jake, a quixotic young man with a history of schizophrenia who sat on his porch with a shotgun across his lap. Neighbors called the police because Jake, though he had never done anything actually dangerous, had aroused a wary attitude in his neighbors before.

When the police came, Jake was sitting on the porch very nonchalantly, with a shotgun, as I said, in his lap. He did not make a move to lift the shotgun. Jake said later that the shotgun was not loaded, and that the police should have thought of asking whether it was loaded or not.

At this point, the police would not necessarily have thought Jake was telling the truth if he said the gun was not loaded. But Jake and his family were aware that others on the street were worried about his behavior. Jake felt he made his point when the police assumed that the shotgun was loaded, but under the circumstances that was a perfectly reasonable assumption for them to make. Better for them to assume the gun was loaded than to find out to their ruing that it was. This is what I mean by saying that you have to imagine what a reasonable person would think if you were engaged in certain behavior or said certain things.

If you have a point about a medication dose that you want to make, you can punchline the story by saying "They started me on the average dose of twenty milligrams of Prozac[R] a day, then increased it to forty milligrams a day (at which time I had horrendous side effects) and then we finally got it down to ten milligrams a day and that was okay – but now, a year later, the ten milligrams doesn't seem to be enough." This would help in terms of an understanding why you come in on such a small dose, since twenty milligrams is more usual for this particular medication.

My point about this is, there is no single good way of telling the story, or one bad way, but patients so often conceal the jewel of the main point of what they're saying in the middle of something, that I think it might behoove them or family members to think over how they can communicate best. I'm not saying headlining or punchlining is better, I'm saying they're different techniques and may elicit a different response. And, for an emergency room, I think headlining is best.

Now, as to content, I'm assuming at this point that you will be talking to an outpatient provider or an inpatient provider, but that the emergency room phase is over. You really want to think about what you're going to say. I've had a number of patients who are so very aware of the point of their story that the point – the goal of telling it – is what they leave out. For example, I remember a young man whom I'll call Mike who told a story of being invited by friends of his who owned property on the shore of the Gulf of Mexico, to "babysit" their house for them while they were out of town for a while. They presented this as an opportunity for Mike, because he could enjoy the sunny weather and all the amenities of their house while the owners were away.

Mike said that this was in the second half of September, when, as he found out, the hurricane season is waning but is not over. A storm which had been a hurricane in the Gulf but which by the time it got to shore was downgraded to a tropical storm (meaning that its winds were no longer hurricane speed or force) came to the house when Mike was there. The owners had not left storm shutters up, so, winds, still very forceful, blew around the house; at one point Mike sat in the living room which was in the center of the house and listened as panes of glass from the back kitchen door were blown in by the wind. Mike conveyed vividly how frightening this was for him, since he was from the upper Midwest where there are no hurricanes, and the very idea that a wind could blow in the windows of your house was scary to him. He talked about having been for several hours without power, sitting in the dark. Fortunately, the wind blew in only a few panes of glass at the back of the house. Mike was able to close the doors and the temperature in the living room remained quite livable. Therefore, Mike wasn't so much in physical danger as he was frightened. But Mike told a wonderful tale about how frightened he had been.

At the end of his story, I asked him how that affected him now. Obviously, he had been quite scared. Did having been scared in the past affect him now?

Mike was quite angry with me. Could not I see that he was furious with his former friends – he didn't feel friendly towards the owners of the house anymore – who had exposed him to such terror, without even having explained to him in advance that he would be coming down in the active hurricane season, and that they were going to leave the house without storm windows in place. It turned out that Mike did locate a flashlight in the kitchen, and so he was not completely in darkness, and he was lucky enough that the water mains were not affected, so he did not find himself without water. About half the contents of the refrigerator went bad after several hours of being unrefrigerated, but Mike was not actually in want. However, he was extremely angry with the people he described as his "former friends" for not warning him that this sort of thing might happen, not putting the storm shutters up, not telling him where he could find a flashlight or warning him to have a supply of bottled water on hand in case the water supply became contaminated – which, as I said, did not happen. Mike was extremely angry with his friends for not warning him of the possible eventualities, so that he could be fully prepared, including psychologically prepared. He was angry with his former friends for exposing him to the great fear he felt, and for not warning him this might come to pass.

In the context of what I'm saying here about how to tell your own story, my point is that Mike told a wonderful tale of being surprised and frightened; he did not tell a tale of resenting his friends' lack of candor and foresight. He meant to tell a tale of resentment, but what he told was a tale of fear. Because Mike did something a lot of people do when they're telling a story that is familiar to them. He assumed that I understood without ever saying it what his reaction really was, and as he said to me later "Anyone would be frightened in such a situation, and anyone would resent friends who do not warn them that this sort of thing could come about."

Another tale was told to me by Marsha, who was a rather self-contained woman in her early thirties. Marsha told a long story of going home to her family of origin in Connecticut and she told about an entire day, with all the detail. What she left out was that her family failed to greet her. She said something like "There I was standing on the threshold of my parents' house and they said 'Come and sit at the table' and I did so." What she left out was that they took it absolutely in stride and failed to remark upon the fact that she had returned to Connecticut from Idaho, and they did not express any surprise (according to her) at seeing her. She said that they let her speak as everyone else at the table spoke, but she apparently expected a sort of hero's welcome for coming from such a distance, and, not getting quite what she expected, she felt very badly done by. I did ask her when she told me this story, had she said to her family anything to the effect that she expected them to be surprised at seeing her? I said something like "Did you say 'Hey guys, you know I'm back from Idaho, aren't you surprised to see me?'" But Marsha said she "wasn't going to tell people what they should say." She preferred, apparently, to feel badly because they had not met her expectations without ever giving a hint as to what her expectations were – an attitude that is bound to lead to trouble.

I'm going to return to Jake's story. Jake, as you remember, was the man who sat on the porch with a shotgun across his lap, but the shotgun was not loaded. Neighbors called the police and the police asked Jake why he was sitting on the porch with a shotgun. Jake cited the constitutional amendment which allows individuals to bear arms and said that no explanation should be required of him for what he was doing. The police then said that he should put down the gun and move away from it. Jake refused to do this. At the same time, he did not mention that the gun was not loaded.

Fortunately, Jake did not get shot for his defiance of the police. He did get taken to a mental hospital and admitted as dangerous.

Jake told me the next day how stupid the police had been because they did not ask whether the gun was loaded. I countered that Jake was not very bright if he would suppose that the police would imagine the gun was <u>not</u> loaded. Especially when Jake refused to put it down and refused to back away from it – naturally, the police would assume the gun <u>was</u> loaded.

These sorts of failure to communicate – failure to say what you really want to say or what really needs to be said to have the other party understand what is going on in the situation – are all examples of things that mental patients and their families could work on.

Do not be afraid to state the obvious. If you do not state what is going on, the chances are unfortunately quite high that the other party will assume something else. If you want to tell a story of resentment, don't tell a story of fear. If you want to tell a story of feeling neglected by your family who seemed to fail to realize how far you have come to see them, state that, instead of going through describing a meal that is several courses, and a description of a whole day without really mentioning what it is you're talking about. If you're foolish enough to sit on your porch with a gun visible, make sure that anyone who questions you realizes that the gun is not loaded, if that is the case. If you do not tell them, they will assume the worst, and they are entitled to do so.

The last thing that I want to say about how to tell your own story is a matter of chronology. A story may make no sense unless you tell it in the sequence in which it happened. Be careful to put in the little phrases that help out such as "in the beginning of last month" or "last Tuesday morning." And make sure that the sequence of worsening symptoms and your attempts to get help jive with each other. If not, the hearer may assume that the story happened differently from the way it did, and that may lead the hearer to a different conclusion.

As providers, we are a little suspicious of people who change their story when it brings a decision on our part that they don't like. It is far better to tell the story carefully from the beginning. I am well aware that patients may not be in a state of mind to be very sequential and logical; this is why the assistance of a family member, roommate, or friend may be invaluable.

Now I'll give a little bit of information about how providers listen to stories. First of all, let me say something about suicide attempts. If a person does something which might be injurious but which in nobody's mind is going to be fatal, this would be called a suicidal gesture. Perhaps they took four aspirin out of a bottle of a hundred. It is certainly true that you're only supposed to take two aspirin at one time, so that is, technically, an overdose. But no one thinks that four pills are going to kill them. We know that some people cut themselves to "let out the pain" when they are distressed. But when they cut themselves it's usually on the backside of the arm (i.e. the side of the arm that is uppermost when you have the arm pronated so that the back of the hand is towards the ceiling). It is true that people who cut their forearms on the underside (that is, with the palm pointing to the ceiling) are more likely to kill themselves if they cut lengthwise parallel to the axis of the arm. If they cut across the wrist, they are less likely to die than if they cut up towards the elbow. But people who are naïve and who have not been through the mental health system for a little bit, may not know this.

There is such a thing as "trying to kill yourself." You may swallow pills or try to hang yourself but you are rescued, or the rope broke. But there is no such thing as "I tried to jump off the bridge." Or "I tried to shoot myself through the head." You either did or did not jump; you did or did not pull the trigger. I always like to ask the person, if they stood on the bridge ready to jump off for some time and then turned around and went back, what <u>wisdom</u> it was that made them change their mind. Because I find that people will reveal what it is that is their main reason for staying alive at such times. Also, I certainly do not want to be saying to someone who was contemplating jumping off a bridge, "why didn't you?" which sounds as if I think maybe he would have been better off to have done it. I want people to understand that any thought which keeps you from taking your own life when you are at the brink of doing so, is a good thought.

<u>Importance of Diagnosis to the Providers</u>

Let's assume you told your story, and the provider made a diagnosis. By the way, there is as much agreement now between psychiatrists as to diagnosis as there is in any other branch of the medical profession, including surgery pre-operatively. Now we get to the importance of diagnosis from the provider's point of view. Supposing the provider sees Ms. Johnson, a twenty-nine year old secretary, in a rather agitated, depressed state. She is nervous and fidgety, at the same time her thoughts and her speech seem to express negative themes. Question: is this the way she usually is lately and the way she has been for some time, or is she going to flip her mood like a pancake when she leaves the provider's office? If by the history she gives she says she's been in this agitated, dysphoric, (which means sour or bad in some way) depressed state for three weeks, without letup in spite of the fact of having some good news (let's say she was promoted at work or that her boyfriend asked her to marry him as she had been hoping that he would) then we can assume that she must indeed be depressed. If on the other hand she says she's fidgety and agitated because she's in front of a 'headshrinker' and she's not sure what we're going to do, but she recounts having enjoyed immensely going out shopping yesterday with a friend, and she still enjoys imagining that she is becoming the successful person she dreams of, then we can assume that her depressive symptoms are short-lived and what she may be complaining of is the mood instability which is characteristic of a person with a personality disorder.

This is usually not a very difficult differential to make, because the people with personality disorders will make clear their habit of blaming others and always assuming that the cause of any change is located inside someone else – nothing ever happens because of their own decision or their hesitancy. It is often easy to spot the personality disordered person within a few minutes of meeting them because they don't talk about their own motivations with ownership. They may talk about fooling around with a new boyfriend and that their old boyfriend left them "because he's like that." They never seem to want to take responsibility, for example, for having driven him away by their philandering.

The point is that the diagnostician must choose which is the principal problem. Is the main problem depression? Or anxiety? Or is the main problem woven into the very being of the patient, in the manner of the personality disorder? Which one is chosen conditions further thinking about the case.

Let me express a danger here. If a provider diagnoses depression, starts the treatment, and shall we say has to go somewhere, and is unable to complete treatment; or if let us say, the patient moved geographically and faces a new provider in a new city; he or she should review the history well enough to be sure the diagnosis is correct. An incorrect diagnosis can creep into the patient's life and be perpetuated by every provider after that, since the provider who is a "me-too" kind of person is just the kind of provider who does not seek to verify the diagnosis before proceeding with the treatment. In state hospitals, this is quite frequent, and so people can have entrenched diagnoses which are and always have been erroneous. "Metooism", as I have said before in this book is slavishly following a previous provider's diagnosis, without checking it out for oneself.

Sometimes this is not very serious. The difference between a major depression with psychotic features (in other words with some illogic in the thought process) and schizo-affective disorder, which is really two pathologic process weaving in and out, each going according to its own timetable, such that the patient is both psychotic <u>and</u> depressed at a given moment, depressed only at another time, and psychotic only at yet a third time, may not be terribly important. In fact, the diagnosis may be back and forth from one to the other over the years, depending on how the patient may have seemed to present themselves, especially in instances where the provider do not go back and look into the old records. It is actually extremely difficult to find the time to look up old records, because of the way a doctor's day is structured – there is little time that he or she is not sitting in front of a patient, and it can be difficult not only to find the time to get old records, but also difficult, if there are ten to fifteen volumes representing thirty or forty years, to know what to look at.

At the same time, if this is done, it can be very revealing and very worthwhile for the patient and the provider. It can be very instructive to look back over the decades and see how a particular problem first presented itself.

There is another reason why diagnosis is so important to providers. Many people feel that personality disorders are too difficult to treat and that they don't want to be pouring in the energy that this would require. Therefore, they will put all their energy into Axis I disorders and sort of smile wryly and not sagely when it comes to Axis II disorders. It is true that Marsha Linehan brought forth a newly synthesized method of treating borderline personality disorder called dialectical behavioral treatment (or DBT) decades ago. Ms. Linehan wants to be very careful that only well-trained people would be using DBT for their patients, which seems a sensible precaution, but the fact is that there are a great many communities in the United States, far from big academic centers, which have no one who can use DBT. This particular method can be life-saving for people with borderline personality disorder.

Very little of Marsha Linehan's program is actually original. What is original is putting it together the way she did. She has taken ideas from long ago in history and many many different approaches to psychological problems. The major thrust of her endeavor is to get people away from extremes ("I hate it" or "I love it") and get people to be able to say, "Well, the work is good enough, but the pay isn't great" or "Well, I'm sure he has a stable character, but I wish he were more fun." Ambivalence can thus be expressed as "on the one hand….on the other hand…." rather than in extremely favorable statements one minute and extremely derogatory ones the next.

Shana Wibberley Clark, M.D., Dr. P.H.

Importance of Diagnosis to the Patients

First of all as a patient or a patient's immediate family member, you are entitled to the diagnosis. You're entitled to know what the diagnosis means, both as to the nature of the patient's problem and the likelihood of finding a solution to it.

If you disagree with the diagnosis as you are given it, present your reasons. The main importance from the patient's point of view of the given diagnosis is that there are statistics about what prognosis (future) is likely for people with that diagnosis.

For instance, taking one hundred people who have an episode of major depression (which means the episode comes to an end and the person recovers), if they come off their medication, another episode will recur within a year for fifty of those people. The statistics are better if the medication is continued for over a year, even after symptoms abate. For a young person with a first episode of psychosis only one third will develop a psychotic disorder with a down-spiraling course – in other words, at the end of each episode they will recover to some degree, but not to the level of functioning they had before that latest episode. Therefore, these people will gradually, as we say, "drift downwards" in society and may, if provision is not made for them, end up as homeless people on the street who have nothing. This can happen because a person is not able to keep a job or they are not able to maintain a household such that police or health officials do not have any need to interfere.

If such people who cannot function and maintain functioning fairly consistently are not institutionalized in a group home while they are still fairly able to function, they may drift down to homelessness. In the great downsizing of State hospitals (for individual rights, and to save State funds) in which many were deinstitutionalized after years, not enough group homes were built and staffed, and resources to find people who had run away were not made available, which is part of the reason there are so many psychotic homeless today.

Now we're always dealing with probabilities here; there's nothing cast in stone about any of this. But it goes through the minds of the providers. If you don't know what your provider sees as the future of your family member, ASK, and ask for a range from worst to best (as no one has a crystal ball).

It should be said that prognoses are changing, especially for people with psychotic disorders. With the latest medications, an ever increasing number can maintain an ability to function and have a life. This is why convincing them to take their medication is so important. Otherwise they may have a lot of jail time for repeated minor offenses, or never have a family, friends, or decent employment.

CHAPTER 14

IT'S YOUR LIFE

Most people stop trying far short of what they could achieve in terms of mental health. Let's face it, life is difficult, life is painful, and the average citizen, even if he has never gone for treatment, has a lot of "hang-ups" and is not very healthy. Mental health includes flexibility, a capacity to roll with the punches when life socks it to you, adaptability, which is the capacity to find a way to make things work out when what you had thought of or what you had planned does not go your way, and a generally positive outlook, which means an ability to look at life and face the bad and appreciate the good, and so feel a modicum of optimism. A healthy person feels that they are a significant agent in their own life – what they do matters to the course of their lives. That does not mean that a healthy person feels they are or that they need to be in control of everything; anyone who has ever slipped on a banana peel or something similar knows that their own lives are not under their total control. But a healthy person feels that whatever happens, they will cope as well as they can. Ideally (and this is an ideal and beyond the reach of most of us perhaps) this means accepting that today is the day we die, if that turns out to be the case.

Oddly enough, it is through the acceptance of suffering and through allowing ourselves to suffer that we achieve the best liberation from suffering. Because the irony is that the other side of feeling terrible is often accepting the terrible, and so coming to feeling better.

Once again, I will say that most people give up on themselves and their lives long before they have reached their maximum potential. This is primarily because achieving mental health, whether through psychiatry or through some other means, is hard work. Being aware of your journey, aware of where you come from, and aware of the freedom and the responsibilities you have from moment to moment to choose to which part of your thoughts and feelings you will give expression and which you will hold in check, is hard work. Also, it is very hard work to acknowledge that you took a wrong step in the past which may have had far- reaching consequences, possibly right up to the present. It is hard to face the trajectory of the poor judgment you made. And by poor judgment I don't necessarily mean an adult human being standing at a crossroads and deciding which way to go. I also mean a child who is buffeted by circumstances and seems naturally to grow up resenting and disliking certain things and developing either anxiety or an aversion to certain situations or both.

Hopefully, some of our complexities we may be rescued from by a wise older being who will show us that it is a mistake to turn away from life because, for example, someone called a child "fatso" or" four eyes" in the schoolyard. But if this child does not get a correction at a young age, he or she may turn negative on people in general and it can be very difficult to disentangle what actually happened and how a dislike of people and life as a whole built up within this person.

There is one thing I would like to formally advise psychiatric patients not to do. That is, to identify themselves as "mental". It is one thing to say that you have a problem and that you are seeking a solution to that problem. Everyone from Bill Gates to Princess Diana to Mother Theresa to the Dalai Lama can acknowledge a problem. It is another thing altogether to say that you are a sicko. Mental illness is something you have, like blond hair, brown eyes and a great sense of humor.

Unfortunately many psychiatrists are at fault in this way. They see someone who was admitted yesterday for hallucinating in the street, who today is wearing rumpled clothes with a stain or two on them, and they think of this person as in some way inferior to themselves and incapable of change.

I have been a patient in two State mental hospitals, I have worked in five and I have dealt with the sickest of the sick. I can only remember two men whom I was not able to reach by telling them that if each changed his behaviors a bit in terms of not wearing stained clothes, not wetting the bed, not being aggressive to others, he could earn his way out of the mental hospital. Even one of those two men, a very sick individual who I met in Pennsylvania, was someone who when I looked up the medication he took and went over his regimen and history carefully (it took about four hours) I came up with a mixture of medications which made him greatly improved.

There was one other lady in a New York State hospital who was continually psychotic, but she was not willing to take medications, which is another difficulty. Except for these three, most of the schizophrenics I have met can be treated and brought to sanity with today's medications. Since they drift away from the world of the sane possibly within a few days of stopping their medications (if they do that when they're discharged), I am much in favor of treating the disorder. With meds, the person has some side effects (and I, having personal experience with what it is to be overmedicated, have frequently gone into state hospitals and slowly reduced many peoples' medications so they get more independence of thought than they believed possible). But it is much better for the patient to think that they have a problem (for which they need to find a good solution) of having a mental illness, than thinking that they "are" a mental patient. If you undertake the identity that you "are" a mental patient, you will be accepting lots of limitations, lots of ideas about what mental patients can and cannot do. Also, if being a mental patient is who you 'are', then to get well, you must attack your identity.

I still carry a diagnosis, but I am not mentally ill. I am a well patient, which is why I have been able to work as a psychiatrist. Right now, I am also a patient or client in a nursing home because I am hoping to get some return of function on a fractured (in 3 pieces) right arm. For the time being, I am imagining full return of function in my right arm. Perhaps the time will come when I need to revise this notion, and settle for less than full return of function. But I don't know this yet.

It is a tragedy that psychiatry, which is in the business of offering change to many people, cannot always believe that those very same patients can change. People will start to criticize a person for being delusional about their own prospects, if the provider does not see the same future for the patient as the patient does. I prefer my psychiatrist's and Professor Guillemot's take on things when, asked if I would ever return to medical school, said "I don't know; we will have to do is get you well first, and then see what you will do with your life."

And I am aware that for some people, tolerating some side effects may be necessary to appear well; try not to be a person who will tolerate no side effects at all, because good medicine sometimes has some inconveniences to it.

Anyway, it's your life, you are the one who will do or will not do what you want with it, and you are the one who can decide how much you will change. Certainly, there is no universally valid answer, whether to take a medication, with its side effects, or to take a "side effect medication", or not to take the medication at all; but it is a situation that needs to be decided.

It is your life, and what you decide to do, and the energy you bring to doing it, will have a big effect on what you do manage to accomplish. Please do not buy into any negative provider's assessment of your capabilities. Try and stay away from thinking you need to be the best in the world, or the best of the century, or the best of your generation. But if you want, for example to sing songs, be happy if you could play at night in the local café down the street, at least to start. I would like to say to providers, not to buy into their patients' extravagant claims, but at the same time try not to be telling the patient that any life outside the hospital will be impossible. This will only set up antagonism between you and your patient, and let's face it, you are no arbiter of artistic talent nor do you have a crystal ball which predicts accurately what will happen. By all means caution people against any absolutist perfectionist ideas (that they have to be the best in the country, the best in the world, the best that ever was or some such) but do not yourself imagine that the mentally ill have no talents and no abilities. Try to have a sense of humility about your own inability to be a judge.

What I usually do is suggest to the patient that they have to start wherever they are and see what they can get to. This means, if a patient has a twenty year history of being a nightclub singer, they might resume nightclub singing without too much difficulty; on the other hand, if the patient is very nervous at the idea of singing in front of strangers, perhaps the first thing they should do is sing at a local open mike place.

To the patients; if you learn to control your symptoms, either by yourself or with the help of some medication so that you do not seem mentally ill to other people, you may be capable of a great deal more. Please do read the chapter on controlling your feelings and controlling your moods.

It is very important that you realize that you are the major human arbiter of what happens to you in this life. Don't let any doctor, including any psychiatrist or other specialist, tell you that you could never do a certain thing, if that's what you've got your heart set on. Do spend time and energy preparing to do that thing. In other words, if you have your heart set on being an attorney, do hurry up to get your GED and apply yourself to books. People become attorneys these days <u>after</u> they have attended college, so if you really don't like book learning, then perhaps being an attorney is not for you.

But if you are convinced that you would make a good attorney, <u>and that is what you want</u>, do not let others deter you from trying. Now, if you have tried to get into law school a number of times and had a psychiatric decompensation each time just before you took the LSAT (the big exam to take for becoming a lawyer, just like the MCAT's are the big exam for becoming a doctor), then maybe you need to rethink your situation. You may have test anxiety, and this is something you could struggle against. But it would be a hard struggle, and require a great deal of discipline, hard work, and vigorous application to study that is perhaps not part of your nature.

If it is in your nature to be studious and disciplined (if, for example, you had a depressive break at age eighteen in your freshman year of college and you left college and have earned your living quite well in the work world but now wish to return to your studies) do not let the mere fact that you haven't done it already give everybody else the license to tell you that you're not capable of it. I have known some psychiatrists who take one look at somebody, and without even speaking to them say "Oh, he'll never change" – even though we as psychiatrists are in the business of offering people constructive change.

All I can say is, do not let one such as that ruin your life. If someone is busy telling you that you can't do what you like or what you had originally proposed to do, ask them what they imagine you should do instead. If they have no answer, this should make you aware that there are many mental health practitioners who feel it is their job to stop anyone from trying to do anything that would be a real accomplishment, without making any alternative suggestions that are reasonable. I couldn't tell you how many scores of people told me I would never get back to medical school after my manic break when I had been the youngest in my class, in the third (Major Clinical) year in Columbia College of Physicians and Surgeons. They said I simply wasn't "in reality" to hang on to my dream.

Yet I did, and much to my surprise I became a psychiatrist and worked in mental health for almost 22years. It took all the decision, energy, discipline etc. that I had – but I did it. When people told me that in their opinion I could never succeed I turned them off, thinking to myself "so this person is one more who won't help me achieve my goal." I was the first doctor with Bipolar (or manic depressive) illness to get a New York license to practice based on the truth of my having an illness. It took the New York Board eleven years to see it my way, but they did, that's the point.

If your provider is trying to suggest that you should undertake the same course of study, just take a little longer to do it, giving yourself a little extra room because you have a mental illness, that is a sensible suggestion. You should look into the finances of this (obviously it can cost more to take longer to arrive at any particular qualification) and also look into what the requirements are from your institution. Are you thinking of going or are you going to a four year college that requires you to finish all the degree requirements in five years or less? Would they be willing to give you an extension because a major illness intervened? Try to get what your learning institution will do in writing. It may be in writing already in the bylaws or the fine print of the academic stipulations. But you should go into this knowingly. You should also find out whether repayment of your student loans can be deferred or postponed past the usual date, and how you are to go about applying for this. (It's called a hardship deferment.)

But, I'll say it again – do not fall prey to the blandishments of people, whatever they have or do not have in terms of professional qualifications, who say in effect, "You can't, you won't, and you shouldn't even try." The world of psychiatry is just getting around to the idea that some of us may live with an illness which may for years or for decades be quite severe, and yet manage to accomplish and achieve on this world's terms. Doctor Kay Redfield Jameson, a psychologist who has written brilliantly on manic depressive illness and done ground breaking research, admits that she herself has manic depressive illness (bipolar disorder) and she has been a trailblazer for many in the idea that a person who has an illness which is betimes active may still look for professional employment.

I would caution anyone with a serious illness about going into medicine, only because from senior medical school onward through residency, most doctors are still expected to work a nearly impossible number of hours. My illness began when I was a student expected to participate in the night call schedule. But my experience with internship and residency nearly did me in, and I have wondered many times since whether that was the best way to spend my time and talents, being so pigheadedly determined that I would finish and go into clinical practice. As it was, the manic break suffered by an attending in my residency program (this physician had been diagnosed as bipolar, but she refused the diagnosis and refused treatment) caused the program to panic and put me on probation for a while, which put an end to any ideas I might have had of a pleasant job in an academic setting – in other words what most people thought of as a really desirable job. Faced with a lack of really solid recommendation when I finished my training, I started on the road to doing locum tenens work. This is hard work, it is in psychiatry and does pay a good income, but it obliges one to be constantly on the move, constantly away from home, and to have a very geographically unstable life. This in turn makes it hard to keep friends. I would caution anyone against doing this for years on end, as I did.

A counter argument is that I believe I had a talent for cheering up patients and getting them to start working on really getting better. If a person has a small light, they would make best use of it, not by taking it out into the sunshine, but by taking it into a very dark place, where the little bit of light will be appreciated. And I did choose to work in some very dark places, because these were the places where I felt I could make the most difference.

I don't put myself up as an example, because I'm not too sure whether other people would wish to follow me, and I'm not too sure other people would wish to throw their all into working as a doctor. After all, I never married, I never had children – though there were other reasons for this. Perhaps my problem is that I am simply not a person who will give up when I have difficulty achieving something, if I have decided that is what I want to achieve.

I mentioned in another book ("My Money's on the Turtle", published by PublishAmerica in 2010) an attending who, while he acknowledged that I knew my subject matter, could get along with pediatric patients and their parents, and had a gift for handling third parties such as schools or the police, said that if I could not stand the rigors of standard residency training "he could not see" any future for me in medicine. When he said this I was crushed, but I later realized that what he was saying was a reference to his own figurative blindness – not that there was no future for me, but that he could not see it. At the same time, I would like to caution others of the enormous cost that there may be in following their dream against a major obstacle. It's not that I imagine that I would have had a bucolic, easy life had I become a flower arranger instead of a psychiatrist, but I'm not sure that it's a very good idea to throw everything you have into one thing in the way that I did. But it should be noted that many people including Steve Jobs, the founder of Apple Computing, have done just that, as did Edison and others before him.

Every person should have his or her own reasons for starting out or for continuing in a given course of study or field of endeavor. You should have thought out what the alternatives might be and decided how much you're willing to commit yourself to getting where you want to go.

When I was in my twenties, no effort seemed too great to become a physician. I literally thought that I would either become a physician or die in the attempt. Now I have some reservations, because I am living with the long-term effects of some of the choices I made as a young person, which were not at all the usual choices.

But against that I do have the immense satisfaction of knowing that my illness did not "win". I'll never forget the delicious feeling I had when

I was given the keys to a locked ward, and told "You will be starting with us on Monday." I had been locked up a number of times myself as a young person, and now I had the keys! Now I would be deciding who came and went, and when and where they would go! I also decided to be much more benevolent, to focus on the patients' needs and their families' needs much more than on any aggrandizement of mine, and to be willing just to help people along a little in their journey of life, not to consider myself God or God's right hand in deciding what happened to them. I am much more comfortable with a smaller role than the role I think many if not most physicians imagine in their heads. I don't want to give myself the delusion that I am determining what path people take. In my mind, I do proffer a helping hand, to help them navigate life, and some medications, and some philosophy which I think of as quieting down the illness so that the real person underneath can surface and take control.

About Suicide

I think one of the most challenging and potentially the most fun assignments I've ever had is to be the first person that a patient sees when they come around in the intensive care unit after a serious suicide attempt. The patient may be floored to find themselves in the intensive care unit, especially if they hadn't really intended to die. Some people who were supposed to take one pill may take two or three with a vague expectation that they get some sleep, and these people can be quite put out when they wake up in the intensive care unit. The ones who intended to die are quite easy to spot – they are the ones who are extremely anxious or depressed or at any rate majorly unhappy with their lives when they wake up.

As a person in my twenties I attempted suicide three times, and then, because getting psychiatric training as a physician didn't immediately seem to make much of a difference (because getting the training didn't seem to result in quickly attaining employment), and because I found myself penniless, I was suicidal once again at the age of forty-six. All these suicide attempts were extremely close calls – two had hemoraghic shock (that is bleeding to the point where one's life is in jeopardy) and two had coma for a few days as a consequence. So I do have a great empathy for anyone who feels desperate enough to hurt themselves in such a way that they believe they will die.

I will also add that a person who wakes up from a suicide attempt to find themselves alive now has the consequences of the suicide attempt (being known as an attempter among family, friends and acquaintances) to add to all of the problems which were unbearable before they attempted suicide. So the person who is rescued may paradoxically be extremely angry at the providers of care. Somehow, a lot of emergency room personnel believe that even a suicide attempter should be happy and grateful to be rescued, whereas of course the patient may see the rescuers as people who stepped in at the wrong moment and spoiled it all, and who will not be around when the patient has to pick up the pieces of their lives.

I remember the first time I attempted suicide (I cut my wrists and cut all my flexor tendons to my left thumb). I remember feeling very very sad and depressed afterwards, although I will remember Dr. Pacquet forever (he was the orthopedic surgeon who came in to suture the tendons in my left hand, and he was so kind and so thoughtful). I have never encountered any other surgeon like him. But, as I was saying, I felt so desperate to have someone register some sort of happiness or pleasure that I survived the ordeal, that I always begin my discussion and interview with a recently suicidal person by saying that I'm so glad they made it. Quite often, people say "Why should I matter to you? You don't know me. You don't care about me." Now this may be said cynically and with a sneer but in my experience, physicians should not be put off by this. The patient is absolutely longing to have somebody care about him or her, particularly since in a way he or she has been unable to care about him or herself. When they ask me, why do I care (because I don't know them) I say, "Well, if they had called me to say I needn't come to see you because you had just died, I would've missed the chance to meet you, and to me that would have been very very sad. So I'm always glad when I can meet the person whose physical life the emergency room and intensive care staff have been trying to save."

I then give them an opportunity to tell me about what had led up to their doing whatever they did. By the way, I try to have the details of what pills they took, how much, from where, as much as I can, before I go see them, so I'm not seeming like a completely noncaring doctor who hasn't even gotten the story straight. I may ask for clarification of some specifics, but there's nothing worse than saying "I'm sorry you took an overdose of Tuinal^R (a barbiturate)" when in fact the person had taken Valium^R or something else.

I want to get the patient to talk as soon as I can about what matters to them. I remember a young man who was twenty or twenty-one who told me he had a great interest in some French writers like Baudelaire and Camus. Now, both these writers are rather renowned for their cynicism, and cynicism ill becomes a twenty-one year old. At twenty-one a person is just coming into their big doing phase of life and should go about it whole heartedly with all the love and all the energy they can muster.

Dominic didn't know it, but I had done a great study of Baudelaire and Camus and all the post-World War I writers in France, and we went tit for tat for a while about them, and about what they had written. He mentioned several important quotes, and I quoted to him French writers from the eighteenth and early nineteenth centuries who had been of the opposite opinion, the Romantics and people who were certainly far from cynical. I suggested he read a particular book which I recommended to his family; I told him why I wanted him to read it. So perhaps I was a good doctor to have been sent to that young man that night, because the end of the story is that as I was leaving him I got him to burst out laughing. It was good laughter, it was not cynical, it was full throated twenty-one year old laughter, so I left him with a good feeling that he would make a future for himself. I always think that if your shell of indifference and cynicism and negativism can be punctured, exploded and discarded in a one hour interview, then it cannot have been that thick to begin with. Plus there were elements of impulsivity in his behavior. People who plan their suicide very carefully, plot its execution, plan not to be found, usually do not come to the emergency room because they escape detection, sadly, and they do die.

One thing I will say about suicide attempters is the following: we always ask about previous episodes of suicidality, including actual attempts, thoughts of suicide and non-suicidal self-harm; by the latter I mean cutting oneself in the upper arm or thigh, which can bleed and will produce a scar but which is in the wrong place to cause loss of life. Some people feel so wretchedly unhappy that the little bit of energy they get by injuring themselves (because an injury sets up injury currents and gets survival hormones circulating) is attractive enough that they will cut themselves in secret repeatedly. They may cause themselves serial scars in parallel lines and may in later life, if they cannot afford to have those scars removed, be wearing long skirts and long sleeves and basically avoiding the beach.

Now back to talking about suicide. I said my little bit once to a young man about "What wisdom stopped you from jumping off the bridge?" And Alan who was just turned twenty said to me "It was a silly reason." I said "My goodness, man, a thought that will keep you from jumping off a bridge where you were standing for nearly an hour – that's not silly, that's a lifesaver!" So he told me "Well, because if I had jumped then I would have died without ever having painted my picture." I asked him what he meant by that, and he told me that he grew up in the country in a single storey house with a very large, very old sugar maple outside in the yard. He said the sugar maple was bright orange red when the leaves turned in the fall, and he used to watch the sunsets over the hill in the distance and the bright orange of the sunset matched the bright orange of the leaves and he said reflectively "You have no idea how pretty that was! You see I keep telling myself I have to paint that picture." Then he said under his breath "And I know my father says painting pictures is stupid..." I then asked him what Shakespeare Picasso and Ludwig van Beethoven all had in common. He said "Well, they were all artists."

I said "Yes, but what I'm after is something else." He looked at me blankly, but with the beginning of a smile on his face. I said to him "When they were twenty, nobody had heard of them either." I told him if that picture was calling him to be painted, then he should set about painting that picture, and if he felt very unhappy as a banking apprentice, then maybe he could find some part-time job that would allow him to keep body and soul together while he pursued his passion in his off hours. I told him I would talk to his father, that the creator of the universe who is always bringing us surprises had given him an artist son, not a son who was meant to be a banker.

And I did have a conversation with his father. I got the father to grudgingly acknowledge that a son who was self-supporting would be satisfactory, and much to be preferred over a dead son. Even he had to admit that not everybody was cut out of the same cloth.

Shana Wibberley Clark, M.D., Dr. P.H.

Of course I don't know these years later what the outcome was, but I was struck by what happened when I told this young man that he had had wisdom not to jump in and certainly complete suicide a week before. I often wondered what the was effect of telling him that the thought that kept him from jumping off a bridge and deciding to come back down and trying to cope with life is NOT a silly thought; it is a lifesaving thought. That was also something that I said to his father: that the thought that kept him from jumping off the bridge was not what a great future he had in banking, but rather that he had to paint his picture.

These are the people that I pray for late at night hoping that my few minutes with them might have started something positive in their lives. Let's now talk about something which I have found deeply disturbing, as most psychiatrists and pediatricians have. This is a phenomenon in which pre-teen or early teen girls (I mean between the ages of say 10 and 15) show some adolescent defiance of maternal authority by running into the bathroom, popping maybe half a dozen Tylenol[R] into their mouths and swallowing them. In three cases I've seen, the young girls did not think there would be any serious consequence to what they had done. They were, as it were, putting their hands in the candy jar as a deliberate gesture of defiance because their mother said they were grounded or because they were told to clean up their room or something like that.

Now, these young women would then come to the emergency room and be treated for acetaminophen overdose. Unfortunately, some people may liquefy their livers after consuming six tablets of Tylenol[R] at the same time, and these people die. You can't live without a liver, the drug is absorbed very quickly and you can't really keep it from being absorbed, and so there's little we can do. We always do give Mucomist[R], which is an inhaled treatment which does help, and which saves the lives of some people who but for the Mucomist[R] would have died. But there are always some who, despite our best efforts, will die.

I have had three times in my life to be looking into the distraught face of a mother, aged thirty-something, of one of these young girls, and say to her that her daughter was going to die and there's nothing we could do about it. Actually in two of the cases I got hold of the child early enough that I said to the mothers "Call out the troops, call every person who cares about your little girl, and that is uncles, aunts, grandparents, godparents, and get them praying, because there's a ghost of a chance she might make it." In the third case I was a witness to, the child had taken the Tylenol^R and no one was aware of it for some time, and unfortunately, all three of them died. I can remember the mother's faces as they looked at me and said "But she only took a few Tylenol^R!" and I said "Yes, you're supposed to take two tablets every four to six hours –" and the mother would almost scream at me "But it was only Tylenol^R!!" And I calmly said she took about six tablets which is three times what you're supposed to take. From our point of view that's a serious overdose." And then I try and prepare the mother before going back to speak to her dying child, and say "You know, before you tell the child that you're so frantic, disappointed and fed up, could you please consider that your child is dying, and would you not like her last hours on this earth to be as pleasant as possible?"

All I can say is, I do not think Tylenol^R or any other brand of acetaminophen should be sold in one hundred pill bottles or five hundred pill bottles. This gives people the notion that it's sugar candy and while I do not think it should be a prescription item because there are obviously millions of people who take it perfectly safely, I think there should be some education by the manufacturers on its appropriate use. Because if I have seen three of these cases, other psychiatrists and pediatricians have seen more.

We need to make schoolchildren and mothers aware that there is nothing you put in your mouth that has no risks. Even water can be risky for a person who is in heart failure and certainly there is no medication on earth which has no risks at all. I do think that pharmaceutical companies should be made responsible for educational programs about overdoses of their products; I think this could be worked out.

I don't think we can get rid of young teenagers' impulsivity; it's part of their development. But I think if they were told repeatedly at age 8, 9 and 10 that all medicines, including Tylenol^R and Aspirin^R, can kill in overdose, and if we told adults repeated that <u>all</u> medications, over-the-counter or no, can be dangerous if given in the wrong dose to the wrong people, we might decrease these tragic deaths.

Now I would like to address my fellow patients about the topic of this chapter "It's Your Life." Having a mental illness in no way excludes a person from having to make decisions, small medium and large, about who they are all their lives. Are you an honest person? Are you a person of integrity? Neither of these means that you should think of divulging embarrassing or difficult parts of your history to those who don't have a need to know about it. But you, like everybody else, must decide whether or not you are going to be honest and forthright to the people who do have the right to make such inquiries. Part of the reason that there is still so much prejudice and discrimination against people with mental illness is that your predecessors have been neither honest nor forthright, thinking only of their potential personal loss that telling the truth would cost them, never thinking of the dignity that speaking clearly when clarity is asked for could give them. I was horrified when I found out that of an estimated 2,000 doctors who do have a mental illness or have been treated for one, in the State of New York, not a single one had been honest with licensure, so that the Board of Licensure felt that there was no one in New York State who was licensed as a physician who had a mental illness, officially. It is of some comfort to me that in New York State as in the other six states in which I have been licensed, I stood up and was counted as a mentally ill person who became a physician. New York State did give me a license to practice, but only <u>11 years</u> after I applied for it.

There is a professional who wrote a very moving book about her experiences as a physician with a mental illness, who said that she could not "die dishonest". Yet she had been perfectly content to live for decades, dishonest.

I decided early on in my mental illness (with my first hospitalization in fact) that I would not shrink from using both my real first name and my real last name in whatever patient roles my illness might get me to. It seemed to me that this was the best way to be able to advocate for patients in future (I did not give up on my becoming a physician for one minute, even when I was in mental hospitals). I always was ferociously honest, and I didn't see why I should change character just because the cost of honesty went up.

I was offered, at the beginning of my illness, to be hospitalized under an assumed name and I declined. Later, I faced many many times when employers particularly would refuse to hire me because of what I had told them.

I consider it an achievement that I have lived to the age of 63 without ever compromising my integrity in any way. Apparently, this is rather rare. I have missed many job opportunities because of it, but have always felt that if to become employed by some organization I am required to be a person of tarnished integrity, then that is not the place for me. I don't sit in judgment of other people who choose differently, but I do wonder how they sleep at night. Of course, this matter of keeping one's integrity, of being honest versus taking the easy way out and failing to mention certain things, is something that is particularly acute for anyone who has a profession for which they are required to have a state license. On these license applications, there is a sentence above one's signature which says "Under penalty of perjury, I swear that the above is correct and complete to the best of my knowledge and belief." In other words, one is slammed against the wall to either lie and perjure oneself, or stay honest. There is no way of sidestepping the question.

I remember when I was hospitalized in 1973 there came into the hospital after me a patient named "Joe". We were told that Joe was a surgeon. The staff would never use his last name, and Joe was excused from any participation in community meetings, which were compulsory for everybody else. I remember thinking what a chicken Joe was because he was obviously trying to protect his identity. I later found out that as far as hospital records were concerned, he was hospitalized under an assumed name so that no one who looked up the hospital records would ever find that he had been a patient there. I wondered how I would handle it if I was expected to collude with another physician over concealing their identity from licensure. I remember I prayed never to have that happen to me, because I would not be able to participate in the group lie. Mercifully, it never did happen. No patient of mine was ever hospitalized under a false name.

Today I can empathize with Joe's reluctance to face the truth and be honest about what happened to him, but I still choose my path, the one of honesty. What strikes me as strange is that no one seems to be upset by the idea of committing perjury, and no one seems to be perturbed by the idea that in being dishonest they are perpetuating the stigma against mental illness. Physicians would not be so frightened of the Board of Licensure in medicine if there were already several admittedly mentally

Shana Wibberley Clark, M.D., Dr. P.H.

ill people who were registered to practice in the State of New York. And I have contributed what I could to this situation, which is to be the first one.

In Chapter 17 I will tell the story of how I managed to vote from inside a mental hospital. Mental patients, if they care to, are entitled to vote, though prisoners are not.

CHAPTER 15

HOW TO MANAGE YOUR PROVIDER

Section 1: Preparing to Visit the Provider

There are three short-term categories of things to talk over with your doctor: one, whether the medication you are currently taking (including especially whatever has been recently changed) is effective for you in decreasing your symptoms; two, side effects (any unwanted, unexpected, or unacceptable effect that the medication has that you may find difficult to put up with); and three whatever forms you may want the doctor to fill out and sign.

I would invite you to consider very carefully which items you need to spend time discussing. First, realize that your doctor or other provider only has a set amount of time for you. Unfortunately and shockingly, in some areas of this country today this means perhaps a thirty minute initial visit and a ten minute subsequent visit. Personally, I have refused to work under such conditions, but they are getting quite commonplace. This is partly because there are more and more patients who are coming around to the idea that professional help can be of assistance in a wide variety of personal difficulties, and also because insurances want to give less and less resources to each individual patient, and clinics, faced with more and more patients and less and less pay per each, are trying to push providers to see people faster and faster. This runs counter to what psychiatry is about, which is a progressive, reasoned change in a person so that the way they live their lives, what they focus their attention on, how they are thinking and how they are feeling change quite substantially. You may for a given session have to decide what is more important to mention -- side effects of the medication your doctor put you on at the last visit, or that form you need him or her to fill out. Before you go to your doctor's office, make a "trigger word" list of the items you want to discuss, most important first.

But you have to deal with the reality that you may only have a quarter of an hour with your doctor. So before you go to see him or her, make a short list of the items you want to have discussed. Remember that I said that if you have a form you want the doctor to fill out you should mention that at the beginning of the session. Otherwise, if you mention it and hand it over at the end the doctor must get on to the next patient and may not get to your form for quite some time. The other thing you need to do before you go is to pack your list (which is a list for you only – it needs only to trigger your memory when you see it so that you can move quickly from one item to another without a lot of hemming and hawing), and put it somewhere where you will be able to just reach into whatever you are carrying and come out with it.

Surely the most important point from your doctor's point of view is how you are feeling in terms of your symptoms – i.e. if you are taking the medication he gave you, are you feeling better? The best way to phrase this, if you're having a significant side effect, is to mention the side effect first i.e. "I'm having problems being sleepy, though I do feel better on the medication."

Section Two: Going to Your Provider's Office

My point here is that you should make a habit of arriving in your doctor's office five to ten minutes early, even when you don't have any history forms to fill out because you're not a new patient. It is not the wisest thing to announce yourself to the receptionist if you need to go to the bathroom first, because the receptionist will assume that you're in the waiting area between telling her you're there and whenever the doctor comes to get you, so the best thing is to go into the bathroom, do what you need to do first, and <u>then</u> announce yourself to the receptionist. You don't want the doctor to come out looking for you when you're in the restroom, because if he doesn't find you waiting immediately, he may take the next person who is there very early, and you will start late and may not get as much time as you would if you were in the waiting room when the doctor was looking for you.

Also, going to the restroom will give you a moment to recover from whatever happened on the way – you had an argument with the taxi driver, someone on the bus was rude, etc.—get out your list, and focus on what you need to say to your doctor.

When I was a patient it took me a long time to learn this point, so I would go into the doctor's office full of my indignation about what the cab driver had said to me, or the argument we had when I did not have exact change for the fare, or what have you – and I remember when I was new to being a patient, this minor mishap could mushroom into something that took up the entire session with my doctor. After a few minutes of talking about this, he would say to me "Well, I hope you have a better time getting here next time," and that would be the end of the session. Remember what I said in Chapter 12.

Part 3: The Session With Your Doctor Itself

Think about the wording you would like in the doctor's part of the form. If you would like the doctor to say that you have been under his care, but not to mention the diagnosis or the medications you are given, be sure to say so. Some forms may require a diagnosis. For instance, many companies who would give you a form to fill out for sick leave would require the doctor's signature and the diagnosis on the form from a doctor. The diagnosis, particularly how it is worded, is the doctor's business. This is not a part of the form you should be writing anything in. But if you don't want some particular item mentioned, be sure to say so. You might point out that people at the school who gave you the form to enroll in the course that you want are not particularly expecting the enrollees for this course to be psychiatric patients, and all they may want (since they're not giving you leave from work, they are simply allowing you to take the course) is a general reassurance that you will not be likely to faint or collapse or have other physical difficulties in class. If there is a specific thing they are asking for (such as for example if you will be required to do what for some might be feats of strength or feats of balance), show your doctor you are capable of these, or give him some evidence to back it up (i.e. you took a similar course at your local community center last year.) If the course is something that is difficult mentally and will require a great deal of homework, it's up to you to convince your doctor you can do this. You will be more convincing if you have done some intermediate steps before you take a very demanding course. For example, if you can take an online course on something and have finished it ahead of schedule (ahead of the deadline for the students in that class) say so. Most doctors will give you the benefit of the doubt if they have some idea that you might be able to get through this class. But they certainly don't want to send into a class someone who's totally unprepared for it.

Physicians do not guarantee anything to anyone; they say they feel that there is a good possibility that the person may finish or whatever. But we know all too well that a person can be run over by a truck overnight, or that they can have a heart attack or stroke when it is least expected. This is a once-in-a- lifetime occurrence for this patient, but seeing it can be a common occurrence for us, so we naturally have a different perspective on it.

If it's the side effects that are the most important, list them in your mind, most important first. I refer the reader to Chapter 10 "The Skinny on Side Effects" for more on this. You may have to decide whether being sleepy during the day or being dizzy at times, is more important to you. Try to be able to describe when it happens and what happens (for example, "I get dizzy when I bend over and come back up again, and also when I get up in the morning or get up from a nap"), or what brings it on ("I get sleepy about an hour after I finish lunch.") If there is something you can do to make the side effect more tolerable -- such as make the dizziness from bending down to tie your shoelace more bearable, by putting your foot up on the chair so you don't bend down very much, or remember to bring your head back up from bent over slowly, or if you have to rearrange your lunch time so you have time after lunch to be sleepy, if you can do that) then perhaps you have dealt with these side effects and they are not a priority to bring up with your doctor.

What You Should Tell Your Employer or Your School

Let's face it, prejudice against mental illness is rampant in this country and quite unreasonable. By 'unreasonable' what I mean is, that the American public has not gotten ahold of the idea that people can take psychiatric meds and control their illness and so function quite well for an extended period of time. Others take medication for symptom relief so they feel better interiorly, but their illness or suffering is mild enough so that it does not drastically affect their abilities anyway. Both of these groups of people suffer from the general perception that people who take psychotropic medications are "crazy" or untrustworthy or some other negative.

I myself have not done what I'm advocating in this chapter, which is to limit very severely the amount of information that your employer or your school may have. I have not done this because doctors are expected (at least theoretically -- in practice people don't usually do this) to be candid about their state of mental health, and to mention anything that might impair their functioning. Some hospitals ask if the applicant has ever been treated for something that might impair their functioning.

This is actually an illegal question, since it may have little bearing on one's present ability to function. The fact that twenty years ago, after the death of your child, you had a bout of depression, does not mean that now, 2 decades later, you are not able to perform the requirements of your job. Senator Eagleton, a Vice Presidential hopeful in 1972, fell out of consideration as a candidate when it became known that after the death of his wife years earlier he was treated for depression. I remember this, because it happened just at the time I was admitted to a psychiatric hospital the first time myself. I was glad I had no political ambitions.

The trouble is that people do not realize that having a malady treated can mean that it does not interfere or interferes very little with one's daily functioning. Senator Eagleton had functioned well for years as a senator after his depression, but nonetheless he was excluded from being Vice President.

Now to what your employer or school should be told about your mental health status and treatment. They should be told that you are under a doctor's care and that a reduction in your course load would be advisable, or that the doctor believes you can finish the term satisfactorily or whatever. Anything the doctor can put in such as "based on his excellent performance last year" is all to the good. Have a very practical, forward-looking letter.

One last word. What, you say, should I do if I am unable to do more than feel the symptoms that I feel, show up to the doctor's office on time, and give him a description of what the medication he gave last time does to me or for me? what if I am, because I am mentally ill, not able to do all these things to keep my doctor in line?

That is an important question. First of all, all of us, mentally ill or no, have times in our lives when we don't function as well as we do other times, and when we wish that somebody else would "make" us better. But that is not really what will get you better. If you don't have the ability to be organized yourself, I suggest you might get a case manager, and once you have a case manager, follow his or her lead. If you have a concerned family member who shows their appropriate concern without smothering you and without "oh-there-you-go-again" fatalism whenever you slip a bit, then perhaps they can help you. The most important item, I think, is how motivated you are as the patient, how determined you are to change, so that you will not always be in this quandary. You may find a way to get yourself out of it. Perhaps you see your doctor once a month, perhaps the next visit is on Friday, so maybe you can appoint some time on Tuesday or Wednesday to make your list, to make the best possible use of your time with your doctor.

Unfortunately I'm going to have to ask you to jettison the idea that anyone or anything is going to "make" (with its connotation of almost brute force) you better. Many many people slip into being chronically ill, perhaps not because they really have to (their illness may not be that bad, and their resources to fight it may not be that poor) but simply because they themselves and everyone around them expects them never to "get well".

I would like to suggest to you that being well is a continuum; there is a spectrum, from people who have never worked or never had families to people who have families but are not consistently able to put food on the table, or who have had many jobs but have never held one for a period of time, all the way up to someone who is able to take the stresses and strains of being president, and even among presidents, there is the apparent balance and reason of a Mr. Obama compared to the paranoia of a Mr. Richard Nixon.

I am not saying that everybody is ready to be president or ever will be. But I am saying, and I hope with some force, that many people could function better than they already do if they thought about it, and if they really decided to bootstrap themselves up to better functioning.

If you need your provider to talk to or correspond with your employer, your school, your university, or with other people that are important to you but are not family, I would suggest that you say to the provider that they should reveal that you are under their care, but they should certainly refrain from mentioning exact medications. A boss may not be able to evaluate what the probability is that you will be able to work for him with only the usual amount of absences and interruptions. But the boss may have some notions about people who take Thorazine[R] or Haldol[R] or Prozac[R] or some other medication that your doctor mentions. I do it this way: "John Dokes is under my care. I am his psychiatrist, helping him with for his difficulties with social situations (or work situations). He takes medication regularly (if that is true) and in the last six months has attended seven out of eight scheduled sessions (or whatever is true). He is very interested in improving or perfecting his work attendance (if that is true) and in my view has a very good prospect of doing so."

If I then get a call from the employer asking for the diagnosis or the medications, I ask the employer why he wants to know, since he, the employer, is not equipped to evaluate what the diagnosis means or what the medications mean. Therefore, say I to the employer, why would such information be of interest to him?

I usually then ask the employer why he's calling me, since I did already put an estimate of John Dokes' prospects in terms of improving his work performance in my letter. Sometimes the employer has a very good reason to talk to me – for instance he might want to know if giving Mr. Dokes a steady schedule, the same every week, would help his work attendance, versus his current schedule which varies by shift change from week to week. That is an excellent question. It is usually better for someone who is a psychiatric patient to have the same schedule every week, since adjusting to phase changes with a different schedule between one week and the next can be very difficult for psychiatric patients. I may say "for my patients" and avoid mentioning that I am a psychiatrist. Usually, the letter says that I am a psychiatrist. Also, I may refer to difficulties in the patient's home, but I never refer to specifics.

I point out to the employer that from his point of view what is most important is, will Mr. Dokes be able to work better than he has in the past, or maintain his good performance? And I do give my best appraisal of that.

If I am not able to say that Mr. Dokes has attended most of his sessions or that he takes his medications regularly, I may say something like "Mr. Dokes is experiencing difficulty in adjusting to a particular regimen and may have some continuation of that difficulty until we get everything settled." I always go over with the patient what I'm going to say and I try to put a helpful construction on things, but I do not make falsely optimistic statements. I may say, for example, of someone who has changed jobs a great deal in the past, "Mr. Dokes is currently interested in continuing to work for your company." This statement does not say anything about how long he is going to remain interested in working for that company; I do not say something positive that the patient has not expressed. At the same time, I do not shoot down a patient of mine simply for being a patient.

Some people who have stable symptoms and who take their medications faithfully can be among the most reliable employees a company has ever known. Because, they realize that changing jobs might be ill-perceived and that job performance in terms of number of years working for a firm can speak for itself as showing the patient to be very reliable and trustworthy. There have been studies done which show that people with disabilities (including physical disabilities), when they do find work, are more reliable as employees than their non-disabled counterparts, for the simple reason that a disabled person who has a job will value it more than a non-disabled person. Also, it has been shown that people with physical disabilities are less likely to have work accidents than people with no physical disabilities. This is possibly because the person with a disability already has one physical problem, and would not relish having another. And, for disabled people, living with a disability is a reality, not some vague unreal possibility.

I have been surprised a number of times in my career at the willingness which doctors have had, once they have a signed release form from the patient that allows them to be in touch with the patient's employer, to release diagnostic and treatment specifics, (which is particularly unwise if the patient himself or herself does not know and understand his or her own diagnosis in all its details.)

More than that, the prejudice against the mentally ill in the general public is so strong that I think it is very unwise to let a person who is not trained about mental illness have any juicy details, and so I do not usually do this, although sometimes it is unavoidable. I would like other providers to consider this approach.

Section 4: How to cope with officials

Because of the time constraint problem, and because nurses, therapists, a lot of people think that I'm doing nothing if I do not have a patient in my office who has an appointment with me, I will sometimes ask the patient to make another appointment for me to do a form. During this period of form filling, the patient will sit quietly and occupy the patient's chair while I fill out the form. I am then free to ask any questions that might come up such as what was the longest job ever held, or when precisely did a physical limitation hit.

If the doctor says "I'll get to this later" be careful not to let him or her. Don't be afraid to say, "I think we should do this now because I have to turn it in to the government office tomorrow" if that is true. Actually, it may be wisest to make an appointment perhaps two weeks before the deadline.

If you leave the form to be filled out with your doctor, it is quite possible it will not be filled out in a timely manner and it is also possible that you will never hear when it *is* filled out. Since you are the party most concerned, it is much better that you take the form with you. In those cases where this is not allowed, ask your doctor who in his office you may call to know if the form in question has been mailed out. Usually, in most practices, the fact that a form has been mailed out on your behalf is recorded in your chart. In a well-run practice, a copy of the form will also be in the chart, in case officialdom has any additional questions to ask. It is much easier for the doctor (I speak from experience here) if a doctor get a question from a government official about his or her answer on question eleven (I'm making the number up) if you can refer to the chart and know exactly what you did write on question eleven. Then you can have a reality-based conversation with the government official. People who work for the government seem to think that the doctor should be able to instantly recall any answer on any form for at least several months – and of course this is not the case.

So, a well-run practice will have a copy of the completed form and the notation somewhere of when it was sent out. What you need to know is whom you can call to ask for that information. If you get the feeling that they won't write in the chart when it was sent out, offer to stay past your visit time waiting in the waiting room until the doctor or secretary says that your form has been completed. But don't just get up and walk out and assume that all these clerical tasks will happen. In many busy public clinics, it is very difficult for a provider to find the time even for the most necessary forms. And the only way to be sure that your paperwork is taken care of is to stay on top of it yourself.

If you say you're going to wait in the waiting room until you hear that the form has been done, listen to what the provider says. If he says "Oh I'll do it tomorrow at 7 a.m. because that's when I always do the forms" then stop by early tomorrow say 8 or 9 a.m. and ask if it has been completed. Tell the doctor you're going to be asking at the front desk at 8 o'clock tomorrow so that the doctor communicates with the front desk about your form. Also tell the front desk that you will be asking for it so that they understand what's going on. You can also gently inquire if the personnel at the front desk today is going to be the same as tomorrow. Sometimes, the person that you made a connection with is on vacation the next day and no one else knows what on earth you're talking about. Try to avoid this problem.

I realize that this is going way beyond what most people tell you or do do for their own government papers. But you have to realize it is your future, and you are the person most affected. Therefore, it behooves you to take an interest in what's going on. It could be that the office will 'get around to it' in three weeks – but by that time that wonderful apartment you were hoping to apply for will have been assigned to someone else. Therefore, going at it with determination and decision is appropriate.

If the patient, because they are mentally ill, is unable to negotiate for themselves, this is a point at which family members can be invaluable. Don't ever be insulting to the provider or anyone in the provider's office, and don't make snide remarks about how slow the government programs are. Just keep gently pushing to the next step, leaving people plenty of room to say, for example, on a Friday, "Doctor X is on vacation next week" or "Ms. Y, the office manager, is on sick leave for foot surgery and will be back on such a date." You have to realize that other people's exigencies may well hold up your progress. This is life. If you and your family members handle this well and are reasonably polite, the staff will be all the more eager to help you get to the housing or the job training program or the free medication for the indigent (poor people) or whatever is the topic at hand. If you handle this badly, it is understandable, but when you say "Oh no!" or make a sarcastic remark when you hear that someone is going on vacation or someone is out of town for a funeral or whatever, you are not making friends, and the very people who could most help you will feel less inclined to do so.

It is my experience that in the grand scheme of things, while somebody else's foot surgery might hold up your getting a particular apartment, the universe works these things out and you'll get something nice at a later date.

What is not a good idea is to be not participating in your own care and simply dropping off a form at the doctor's office without any concern whatever about when it will be filled out or when it will be sent back or how you will continue with the next step of the paperwork. If you are nice, pleasant, and concerned, it may be that the staff will outdo themselves in being nice and pleasant and concerned with you. Staff often find it refreshing to find someone who has a good reality orientation <u>and</u> an interest in the paperwork that is done for the patient. We have millions of people who want things, but who cannot be persuaded to go and get the form, let alone deliver it to the provider's office and take an interest in how it is going to get back to the proper functionary.

The same sorts of precautions can apply to the government official. When you contact them, you should ask to whom the form should be returned, hoping for at least a first name. Government officials may be reluctant to use their last names because they don't want irate citizens looking them up and bothering them at home. But a first name and a job title is fine. Just something so that when the office of that government department receives the communication, there is no delay in getting it to the right individual.

Another point is about time delays. If the department that handles housing applications or job training applications tells you at the outset that you should expect your application to be processed six weeks after you return it, keep a record of the date it is returned, pick out the date that is six weeks from that date and say "So you mean I'll get an answer around August 27", mentioning the date that is six weeks from that date. They then may say "If it goes past the end of August, I would call us back." Keep a notation of the person you spoke to, and then on the second of September you call the office and you say "Mary Jane told me on July the fourteenth when I delivered it that I should expect a reply within about six weeks, which is August 27, and that if things went into September and I still didn't hear anything I should call you." This establishes to the next official that you are a person who listens to what his co-worker told you. This may not get you the reply you seek, but it's a lot better than just to say "Oh gee, I came with this form sometime in the middle of July and it seems like a long time and I wonder if you guys have had a chance to process it?" A co-worker of Mary Jane's would be very reluctant to tell you that the expectation she created by saying that it should be done by about August 27 was phony. At least the co-worker will go look and see what has happened with your form. Whereas the "Oh gee I dropped it off in July" approach will have the functionary saying to you "you have to be patient", and not even bothering to get you any additional information.

If the official says to you "I'm so sorry but Mary Jane was in an accident three weeks ago and she's still in the hospital", you should say "I'm so sorry" and look sorry and sound sorry and think a minute about Mary Jane and her family. If you are a kind considerate human being, it becomes difficult for the person facing you to be totally unkind and totally inconsiderate. Whereas if you say "That ain't my problem" or "Oh boy, watch the officials make excuses" you may make yourself an enemy.

Again, this is a situation in which the help of a family member of the mentally ill person can be most helpful. If you have a family member who is mentally ill and you find being with him or her a difficult experience, a gentle inquiry as to whether they are trying to get any help with housing or with job training or with medication could reveal that they are in the middle of one of these quests. Then you have something that is not very difficult that you could do to help your family member. And, when you get even a partial result, your family member should be very glad of your help.

Realize that no one was put in this life to sign your papers, and always be willing to consider the feelings and the reaction of the person in front of you. A great many people are longing to help someone if they feel that the help they give would only be noticed. I don't mean by this that you have to buy people flowers or chocolates. But if an official does something wonderful for you a simple thank you card might be nice. From a provider's point of view, the world can seem to be full of demanding, ungrateful, exigent people who are on the edge of exploding into abusive language, and this generates a certain understandable unwillingness to do much to cooperate. People hide behind "the system" or "the rules" because no one says to them "Look, see me, I'm a human being, and I can see that you are a human being too." If an official tells you that something you want very much is impossible or is disallowed or is discontinued or whatever, look nonplussed (but not angry) and say "Well, what would you do if you were in my shoes? I need housing, I must move out of my house in X weeks, and you're telling me I'm not eligible for this program. You know the system – do you know of any other program for which I am eligible?" and then listen to what you are told.

Don't try to throw your weight around with officialdom. I'm assuming that if you really could throw your weight around, that would have been done for you by your uncle the senator (or whatever) already. So if you're just a regular person like most of us, don't try to be impressive. It will fall flat and will not win you friends. Always be pleasant with people – you never know, an official you meet today may be in charge of the program you want to get into tomorrow. Officials in bureaucracies move too, and you never want to make an enemy of the person you may most need in the future. Keep careful records of when you spoke to someone, what they said etc. so that you have your own history of your experience in trying to get this. It really doesn't help you if someone asks you have you ever approached this program before and you say, "Oh gosh, I have no idea". The feeling that this engenders in an official is to say to you "Well, Mr., I have no idea either." And that's not what you want.

Many people may have the benefit of a case manager. Some case managers even pick up the client/patients at their houses and take them to appointments. This is more likely to be true if the patient is simply not together enough to be with it and make sense. But if you do make sense, there is no harm in keeping documentation of what happens. This need not be an awful lot of papers – it may be something as simple as application for city housing: 1) Went to the housing office on (date) and got application forms; 2) Saw my doctor, Doctor X (name and address) on such a date, and gave him the application form; 3) followed up with his office manager (name) on such a date and found that the form had been sent to the housing office on (date); 4) Four weeks later called housing office to hear about progress of application. Spoke to Chris. She stated that the average application takes about six weeks to process, so I said to her that we should be finished in another two weeks on (date); 5) On (that date), not having heard from the housing office, called Chris again. She looked up the application and stated that a favorable response had been determined, and the letter was sent out to my present address on (date) 6) Received the acceptance from the housing authority on (date); went to housing authority on the day after receiving the acceptance to discuss with them precisely what accommodations might be available. 7) Put my name down for apartment seven at (address); 8) (date three months later) they said I could move in, the move in date will be (date). Each of these entries is written on the date it occurs and as you can see each entry is just a few words, so you do not have to be a writer to keep a record of your progress.

If I seem to stress these points heavily, it is because in the early part of my forty years and counting as a mental patient, I fell afoul of each one of these points – there was nobody to show me how to do things, so I did it the wrong way, and paid the consequences. That is why I am trying so hard to show you, my reader, how to do it right.

I think I have learned something in all these years, because when it came time to claim Social Security Disability I had learned how to get the papers to Social Security quickly. Therefore, Social Security, armed with all the proof of my disabling condition which I sent them, granted me disability fast.

I will finish with one more observation, that it is possible under the Freedom of Information Act which was passed I believe in 1974, to get copies of all reports from doctors, interpretations of X-rays or other studies, and if you request these reports close to the time the examination is done, you should have no difficulty getting them. In fact, many X-ray and MRI places today will offer you a free CD with your X-ray or MRI on it. I would strongly advise people to keep paper and CD copies of their own medical record, because then, when needed, you just go to your own file drawer and make copies of your copies to send out to something like Social Security Disability, and you don't have to wait weeks and call many many people to get these medical documents sent. This also eliminates the problem that the sending entity says it went out the door, whereas the receiving entity has not received it (probably some clerk put it in the wrong file, or it is under something else and at any rate does not get into your file). There is also the matter that after some variable period of years, hospitals may destroy medical records, so it is without doubt better to get copies of pertinent things when you leave the institution, and keep your own records for yourself.

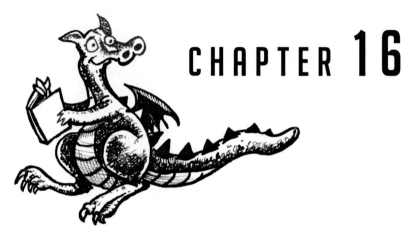

CHAPTER 16

MOTIVATION AND HOW TO ENHANCE IT

Motivation is the engine of change. It is what takes something from being merely a dream, a possibility, even a plan, to being a present reality. A person who is highly motivated, even if they lack other resources such as time, or money, or good health, to devote to getting what they want, may nevertheless get it because their motivation is so strong that they are always looking for opportunities to progress toward their goal.

Motivation is one of the things that a prudent psychiatrist will assess from the first meeting. This is because if a person has a deep-seated conviction that they will not get better, that they will not get what they want, then this negative motivation will be a great obstacle to overcome before they have permission from themselves to get better. Therefore, it is wisest to work on the motivation factor from the beginning.

Many if not most psychiatric patients could use some work on motivation. This may be part of their illness (amotivation – the lack of any kind of motivation – and avolition – the lack of power of the will – are part of the negative symptoms of schizophrenia). Remember that the things which would have to be added to normal experience to arrive at the experience of people with schizophrenia are called 'positive' symptoms, (such things as hallucinations or delusions), and the things which have to be subtracted from a normal person's experience to arrive at the position of a schizophrenic are part of the 'negative' symptoms (such as amotivation, avolition, alogia which means not talking) and general indifference.

We know how to control positive symptoms now, but not the negative ones. Lack of motivation may also be because the person is overmedicated or still so anxious or so scared or so depressed that they don't seem able to make a move. Falling into the mental health system can be a rather overwhelming experience and the person may be thinking, what on earth is going on? Why am I in a mental hospital? What happened here? For any or all of these reasons, the patient may appear to be very poorly motivated. Further, if they have been subjected to providers whose basic attitude is "You will never change", this negativity can be difficult to counter.

Some of these patients may be indifferent to the fact that they are rewarded for behaving in pro-social manner. People who get washed and get dressed in the morning may be rewarded with the right to go for a walk on the grounds, people who handle the daily frustrations of life (and frustrations abound in a mental hospital – something as simple as getting a stamp to mail a postcard or pay a household bill can be a major undertaking when the person cannot get it themselves.) Those who handle these frustrations without yelling, threatening, pounding a table with their fist or showing their exasperation to any marked degree, will do much better than people who engage in these behaviors which collectively are spoken of as "anti-social".

If you have a family member who is locked up in a mental hospital, and they ask you for a stamp, have the kindness to get it to them as soon as you can. In fact, having a bunch of stamps or, if you have access to their living quarters and they can tell you where they keep their stamps, just taking them the stamps they have can be extremely helpful, as can bringing any other common household items. It can be extremely difficult, for example, in a state hospital, to get some deodorant, and there are definite social consequences to not using one and so being stinky. This is something for which an outside friend or family member can be very helpful.

Now back to motivation. I think the best thing to do is to ask patients how they're doing. If they seem preoccupied with depression or anxiety or hallucinations or delusions or some other mental health problem, then perhaps harping on their apparent lack of motivation is not a good idea. But if they seem to have settled into where they are, then a few questions such as "Where do you expect to be, come Christmas time?" (if it is summer) or "Where do you expect to be by summertime?" (if it is winter) may be appropriate. If the person says "Well I don't know, but I sure would like to have left here by then" or something similar, the next question is "What do you think is still keeping you here?" If the patient can identify a specific behavior which is less than optimal, then perhaps check with the staff and see if that is the behavior which is the limiting factor. Patients can sometimes forget to tell you about the screaming match they had with the staff member that morning, if they feel justified in what they said. If that is the case, the thing to do is to sit down with the staff and sort out what happened, sort out how you can help the patient. This might be best done without the patient, if the patient is very fragile or very apt to get angry easily. If not, if you think the patient can take the conversation, it might be very instructive for him or her to hear it.

If the patient can't answer you as to why they are here, but does evince some desire to be elsewhere, then I find it useful to ask them what about their behavior or their presentation signals to staff members (who do not know what is going on inside their heads) that they need to be in the hospital. Perhaps it should be directly said that thinking about where the person wants to be in a few months is not appropriate when they have just been admitted to the hospital. Let them get settled into their new environment and let them begin to get over the mental experiences (which are usually painful) that got them there in the first place. Only when their internal temperature becomes calmer is it wise to ask questions about their future.

Much of the rest of this chapter is addressed to a friend or family member or volunteer who would like to help the patient. Please be aware that the state hospital system is geared to get somebody well enough to go back to jail, or geared to get somebody placed in a mental health group home, but is not particularly geared (and I'm very sorry to say this) to work with people so that they will get out of the hospital as _fast_ as possible. (Hospitals in the private sector, on the other hand, are geared to discharge as per insurance when the patient _seems_ better, whether or not they really are ready to go.) Nor is the system particularly geared to getting patients back to school, to a job, or to what most of us would consider a functional, if imperfect, life. The mental health system is geared to perpetuating the mental health system, and to do that it will hold people back rather than taking a chance and promoting someone to life out of the hospital, let alone to an independent life out of the hospital, or at least one with some elements of independence, let alone to the life that the patient really wants. This is not to be viewed as an evil design on the part of individual mental health workers – it is simply what happens with every bureaucracy – the bureaucracy perpetuates itself, and may be more concerned with itself than with anyone involved in it, be it worker, consumer, or family.

Personally, I did not have any family members who did much to advocate for me. My mother did at times, as for example when she sat for a day and a half in Professor Guillemot's office and got him to take me as his patient. But my mother was frequently not around when outside intervention would have been very useful. I can tell you that except for the first few days after most of my admissions, I would begin to advocate for myself. This went to subtleties such as learning the names of the staff, since most people will pay attention if addressed by name. I would work as hard as I could to get the privileges, first to go off the ward in a group, then to go off the grounds in a group, then to go off the ward on the grounds alone, and finally to go off the ward and off the grounds alone. I can tell you that it is extremely difficult to advance in such a way that the progress is noted from the inside of a mental hospital, and so a family member or friend who can visit them with some regularity and take an interest in their progress, asking staff if the patient is ready for the next step, is very helpful.

Now as to some strategies to help less motivated people become more so. First of all, if the person wants something – be it increased privileges to go somewhere, increased visiting time, extra ice cream at dinner (provided they are not diabetic) if the client or patient wants something, you can make a bargain with them. Be explicit about such things as how much and by what time they must do something to earn, shall we say, that extra half hour outside. Be explicit, but not too rigid; always think about what it would be like if you have to tell them they have failed their part of the bargain because, shall we say, you have said that they needed to get something done by five p.m. and they run after you as you are leaving at 5:10 to say they just finished it.

Do you really want to tell them they didn't meet their part of the bargain because they are ten minutes late? On the other hand do you really want to come over as a softie, a pushover who doesn't realize they are late? Be careful how you phrase this. My favorite tactic on something like that is to say it has to be done by four, knowing I will be in the building until five, and then if it happens to be 4:10 I can say "Well, you are ten minutes late, but I will let you have it anyway." If you are going to do something in return, then get the order book or get out your appointment book or do whatever you need to do to register with them, at that moment, that they're going to have what they bargained for.

You are trying to build a relationship with this person and you cannot expect a mental patient to trust you if you forget your side of the bargain, nor can the mental patient be expected to understand the thousand and one things crowding in on your mind. If you go as a volunteer to visit a mental patient, and they do something which you have agreed earns them some extra privilege for the next visit, make sure you write it down in your appointment book while they are sitting there. This reassures them that you take them seriously, and it also is likely that you will remember, or that if you forget they can point it out to you, and seeing an entry in your own handwriting about it in your appointment book, you will then remember.

Don't ever promise one stamp and then forget it. The patient is desperate for that one stamp, and your casual forgetting is a betrayal to them. You promised! Now their rent check will be late and they may be evicted!

There is no excuse as a mental health provider, family member, friend, compeer, or whatever, for not paying attention. There just is not any excuse. If you have some family emergency which you need to pay attention to, then you should explain that to your mental health client and tell them you will get back to them as soon as possible after the resolution of your emergency, giving, if you can, some estimate of when that might be.

I personally was an attending for about thirty patients in the New York State sex offender treatment program (this is the post-incarceration program in which it is attempted to teach these offenders before they go back on the street some more desirable habits of behavior). I do not propose to discuss in this volume whether it is possible to teach a recidivist sex offender better behavior, nor the legal ramifications of holding a sex offender against his will in a treatment program when he has already fulfilled his term of incarceration for his previous crimes. What I do want to talk about is something about how to get the respect and collaboration of these people (assuredly, a very difficult population to work with).

I had told Mr. Tobias, (not his real name) one of the patients, that I would see him the next day. But when the next day rolled around, some patients on another floor were getting into a physical scuffle and it was my responsibility to end the scuffle, see to it that any injuries were taken care of, and review each participant's behavior with an eye toward not having it repeated. Therefore, I did not get to see Mr. Tobias that morning. In the afternoon, we had an urgency in the admissions, which we handled by rotation, and I was responsible for that as well. So, once again I did not get to see Mr. Tobias.

So, as I was walking down from my usual floor past Mr. Tobias' floor, I stopped off and asked to see him and admitted that I had failed to see him that morning and that afternoon. I apologized and said that after rounds and some other formalities, he would be the first patient I would be looking for the following morning.

Mr. Tobias was quite overcome; he said, "A doctor is apologizing to me?!" Mr. Tobias, though we may not feel much respect for his multiple criminal offenses, is a human being, and as a human being is entitled to be treated respectfully and well. I take what I say I will do very seriously, and if I do not fulfill what I said I would do, I consider that I owe the other party an apology, and every reasonable effort to rectify the situation.

When I was a patient (though I have never done anything criminal in my life) it was very disheartening to me when a doctor, for example, promised me a change in medication dose, or a pass, and did not get around to writing the order for it by day's end. Also, I learned a certain distrust of physicians who would promise to "see you tomorrow" and think nothing of not seeing you for a couple of days. It certainly puts a person in their place – you realize you are not the one with any power in this situation – but it also leads to a fine disregard for not only that individual, but others of a similar rank, and eventually for the whole mental health system.

Such behavior has no place when you are trying to help an unmotivated client become motivated. They will very quickly get the idea that you don't care, and so they don't care either. And, actions do speak louder than words in these situations.

I would suggest; 1) promise less than you think you can deliver; 2) keep a careful record of your promises and your bargains; and 3) keep the parameters of what you had promised clear and easy for you and the client to understand. Do not let yourself get caught in the ambiguity of what you had said. For example, if you are seeing a patient in your office, do not say "I will give you a pass starting at two o'clock and you are to be back here at four o'clock." What you mean, I think, is that the patient may leave at two o'clock and is to be back <u>on the unit</u> by four o'clock." Otherwise, the patient may interpret 'be back here' as meaning 'be back on the grounds somewhere'.

If in talking with the patient you are not able to find anything that they want (and don't forget to ask, if they look listless and disinterested, things like "Where would you like to be right now?" Or "What would you like to be doing right now?" And let people dream of the impossible. Let them say they wished they hadn't smoked pot the other night or whatever unreality they want to express without immediately chiding them for indulging in unreality. I have seen clients say "I wish I hadn't smoked the pot which made me strip off and jump into the fountain" only to have the mental health worker say "Well, but you did, didn't you?" so that the person can't even express regret without getting an instant reprimand.

But if in spite of these maneuvers you are unable to elicit any direct answer from the patient, then you can say "Well, why don't we just sit here awhile. Please realize that I have to go at four o'clock." And then at ten minutes to four you say, "Well, I guess that about wraps it up for today. Would you like to go somewhere or do something next time?" And leave them with something to think about.

Of course, this means that you have to be comfortable in sitting in silence, doing nothing, with your client. If such an experience makes you uncomfortable or would make you uncomfortable, then may I suggest picking a quiet time including before you get undressed to go to bed or before you get into bed, to sit in silence by yourself doing nothing. At first, you may not be able to tolerate more than a few minutes. By the time you can sit twenty minutes or more in absolute silence, with no music on, no TV, no schedule to look at, just <u>being</u> in silence with yourself, then I think you are beginning to get one of the skills that you do need, to be working with a mental health client.

The reason it's important to be able to sit in silence is that it is important to be able to at once call their bluff when they say they really don't want to do anything, and to let the client realize how much autonomy and how much control he does have of the situation. If he doesn't want to go anywhere, then you aren't going to force him. Don't forget to bring up the possibility of going somewhere on the following visit. Sooner or later, he will take you up on your offer, and express a desire to go. That is golden.

It is also a golden lesson for most mental health clients to realize that even though they are sitting in their room doing nothing and saying nothing, a person who has volunteered to help them does not resent them, but stays by their side. There are no beautiful words and mission statements and statements of intent that will be the equivalent of saying in effect to the person "You and you alone are worth my time – whether or not we go anywhere, do anything, or even have anything to say to each other – you alone are worthy of my coming here." If on the following visit the client still doesn't want to go anywhere or say anything, put in the time; I can almost guarantee you that after five or six weekly visits of sitting in their room saying nothing the client will say "Mrs. X, it's awfully nice of you to come here, but this is awfully boring. Couldn't we do something?" or words to that effect. It's just that it takes some clients longer to get to the point where the boredom factor is prominent. And it may be a lesson to you, as a middle class busy person, how difficult it is for you to sit with someone in silence, doing nothing. <u>Doing</u> nothing, but <u>being</u> with that person.

If the client says at a certain point "I am thirsty" this is an expression of a need or want, so, as with any other expression of a need or want, you can say "Why don't we go down to the kitchen together and see what is in the fridge?" – and so you have gotten them out of their room.

But peppering the client with constant questions about "Why don't you get washed up?" "Why don't you get dressed? Where do you want to go? Oh come on – surely you want to see something, it's been three weeks already, and you don't do anything at all when I come here." This is not helpful. This is you expressing your frustrations and you're not volunteering in order to express your frustrations. The client is not there to meet your needs. You are there to meet the client's needs.

Another question of motivation is what happens when the patient's behavior is somewhat controlled, so that he could move out of the hospital to a group home and possibly to a part time job. Now the objective is to keep that person interested enough to a) stay on their medication and b) put into play those basic social skills (such as walking away when upset rather than screaming or throwing things), which they demonstrated they could use before leaving the hospital. Keeping the patient on their medication can be difficult, which is why we have depot injections such that one injection every two to four <u>weeks</u> can be enough to keep them sane. Most people do not like to admit they need to keep taking their medicine, so these folks, even with a case manager to drive them to the clinic, will "disappear" on the morning they are supposed to go. If the patient can see the group home and part time job as a stepping stone in a progression to earn greater independence <u>which</u> <u>they</u> <u>want</u>, they may stick with the program. But the mental health system, having placed someone in a home, is very reluctant to encourage them to think of progressing beyond that (it's a lot of work which might prove pointless if the patient does not succeed.) Psychiatry, as a specialty, encourages change, yet the psychiatric bureaucracy is unwilling to take a risk to give a patient a chance, and many psychiatrists are lazy, unwilling to think outside of the box, unwilling to let the patient try something new. This is why caring family can be so important.

Now I'm going to tell stories of what happened to me in the cases where I did not understand and apply the material in the last two chapters. First, I will admit that as a physician I once neglected to write a weekend pass for a patient. The doctor on call wrote the pass at the behest of the nurses, the family was willing to wait, and I'm very relieved to say the family waited only approximately ten minutes. This is just to say that I was not always above forgetting things myself, though I tried hard not to.

My patient story is about being granted a pass (meaning the doctor agreed to it, but did not write the order when he did so) to go with my friend Jeanne out from the state hospital to spend the night in her house and come back the next day. Overnight passes have become rather rare since, since insurance companies, including Medicaid and Medicare, have taken the stance that being able to go on an overnight pass means that the patient is ready for discharge. Overnight passes are still permitted from state hospitals, for patients to try out a placement in a group home. Just before they are discharged, they may be sent two or three times out overnight or over a weekend to "visit" the group home, to make sure they could cope with it. This is because these patients may have been hospitalized for months or years, and the adjustment that is asked of them to live in these communities may be considerable.

Let me get back to my story. Jeanne came when she was expected at four-thirty p.m. But the ward attending had left for the day, and had not written my pass, which had been agreed to at about eight o'clock that morning. The same head nurse was on duty who had been in the meeting at which the pass was agreed to, and I asked her to get hold of the doctor on call. I knew very well that if I spoke to him, he would not believe me if I said I had a pass. But she knew I did. The problem was that the doctor on call had a string of three medical emergencies to deal with before he could get to writing my pass. I remember having dinner in the mental hospital, and after dinner Jeanne said to me that she might as well go, since we weren't leaving today. I said to her then as I had said before "It's just a matter of waiting it out. I will get that pass and I will come out with you."

At about a quarter of nine I did get the pass and I did go out with my friend. Unfortunately, because it was late, we did not have the nice friendly evening together we had been thinking we would, but I did get my night out of the state loony bin, and I did come back the next day on time. It was a very strange feeling that I had while we were waiting because of course one has to be patient with the staff; (pacing, swearing or other signs of impatience would register with the staff that I was not ready to leave the hospital, even for a few hours). I have seen many patients have a privilege granted to them, then be asked to tolerate a delay when they are due to receive it, and because they cannot tolerate the delay, the privilege is cancelled. I used to say facetiously that mental patients are not allowed frustration – at least they are not allowed to show it. I also felt very odd in that my friend Jeanne was having more trouble waiting than I was, or so it seemed, though she was in my room with me. I had to continually reassure her that we would win if we just bided our time and hung on. I did ask a few times during all those hours, and I did have the head nurse call the doctor on call a couple of times and remind him that we were still waiting for the pass. Finally, we did get it and we did go.

I cannot pretend to such a happy outcome when I was in another hospital in New York City. The doctor had some news for me which he was anxious to give me, and so he pulled apart the opaque cloth curtain that I had pulled all around the bed because I was getting dressed. I remonstrated with him that he should not come into a lady's quarters when she is in a state of undress; he replied with perfect indifference to the feelings of the one who was mentally ill in this situation, that he didn't mind seeing a naked patient, he'd seen naked women before. I pointed out that I did mind, since his seeing me naked was in this instance an infringement upon my dignity. I also pointed out that though I thanked him for his news, he could have left me a written message at the nursing station. I finished with a rather haughty and not very kind reference to his indifference to the feelings of his patient. I don't know if he learned anything from the incident; I do know he never broke in upon me as I was dressing again.

The zeal of providers, their effort to whole heartedly, sincerely and repeatedly hold forth the possibility of major change to <u>every</u> patient, without prejudging who is "ready" to change, is extremely important. When dozens of people have said or have silently communicated their conviction that meaningful change in your case will never happen, it is only human for most people to react with a lack of motivation. So, we professionals need to clean up our act, big time. Then we may find the patients improve more than most of us had thought possible.

I'm going to close this chapter on motivation with a true story that occurred when I was working in a state hospital in New York State. It was about the middle of December, and I was going through the list of patients' names with staff to decide who would get what privileges for going home to their families to celebrate Christmas. There were three patients who had been there for fifteen years or more whose recent behavior had been not good (in terms of refusing to cooperate with the schedule, yelling and screaming for no good reason, slamming doors etc. – poor behavior, but nothing really dangerous). The staff told me that these three patients should not be allowed out over Christmas, even though all three of them had a personal tradition going back many years of going to visit their families for the holidays.

I came up with a different idea. I said I would write the passes, and tell the patients that whether or not they would be let out according to the conditions set forth in the pass would depend upon their behavior between now and December 24. (Christmas passes usually had patients picked up on the 24th during the day, and returning on the 26th). The staff were very reluctant to allow me to do this, since they thought that past behavior should already cause a forfeit. But we all know patients' memories are of short duration, and to penalize them in the future for something that occurred two or three weeks ago doesn't make sense. It doesn't lead to behavior change.

I told each patient that whether or not they went home for Christmas would depend entirely on their behavior between that date (which was about December 12$^{th)}$ and the 24th. I confess I wanted them to succeed, so I would remind them periodically and I remember stopping a physical fight between two patients because I said to the one who was one of those three that if he threw a punch now, he should say good-bye to a Christmas at home, whereas if he walked away he could still go home on Christmas Eve. Luckily for me, he heard me and chose to walk away.

All three of them "earned" their Christmas leave. I'm not too sure whether this impressed the staff very much, because of course after Christmas we did not have anything as attractive to hold out as a possibility if they behaved well, and they reverted to a large extent to their poor behavior. But to me, this proved my point that most people, even people who were quite obviously mentally ill, can choose the consequences that they would enjoy and control themselves in function of what possibilities showing self-control would offer them. Oftentimes we don't have something we can use to give a person an incentive to be cooperative. I choose to call this giving them incentive, rather than 'bribe' because it operates very much like an incentive. I was not asking them to do something they should not do, which is what bribery is about. The incentive must be attractive and must be important enough and close enough in the future to be meaningful. You couldn't use the idea of going home for Christmas as an incentive in the beginning of November; it would simply be too far away.

But for me at least, the fact that all three earned their Christmas passes meant that most people can choose among a set of consequences which one they want. Note that as a staff member, my getting exasperated with them would serve no purpose at all, neither for me nor for them. I think a lot of the staff of state hospitals in many places need to work on having more patience and having a longer fuse. They keep expecting severely ill patients to have the same memory of what they were told this morning or yesterday or last week that a person with normal thought processes have, to their downfall. I was proud of my three patients, and they all enjoyed their Christmas at home very much.

CHAPTER 17

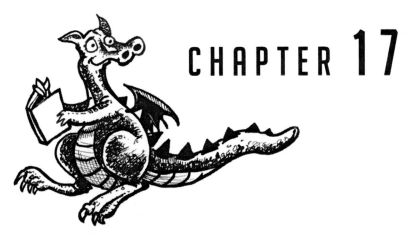

EFFORT IS NECESSARY FOR A FULL LIFE

Effort is, in my considered opinion, as necessary for a full and satisfying life as is anything else, including food, water, shelter, adequate temperature and sufficient clothing. I know this is not perhaps the usual method of looking at it, but I have seen the spiritual and psychological rot that sets in when a person is not attempting to accomplish anything from close range many times. This spiritual and psychological state of ill health can arise because a person has given up hope and is being warehoused in a psychiatric facility or a prison and has lost all interest in interacting with the environment because the environment is impoverished. It can also occur when the person has a surfeit of wealth, and could have anything they want, so, presuming they could have it easily, they want nothing. I will readily admit that this is not what usually happens to people who fall into an environment that is either too poor or too wealthy to offer them what they need. But it happens often enough, especially among long-term psychiatric patients, so I want to talk about it.

I would not want the reader to imagine that this is only the lot of very chronically ill people who have been too sick for too long a time to respond to normal motivation. It does happen in that setting; I have seen it also as the result of what happens in our well-meaning welfare state. A person who does not have great depth of soul is declared permanently disabled and given a subsistence by the state. And it takes a very short time for that person merely to be marking time and waiting for Godot, attempting nothing.

To put it succinctly, a person should be endeavoring to do something. That something can be as various as people are. It can be increasing the time that the person is able to ride a bucking bronco without falling off, improving a routine as a circus clown, improving the ability to draw a likeness in a few deft strokes on the sidewalk, improving the ability to draw a likeness such that, shrunk down to the size of a postage stamp, it is still visually eye-catching; it can be any number of things.

I wouldn't want the reader to imagine that I think every person should be strapped into a lock-step job which does generate a minimum wage paycheck but is of no interest to the person, and that their longevity in that job is their accomplishment. Some people may be locked into a boring job, and their longevity in that job <u>is</u> an accomplishment – but the accomplishment is key for bringing up their kids, or sustaining a spouse while the spouse got further training, supporting aging parents, supporting the grandchildren, or otherwise contributing to the stability and the welfare of another human being. In such a case, the person's achievement is, that they contributed to the welfare of someone else for a number of years. And that is a fine and beautiful thing.

What I really want people to understand is that if, because of medical disability, unmistakably genuine, or perhaps just a little finagled, they stop having a goal, stop having an objective when they get up in the morning, stop having a hope that maybe today they can be better at whatever it is than they were yesterday – people in this situation are really in trouble for the spiritual and psychological decay that I referred to above. They may fall victim to chronic pain because the mind, stripped of a legitimate objective, will focus on other difficulties and make <u>them</u> into a significant obstacle which would justify their having no interest in getting up to face the day.

I once knew a lady who inherited a house with an extensive front yard. At first, she cursed her luck because she really hated taking care of the grass and bushes in the front yard. Then she had an idea. She decided to plant flowers there, and she made the flower beds function in such a way that as one flowering plant came into bloom and then passed its prime, another came into prominence, and so she had flowers which went from the earliest part of the growing season until the very end. She also made sure that the plants which remained in winter looked attractive, variegated and interesting. At first, her neighbors were a bit askance at the ambition of her plans as a gardener. Then she began to have a bit of a reputation. People would walk a few blocks out of their way to pass by her place. Her summit of achievement occurred when a local guide book mentioned that it was worth a twenty mile detour from the local highway to pass by her gardens.

She never thought of making her garden beautiful for the sake of other people who might pass by or who might detour in order to pass by. She was thinking only of making a beautiful garden, since life had given her a garden. But, as she neared the end of her life, people would come by her garden to see it and then contribute a dollar each to perpetuate the garden and to support the local food bank. Her contribution became one of the mainstays of a thriving food bank, and that is how she left this world. She also taught a number of young people how to garden, and they enjoyed it, and she donated her house, when she died, to the town, with money to perpetuate the garden if people could be found to do it. People were found, and so for quite a few years after her death the gardens continued to be lovely.

And this was from a lady who, remember, used to curse because the house she inherited had a large front yard. She started out planting flowers because she enjoyed that, though she did not enjoy mowing lawns and keeping the grass from encroaching on the bushes. She said to me, when she was my patient briefly because a young nephew was killed and she suffered over the senselessness of his death, that she had started out thinking of the garden as needing restraining, and then came to appreciate the growing possibilities and the flowering of the shrubs and wanted to help them show themselves to their best. And it wasn't that she had anyone stopping the people as they went by her house to collect the dollar, it just became the done thing; and everybody contributed because they felt the flowers were so lovely that they wanted to help out and join in the fun of being among life's helpers.

The reason I'm telling this story now is that it would have been impossible if the lady had stopped at "I inherited the front lawn, I don't like to have to keep it up, I don't want the effort." Because she was able to redefine the effort she put in the garden as not, as she said "restraining life and cutting it back and telling it to keep in its place" but "helping it to flourish and bloom and be beautiful." It took on new meaning for her and the meaning benefited her and countless people who saw it, as well as the recipients of the food bank and the town in general.

This is an extraordinary example, but I do believe that everyone has a choice to make between refusing to make any effort at all, putting forth effort reluctantly, or finding a way of seeing the situation that they can put their heart into, and their passion, and do something lovely. And, of course, we join the forces of creation when we are doing something lovely.

I've had patients who were street people and street musicians; I had one patient who managed, with the help of his Congressman, to sell one of his small pictures (he was always doodling, and always in miniature) to the Post Office. I'm not sure that this changed his life very much, because he defined it in his own mind as a 'fluke' that such a nonentity as himself would have hundreds of thousands of his image reproduced on a stamp, but that's because that's how he chose to interpret it.

I had another patient who drew pictures on the sidewalk in chalk. He was not the least upset that within an hour they were much faded, and were almost completely gone in two hours. He drew them on the sidewalk in Philadelphia where many people would see them, and that was his recompense. And he drew in a district of heavy foot traffic where he thought "at least for a few seconds I make people think of something outside themselves, and think of something lovely". This was his mission, and he was happy to do it. The idea that there was no permanent record of his work bothered him not in the slightest because, as he said "nothing is truly permanent on this earth".

The people I feel sorry for are those who, if they get sidelined such that no one is expecting them to do anything, slip into a sort of death- in-life and don't engage in life. People who have slipped out of a very productive life may take a while to regroup and redefine themselves. But there are those who never do redefine themselves and never do regroup, and these are the people that stare at nothing and that are not animated by any desires or any willingness to make an effort that might enhance their interactions with others.

I think the psychiatric professions (I say professions because I include psychology, nursing and social work with psychiatry in this) have contributed to this, because many practitioners think for example in the case of a patient who was hallucinating wild, destructive hallucinations, that if the patient is now calmer, not hallucinating, and not destructive, that their job as professionals is done.

I would submit to them that a professional's job is not done until the patient is turned back on to live a life. This may well not be a life which requires a calendar with engagements written on it or a social secretary, but it should be a life nonetheless, in which there is some effort being made to try to change themselves or the environment for the better from the point of view of someone.

If all seven billion of us were able to contribute a little bit toward improving the world, the world would become a much better place, and no one, while they are drawing breath on this earth, has the right (in my point of view) to totally forget that they are part of the human family and that we need all the members of our family to be as functional as they can possibly be. Not to mention that people who have spent a long time tuned out of life in this fashion have a very high rate of depression; disconnection is the worst thing that can happen to anyone who is still alive.

So, we in the helping professions must try as hard as we can to reconnect people, to help them find something that has meaning to them so that they can contribute to the fabric of all of us, and be happier doing so. Effort, in my view, is as necessary to living a full life as anything else you could mention.

Some parents and siblings of young people struck by a mental illness may go overboard in an attempt to be kind and considerate. Schizophrenia is an illness that has its highest likelihood of onset in the mid-teen, late teen, and early adult years. This has several consequences, not the least of which is the fact that the schizophrenic patient may not have arrived at full maturity in terms of being able to make stable choices, to choose wisely among different options, to have a good sense of what is important, and to be reliable as the adult world expects a person to be reliable.

For instance, the patient may go on to their mid-twenties, thirties, or forties, and still not have developed an adult work ethic, or the ability to count backwards from an appointment time to figure out when to get up ("I have to be there at 10, it takes 45 minutes on the bus and 15 minutes to get to the bus stop, so I need to get out before 9, (say 8:45) and it takes me

1 ½ hours to get up, shower, have breakfast, dress – so I need to be up by 7:15 a.m.") This may not be because they are lazy; or it may be that when they first became ill at the age of fifteen, they had a teenager's perspective on the importance of work. Or a teenager's apparent inability to focus and get going in the morning.

Parents, siblings, or providers who have no positive expectations of the patient, including that he or she should learn an adult work ethic, are not doing the patient any favors. I'm not speaking of times when the patient is obviously floridly psychotic, hallucinating, doing bizarre things. I am assuming the patient has had enough medication aboard and enough time for it to be effective, and enough therapy that they can behave quite acceptably.

The family has an immense impact here if they choose to. They should not expect a person with a major mental illness to keep even with their contemporaries in terms of the speed at which they learn, but there should be some positive expectation that they will learn and that they will get to understand what constitutes adult behavior.

Teaching people by showing them consequences is what I think is best. I tell my schizophrenic patients point blank that every episode of schizophrenia (I mean an acute episode in which they are hallucinating, behaving wildly, etc.) will cost them a few IQ points because an acute episode of illness seems to be toxic to the brain. I tell them that after several such episodes they will begin to lose some of their intelligence. If they are in an in-patient service, or if they have been in an in-patient service in the past, I remind them that they may have seen some old codgers who were not very bright who had the burnt-out kind of schizophrenia. I explain, that's what happens to people when they don't pay attention to their medication regimen, and repeatedly have breakthrough acute episodes of psychosis. I then emphasize to the patient that they way to avoid being old before their time is to a) take their medication and b) complain constructively about any side effects they may experience to their provider.

My point here is that a good life may come for those who put in the effort. Doing nothing when you wake up in the morning day after day (not just a few days on vacation) never got anybody anything interesting in life. This is something that wealthy people do not always understand. They think that if they don't need to make more money, then they should be partying and relaxing continually, that it is fine to spend their entire lives in vacation mode. In my view, such people miss out. When they get old, they have nothing meaningful to remember as their contribution to the world's solutions.

Families who allow their mentally ill members to go through life without any striving, (and I mean striving beyond the basics that we all have to do just to go on living which are called "Activities of Daily Living" or ADLs -- keeping your body and clothes clean, getting and preparing food to eat, and cleaning up -- people should be expected to do that, or to learn to do that), are fostering having family members who miss much of life's satisfaction. Again if a person fell ill at the age of fifteen, they may have been in a rebellious frame of mind in which they didn't do their own laundry and they didn't clean up their own room. However, this is not an excuse for them to be perpetually dependent on someone else to do the basics. They can learn to clean up after themselves just like other people can. At least, I think that is the attitude to take. If the attitude of those around them is that they cannot learn and they will never do anything meaningful, this is stifling to any hopes they may have of making a contribution and having a life with meaning.

Parents who go to their children's apartments and clean them up FOR them are not really doing a good thing for their offspring. What they should do is clean the place up WITH them, so that the younger generation learns how to do it for themselves, and then have them clean up with progressively less supervision.

I know this can be extremely difficult and exasperating. I also am aware that the parent may still be grieving over the fact that their wonderful and much loved son or daughter now has a major mental illness. But to hasten to do everything for the patient so as to be able to forget that the patient needed help, is not a good thing.

Show the young person how to do it, and tell them that you are showing them so that they will learn. Build into your activity the idea that you are not going to be doing this forever. Remember to praise what patients do, even if it isn't perfect. Think about their progress, not about how much further they need to go.

It is often a question when a person develops schizophrenia or for that matter bipolar disorder or major depression what kind of help they should receive and what should be expected of them. What I am encouraging people to expect is a learning curve, even though it may not be as steep as it would for a normal young person. Also, if it is at all possible, I like to see young people who have had a nervous breakdown in the middle of a course of study, be that high school, a community college, a four year college or whatever, resume their studies, if at a slower pace.

There is no question that it is much harder to go to class, take notes, study and write papers, take examinations, and so forth if you have a major mental illness than if you do not. But there ought to be more frequently an attempt to find something between going back to school at the same pace as people who do not have a mental illness, and giving up school altogether. It makes a person sad to have to slow down their curriculum and therefore be unable to graduate with the rest of their class, that is true. But there is a special feeling of wondrous achievement when the person who has had to slow down does complete their degree requirements and take their degree. To have been affected by the mental illness is hardly surprising; what I am advocating for, is the idea that being affected does not mean giving up.

I personally lost many years in pursuing my professional goal of becoming a physician because of my mental illness. I was originally slated to graduate in May 1974; I graduated from medical school overseas in January 1981. Because I had great difficulty dealing with the hundred hour work week killer schedule that we in the United States seem to find necessary for young doctors, it was not until January 1997, sixteen years later, that I had finished my psychiatry residency.

Along the way I got two other masters degrees and another doctorate, an applied doctorate in public health. So I was still working on climbing that mountain, it's just that I had to take a very roundabout route, climbing very slowly, but I did reach the summit eventually – the end of clinical training and the ability to work in clinical psychiatry as a physician.

As I have said before, we tend to give up on ourselves and on others much too easily if we are not able to complete a course of study or training in standard fashion. Yet if we persist, a way may be found so that goals can be reached.

There were many times during my training when I felt I just couldn't do what I had in front of me in terms of, say, four examinations in six days or something like that. I prayed hard and dove straight into the next task.

As a good friend of mine says, "Just do the next thing" -- meaning don't think about whether you can or you can't, just get started and keep going on whatever you know you must do.

I am very glad that I did finish what I set out to do. I didn't set out to become specifically a psychiatrist, psychiatry found me. I know I would never be able to do what I call with only a little exaggeration the "forty hour shift" again. This is waking up and starting shall we say on a Monday morning at seven a.m. going through all day Monday, all night Monday night, all day Tuesday, and finishing Tuesday evening perhaps eight or nine o'clock at night. I could not do that again, and I'm very glad that I no longer have to. At the time, it nearly killed me. It is very difficult to hang on when you have a mental illness and you are horrendously sleep deprived. I would not recommend it to anyone else. But at the time, the Horsemen of the Apocalypse themselves could not have dissuaded me from the course I had set myself, and I did feel a kind of eerie elation when I had finished it all. It was eerie, because so many of the people who told me that I could never achieve what I wanted were dead and buried. It was spooky too, because very few people that I knew then had known me long enough to realize that this was the achievement of my number one lifelong dream.

I am now going to tell the story of how, as I put it above, psychiatry found me. On Easter Sunday, 1987, I found myself in a horribly manic state and convinced a friend to take me to the local emergency room. At that time, there was no separate psychiatric emergency room; psychiatric patients were mixed in with the people with heart attacks, gunshot wounds, or whatever. I did not have the sense to take some extra medication before I left my lodgings. I should have realized that it would be hours before I was given anything.

I believe I have said before in this book that a person with a heart attack, a gunshot wound, or other obvious physical emergency, is treated as soon as they get to the hospital, whereas treatment is denied to psychiatric patients on the grounds that "they will get treated wherever they go" (meaning that they are unlikely to be hospitalized here and will be sent to another hospital, so let them be treated there). This is illogical, nonsensical, uncaring and I would say inhuman. It is a practice that should be stopped.

I walked into the emergency room and gave all my details (name, address, telephone number, etc.) and told the doctors that I had bipolar disorder and was manic – as if that were not obvious. I also told them the name of my outpatient doctor. I asked them for some medication since mania can be very painful. But even though I walked in on the stroke of noon, I had to wait until after twenty minutes to nine at night, when I finally got to the state hospital, and was seen by the admitting doctor, to get any medication – any treatment – at all.

The psychiatrist in charge of the psychiatric cases in the emergency room told me before I left the emergency room that "you are a disposition problem". I wonder how many other people he said that to, not that they had problems, but that they were a problem. A patient is not a problem, a patient may pose a difficulty for the staff. The difficulty they had with me was that my private sector doctor was trying to get me hospitalized where he had admitting privileges, but my insurance would not approve, so my case was refused.

Finally, I got to the State Hospital at around dinner time, and after waiting several hours, I did see the admitting doctor there who wrote some medication orders. I was told that the medication had been ordered, but that it was after hours, so I would not get any treatment until the next morning.

No person with a heart attack would ever be told that treatment was unavailable until the next morning, nor would a diabetic ever be told that they could not have insulin right away. At the time, I was so much in pain from my illness that I literally got down on my knees and begged a nurse there to get me some medication that night. This was at something after eight o'clock. She did manage to get somebody to go down to the pharmacy and get me the medication I needed, and I was finally given it at twenty minutes to nine. So, having walked into an emergency room at noon obviously in need of treatment, a person whose diagnosis left no doubt, I finally got some treatment at eight-forty p.m., nearly nine hours later.

Things may have improved somewhat since then, but old habits die hard and many times when I was a psychiatric attending myself, I noticed that while people negotiate which hospital they are going to go to that will be accepted by their insurance, and by what conveyance they are to get there (for long distance rides it may take an ambulance a while to be available) the last thing that people are actually thinking about is the welfare of the poor human being in question – the patient.

I lived in the State Hospital as a patient for six months exactly, though after only a few days there I got a daily pass to be able to walk to the University which was just down the street about a quarter of an hour on foot, and work on my Master's thesis. For a year after discharge, I lived in very meager accommodations on South Avenue and earned a bare living doing market research, though I was paid more than others because I was able to call some VIPs in the scientific world and get the opinion of the head honcho himself. Nonetheless, it was a hand-to-mouth existence.

Then I went to New Orleans in the late summer of 1988, with all I possessed in two suitcases and about four hundred dollars in cash on me. I had been accepted into Tulane University's Doctor of Public Health program, and I left without a real address to go to (I stayed in university-owned housing for a short while until I found my own place which was nearly an hour out of the city in a housing development in Metairie, a working-class neighborhood.)

Just before I left New York State, I was contacted by attorneys who were handling the estate of my father's older brother. Uncle Ward had just died and had left my sister and I, as we were his only living relatives, a bequest of $20,000 each. Uncle Ward left the bulk of his vast fortune to a dog and cat hospital, which, since he had never had children, he had always been planning to do, and I suppose some people would have worked up a resentment that they were not to inherit more than a crumb. But to me, the $20,000 bequest came just at the right time, because I had been exercised in my mind for some months about how I was going to pay off some $10,000 in debt on the defaulted student loan from my medical school. The loan had defaulted when I lost my internship and I wrote the lender asking for a hardship deferment on the grounds of having been taken off the payroll, the lender checked with the official in the hospital, and since she had not been told of my losing my internship, she said that I was still an intern. The lender then sent me a letter which literally began "You are a liar and a cheat." I thought at the time that I could take them to court, but I was so demoralized that I didn't know what to do. Of course, it never occurred to the lender to question the hospital official, and apparently the person who wrote the letter had never heard of writing a refusal for hardship deferment by saying "Dear Dr. Clark, we are unable to grant your request because it is our understanding that you are still an intern."

So my uncle's bequest came at just a wonderful time to solve that problem. I had asked the Lord many times in my prayers what I should do about the defaulted loan because obviously I would not be leant student loan money again (to pay for the Tulane doctoral program) if I did not make good on the prior loan. All I got in reply was "Don't worry, I'll take care of it." I'm just telling my readers, if you get as the answer to a prayer something which says the Lord will take care of it, realize that He means what He says.

For the first year in Louisiana I lived on my uncle's bequest. Then I applied for a license to practice in Louisiana, and how I got that is a story in itself. Then I asked my local psychiatrist, who was actually a child psychiatrist trained in Boston, if he knew of anywhere that I might get a job to help make ends meet. He told me he had just left the employ of the State of Louisiana, because when he did not have the parents' consent, he took a child patient out into the parking lot and gave him medication there. Of course that is something he should not have done, in the sense that not having the parents' consent means he did not have the parents' consent. I can empathize with the doctor in that apparently the case was a simple one which would respond very well to medication; but we all have to deal with such instances, and doctors as a group need to become better persuaders to get consent.

He gave me the name of Doctor Arthur Strauss, who was the chief of the Louisiana State Psychiatric Clinic system, and just told me that I should not mention his name to anyone in the state program.

I got home from my doctor's visit and wondered if I should call right away, but I got a little message in my head which said "No, don't call now, lie down to have a rest (which is what I was thinking of doing), and I'll wake you up." So I laid down and fell asleep and awoke rather suddenly about an hour later and the voice inside my head said to me, "Call Dr. Strauss now." I got up to go to the bathroom, but the voice said, "No, call him <u>now</u>" so I dialed the number I had for Dr. Strauss and was very surprised to find that he answered his telephone himself. Almost the first thing he said to me was that he never answers the telephone, but the secretary was out that afternoon and when he heard it ring he felt, "Well why not answer it – after all, it's somebody who wants to talk to me," and he gave me an appointment for a job interview for about a week later.

During that week I found out what had happened recently. Apparently, the Governor of Louisiana had decided to cut the mental health budget, and had slated about half the state clinics for closure to save money. This is not a good thing to have done in Louisiana because in that state, about ninety-seven or ninety-eight percent of mental health services are delivered in the State Clinics – the private sector was miniscule in Louisiana in those days, and I understand it is still small. The clinics due to be closed and the dates for their closure had been chosen, and then a man with paranoid schizophrenia, who felt terrible about the coming closure of his neighborhood clinic, expressed his dismay by shooting three bystanders, killing two and wounding the third severely.

A public outcry followed, and the governor found himself unable to follow through on the order to close the clinics. Therefore, an order stay open was sent out twenty-four hours before these clinics were due to be closed. Needless to say, the staff that worked in those clinics had all found themselves jobs elsewhere. Therefore, the clinics were really hurting for doctors, and so the state was hiring doctors with licenses who had not necessarily even a day's experience working in psychiatry, to staff the clinics.

I was put, as the only psychiatrist in the place when I was there, in the child and adolescent crisis unit. When a properly trained child psychiatrist was found for the position, I was moved across the river to a clinic for adult outpatients.

I worked in the state clinic system from late 1990 until May of 1993, when I graduated with my Doctorate in Public Health and moved to Philadelphia to begin psychiatric residency training.

Let me say that Dr. Strauss took me out to lunch a couple of months after I had begun working in the child and adolescent clinic and said that he came home every day from Baton Rouge (where he had been negotiating that if the clinics were to be kept open, could we have our operating budget back please?) and read through every single one of the cases that I saw.

He said he felt my descriptions were so vivid that he could see the child and the parents. He said he felt I had a real talent for psychiatry, and that he would like to help me get into the training.

Shana Wibberley Clark, M.D., Dr. P.H.

I thought, when I first heard him say it, that he could have knocked me over with a feather. I was so taken aback – and I had to struggle with myself for over a year before I would apply to psychiatry residencies, because the idea of not only being a recipient of mental health care but being a <u>psychiatrist</u> was just overwhelming. I really did not want to be one of <u>them</u>. But over the next year, I persuaded myself that perhaps the best thing I could do with my life was to help out the other patients by getting behind the scenes and figuring out what on earth make psychiatrists tick.

So I say, I didn't find psychiatry – it found me. I will add that when my friends found out that I was applying for a psychiatric residency they were not a bit surprised because they said to me "Shana, you are usually far less interested in the physical disease that someone has, than in how they feel about having that illness – how it changes their perspective on who they think they are, and what they think of their lives." Many people had this reaction, so perhaps in truth I was the last to know. And the fact is, as soon as I had started working in psychiatry, I fell in love with the work.

CHAPTER 18

CONTROLLING YOUR MOODS

I'm going to start on what may seem a discouraging note by stating that bipolar disorder patients, the ones with the most up-and-down feelings and moods anyway, frequently have substance abuse disorders. The statistic is that about 50% of people with bipolar disorder also have a co-occurring substance abuse disorder and about 50% of those with a major substance abuse disorder have co-occurring bipolar disorder. A huge problem with substance abuse disorders is that when people are abusing substances, they are not taking meds, or at least not taking them responsibly, and their inclination to act out and give immediate vent to whatever strong emotions they may feel is well-known.

Psychiatrists often state that when substance use disorders and mood disorders such as bipolar disorder occur together, the thing to do is to treat the substance disorder first, and get that under control, partly because the moodiness of the individual may look very different once they are divorced from their substance use and also because any mood disorder treatment is vitiated, as I said, by the use of substances. The rest of this chapter is going to consider the bipolar or depressive patient (that is, a patient with a major mood disorder) who does <u>not</u> have a substance use disorder of any seriousness other than caffeine or nicotine.

The first thing that a person needs to realize before they can control their moods and feelings, is that if they don't want to control themselves, really want to, they never will. For those that don't really want to control themselves (rather than let it rip whenever they feel anger or excessive hilarity or excessive explosive crying or some other mood disturbance), I will say this: how you behave in society affects very much how other people perceive you. People may well attribute your obvious mood problems to an illness, but they may also say in effect, "Oh, he's not one of us, he's mentally ill". And you may not like what it does to your life to have people around you, particularly people outside your family, thinking of you as mentally ill. If you reply that they do think of you that way anyway and you believe that no improvement is in sight, I would ask you to read the following few pages. If your attitude is "Well, but when I get a feeling of anger or of elation or of despond, I simply <u>must</u> go with my feeling," with no idea that you wish you could do otherwise, (or learn to do otherwise), then until you come around to the idea that it's really important that you learn to control your feelings and your moods, I will leave you to your fate.

I would just ask you the following question: surely you realize that you're not having a very good time when you are in the throes of some mood state or feeling state, and surely you realize it would be nice to get to a more even-tempered, more equable state of mind?

If you find that you get angry over anything that goes against you, including things that are trivial, and you recognize they are trivial, but you do not understand how you could do otherwise than become enraged as you do, then perhaps you could ask either your therapist or your prescriber for a referral to an anger management class. Most large clinics, including county clinics, have anger management classes for anyone who seems to need them, provided you are a patient at that clinic.

The essence of anger management treatment is first to have you become aware of when you are just <u>starting</u> to get ticked off. The capacity to watch one's self and become aware of one's own voice, hands, body language and behavior generally is called an 'observing ego' and is a very important faculty to cultivate. It has been advised that you get in the habit of watching your respiration. Slow down your breathing when it seems to become accelerated and/or loud. This will actually have a calming effect on you and it will also transform other people around you so they will not be thinking of an emergency room visit or a hospitalization for you. You may have to stop your mind for a moment or two to deliberately slow down your breathing. Next, learn to watch your language. It is perfectly okay to say "I find your attitude unacceptable." It is not okay to use a phrase with profanity in it. Also, if you can learn to keep your voice level and keep it low and slow rather than competing for loud and high, this will be appreciated by everyone else, and it will also have a good calming effect on you.

There are undoubtedly some situations in which it is wiser, and, in my view, more courageous to just walk away. This is particularly true early in your treatment when you may be with some friends and acquaintances who do not value being calm and avoiding anger as you do, and who may be mouthing off, as they have for many years, and expecting you to do the same. If you have been in a 'shouting match' relationship with someone for some time, it is particularly difficult to avoid getting into a shouting match again, because that person knows exactly what your triggers are and how to say things so as to 'get your goat,' so to speak.

You need to get to the point where you value staying calm more intently than you value scoring a point off your old shouting match partner. As long as you are trying to outsmart him, or shout him down, you will never get control of your own anger and you will be merely reinforcing an unfavorable social reputation for being someone who gets into shouting matches.

Now I'm going to say something about controlling the moods and feelings when they are your own internal moods and feelings which are not necessarily very obvious to those around you. If you have gotten to the point where these are your concerns, then at least you are no longer spoiling your work prospects or your social future generally. People can be very mean, and there are people who will enjoy seeing you packed off to the emergency room while they regale each other with stories of your past anger. I had a favor given me years ago because I moved around so much, and the people in my new place did not know my past history, so there was no-one to say things like "Oh, she always yells at people." So now, let's get to controling your interior feelings and moods.

First of all, get to know yourself. Are you a person who feels depressed in the morning but whose mood improves by the middle of the day? Are you a person who has difficulty getting through a particular time of day? Such as the time when your husband came home from work, and now that you are a widow this is particularly difficult for you? Are there particular setups in your environment which will cause you to have a feeling which if you indulge it might lead to uncontrollable crying? Try and make your external environment favorable to a fairly equable interior environment.

If you feel some discouragement or immense sadness or silliness coming on, perhaps the first thing for you to say to yourself is that you know it won't last forever and to limit interactions with other people during these times. Is there someone in your environment who is friendly and understanding of your difficulty but a little further on in their self-control than you are? Is there someone, essentially, that you might be able to imitate? Can you tell yourself that you will feel better by tomorrow morning and that you usually do feel sad in late evening, so this is just usual? After all, we don't want people in this world who are incapable of feeling sadness, but we do want to keep you from going from sadness to maudlin sadness to serious depression to acting out.

Get to know whatever is the emotional up or down that you need to avoid and develop, with your therapist, a strategy for becoming aware that you are getting into territory where you might have these painful moods, and practice the strategy as much as you can.

For the purposes of this chapter, I'm going to assume that feelings which last over a period of time and which color all one's perceptions become a mood. In other words, you may receive news about a friend which makes you feel sad, but it only becomes a sad mood when sadness pervades your whole world for the time being, and colors everything to the extent that sunshine or your child's happiness does not change your sadness, or a good joke does not seem funny to you.

Now already we have a difficulty. A great many people feel "they have a right to feel their feelings" and they don't want anybody to mess with that. I'm not suggesting that somebody else mess with you, I'm suggesting that you might want to make a change in how you are in the world. Imagine for a moment that instead of going from anger to annoyance to desperation to elation to perplexity back to anger etc. throughout your day, that you could have the same hue of a feeling (that is the same coloration) but at a much lower intensity. So instead of rageful destructive anger, you feel "Oh, brother". Instead of desperate clinging you feel "I do wish you would stay with me". Instead of wild elation you feel a moderate happiness. Don't you think your life would be easier if you didn't lurch over an hour or two from one very strong feeling to another? Don't you think it would be to your advantage to be calmer inside? Don't you feel it would be better for you not to go from "I hate that man!" to "I don't know how to live without him!"?

If you don't see the advantage to you of becoming less severe in your emotional states, then maybe this chapter is not for you. If you do see an advantage to being less extreme emotionally, let me offer what follows.

The first thing to do is watch your talk. By this I do not mean only don't use swear words, what I do mean is, do not exaggerate the emotional content of what you are saying. If what you are expressing is a moderate annoyance with someone, then don't do as many do and say "I could kill him!" Saying you feel like killing somebody only confirms you to yourself as in an extreme emotional state, not to mention that it may be inconvenient in the future if someone overheard you say that. Try to stick with what you actually mean. If what you actually mean is "I find what he said about X extremely annoying." Then perhaps you can stick with that. Learn to tell it like it is, not say it ten times worse.

Perhaps you can admit that you don't really enjoy the feeling of ragefulness (for example), still less do you enjoy having to deal with the aftermath of your rage. If you destroy other people's property, they may refuse to continue their acquaintance with you, or may take you to court, and if you destroy your own, then repairing it or replacing it can become quite expensive. I remember that I had one man who came to see me who listed a whole bunch of appliances he had destroyed, and told me that two days previously he had whacked his own extra-thin flat screen TV, brand new, with his hammer. He looked at me a little sheepishly and said "This is getting rather expensive – could you help me change?" I could and did, and since this man was willing to acknowledge that he was the source of his own worst unhappiness, he became a most contented person, and his wife said he had "turned into a pussycat".

At some point, you're going to come across the idea that if you're not aware from moment to moment of your states of mind and states of emotion, you can't begin to control them. A person who is so angry that he loses all connection to the fact that he is rageful, loses all connection to the possibility of altering his behavior. Men are more often unable to put their feelings into words; women more often may have three or four or five intense feelings at once, and so may have difficulty organizing what they have to say on the subject of their feelings at a given moment.

What I'm getting at is to be able to monitor your internal temperature, as it were, and be aware when something is beginning to bother you. At the beginning, when you are just <u>starting</u> to be a bit upset, is when you have the most control. Can you teach yourself to note the circumstances of beginnings of increased emotion to take to your therapist, but then turn your thoughts to some other subject so that you don't heat up to the point where you no longer have control of what you say and what you do?

I have made mention several times in this book of having had a life which caused me to live for a few months at a time in one community, then move on to another, and then another – because I fulfilled a succession of temporary work contracts. I also did say that this had the advantage that as I moved through life, in each place I started with a new baseline, and whatever I had learned up until that time was where I was starting from. It turned out that this was useful to me, although I would not recommend the nomadic lifestyle to anyone who isn't forced to have it.

But it did bring me some good things in that I was exposed to a large number of pastors, psychiatrists, therapists – and I could understand as few do that how one behaves really is <u>not</u> dictated by one's role in life. Kindness and goodness and gentleness can come as much from a policeman as they can from a therapist; severity and disapproval can come as much from a therapist as they can from a policeman. Therefore, each of us has much more choice about the person we want to be than many of us would like to admit. Just because you've always been an angry person does not in any way mean that you have to stay that way.

Look at the people around you. Is there anybody who stands out in your mind as being less irritable, less fractious, less angry than most of us are? Have you ever been with someone who is less angry than you are? Did you perhaps undergo one of life's petty negatives together – in other words did you both suffer to find the restaurant you were counting on was closed, the weather when you got to your day for a picnic was tumultuously stormy, your library card had expired or some other petty negative which you might not remember in detail a month later? How did the other person handle it? Did they fly off the handle less than you did? Have you ever considered asking them how they managed to keep their composure, or to regain it so quickly?

Be willing to learn from the people around you. Perhaps there is someone else in the family who knows how difficult it was growing up with your parents or the people who were around when you were little. Is there anyone among you who have learned to handle it better? Without even needing to ask them, could you notice how they handle it?

The plain truth of the matter is this: all of us have negative things happen to us from the small to the bigger to the life-changing. But what do we think about? How do we react to these negative happenings? How do we cope with the negativity that lands on our shoes?

I am reminded of a fable which was once brought to me by a patient. It was the story of a woman who lived by herself and kept her place as neat as a pin. She brushed the floor every day and her front porch shone. And then one day a person who was feeling nasty dumped a cartload of horse manure onto her beautiful front porch. Now the reader is invited to imagine the end of the story.

If the lady had a compost heap, the cartload of manure was a gift. If not, she could run into her house, close the door behind her firmly, and complain that she was too depressed and too anxious to come out for several days in a row, and perhaps in a couple of weeks the rain would have washed it away. But the rain would have washed it onto her neighbor's property, and this would not make her neighbor more fond of her – after all, old manure does stink. Or, she could put it in that compost heap or in that fallow place in the garden, or at the very least she could wrap it up carefully and put it in several garbage bags each tied carefully and leave it out to be picked up by the garbage collectors.

My main point is that the only solution here that does not work is the slamming the door and running in the house and being too depressed and too anxious to come out for several days. This is going to cost our good lady several days out of her life, days in which she feels miserable.

I believe it was M. Scott Peck who in the twentieth century put forth the idea that we suffer greatly with unnecessary suffering when we try to avoid our dose of legitimate suffering. Legitimate suffering is the sorrow, chagrin, misery that comes our way because someone we love is sick, or has died, or we cannot afford a necessity which we will suffer to do without. Legitimate suffering is a matter of having to deal with our limitations as fallible human mortal creatures. But we don't want to feel sad, we don't want to feel left out, we don't want to feel whatever the real feeling underneath would be, so we twist our way around to all kinds of saying and doing in order to avoid the real feeling which is a sorrow that comes about because of our personal and mortal limitations. How hard is it for us to accept that we can't manage the cost of transportation to see someone graduate, and so we tell ourselves that the trip would have been noisy and difficult anyway? Or when someone dies, we don't want to feel bad, so we say, "He never would have liked to get any older." There are even people who will tarnish the memory of someone who has died so that they do not have to face the full grief of having lost them.

Now let's try a different approach. Supposing your daily life did not irritate or annoy or upset you much at all? I can just hear people saying that's impossible, that that's not the human experience of life. I agree that to achieve this you would have to have faced up to and made peace with all the conditions of your life, forgiven everyone and everything that has hurt you, and made reasonable efforts to make amends to everyone you have hurt. That is what I advocate, and if you want to know more, try reading my first book "My Money's on the Turtle." However, I don't propose to recapitulate that book here.

What I am saying is that in a daily sense, you are only irritated, annoyed, or negatively impacted if you are at odds with what is happening in your life. The trick to being mostly contented in your daily life is to not put too many restrictions on what may happen if you are to stay in a pleasant state of mind. If you wake up in the morning and have the attitude "If everything that I do or say or participate in or hear about goes my way today, I will be okay" then you have left very little flexibility for fate, God, the quirkiness of life, or minor mishaps to occur without its costing you your composure. Plus, sometimes the only way that our lives can change is by a forceful change of direction, which can perhaps occur only if there is a major obstacle to continuing as we were.

I myself broke my right arm into three pieces this past August. I had a time in the hospital, I underwent surgery, I then spent time in a nursing home, and because orthopedic surgeons as a group are so afraid of being sued that they will not take a case referred to them by another surgeon they do not know, I had to stay living in a motel in Pennsylvania and proceeding with my rehab until my surgeon said I was no longer an orthopedic case and was free to go home to Western New York. When I broke my right arm I did not have a normal left hand with some ability to use knife fork and spoon, so I literally went for four days after the fall without a bite to eat. I had plenty of food but no way of getting it into my mouth. Literally. So that's when I went into rehab.

If, in contradistinction to what I said above about having the attitude that "If everything goes my way today, I will be okay" — which means that with any minor mishap you are not okay, you could have in your head something like "I'm okay if A) I'm alive B) I have shelter, food, water, heat, clothing for today and C) my pain, if I have any, is manageable" then minor problems such as having a flat tire or getting a spot of ketchup on your silk scarf or finding that you arrive at the bank too late, or whatever it might be, will not be something that will make you lose your cool.

I had a patient once who was very much in love with her husband and I asked her, just to get to know her better, how she had met him. She said she was coming home at a run with some rare books which had been in her grandfather's bank vault for some years, and she slipped on wet pavement and collided with a young man. She was very distraught to see her grandfather's books, some of which had very old binding, spread out all over the sidewalk with pages out of the books. The young man stopped to help her, and in so doing he really looked at her, and once he got her books back together he asked her where she was headed, she told him, and that was their first encounter.

Now it is true that if this young woman had not been running she might not have slipped in the first place. It is also true that had not this young man been walking along the sidewalk he might not have collided with her, and had he not been a sympathetic young man who wanted to help her in her obvious distress, they might never have met each other. But the immediate adversity of dropping the books resulted in her getting a very nice and very loving husband. So not all that is an adversity is only an adversity. Some bad things do have a silver lining. And if they don't, well some rain must fall in every life.

If you could see what has happened to you as "some rain" rather than a major catastrophe, even if you have taken the stiletto heel off one of your brand new shoes, that's a pair of shoes, and they may be subject to repair. Or perhaps not, and perhaps in a few years you would have stopped wearing them anyway, and you have other shoes. In other words, look for every opportunity you have to make the unpleasant things that happen to you more acceptable to you. And if you look for every opportunity to see the rainbow after the rain, life will start changing for you. I can almost guarantee you that if you really change the way you see your life, your life will change. Doctor Wayne Dyer says "If you look at things differently, the things you look at change."

I couldn't agree more. If you insist upon it, your feelings will not change. If you wait for outside events to change to be more favorable to you, that may or may not happen, or there may be a change which in some way is not quite what you had in mind. People sometimes, for example, if they have very little money, imagine how beautiful life would be if they had more resources. Some of them do go on to get more resources, but there turns out to be an aspect of their life which is still not to their liking.

Generally speaking, you <u>can choose</u> how you want to feel. You can monitor your state of mind and correct it as you see fit. I can't tell you exactly how to make yourself feel better, but if you genuinely look at your circumstances and say how would <u>I</u> have to change <u>me</u> to make this seem more acceptable, I think an answer may present itself to your mind. Or perhaps you can change those circumstances. Perhaps it's a question of having the courage to make that geographic move that you have thought about for years, for example.

Of course I can't tell you how to control your feelings or control your moods in any absolute sense. There are billions of us on this earth and no one's path is exactly like any other person's. But the principles are there and so we return full circle to what I said in the beginning, which is, do you WANT better control of your feelings and your moods? If so, you can find a way, or you can with some professional help.

Now, if you choose not to invest too much psychic energy in negative reactions to petty annoyance, how do you do that? I have mentioned before that any unwelcome thought you have, you can have as a thought but refuse to "entertain" it. By that I mean any thought you have may come into your head and be marched out of your head again without your engaging it for a long conversation. By "entertaining a thought" I am imagining a thought which knocks on your mental processes and you open the door, see what the thought is, and say "Oh, it's you! Do come on in…sit down…. what can I get you?" And you invite the thought in to make itself at home and to take its place among all the thoughts that you have in your mind for that day. As opposed to, refusing to entertain the thought. This does not mean that the thought never occurs to you, it's just that you say to it "Go right on by, go right on through, I'm not interested in this thought right now."

It is wise to cultivate friendships with people who are a little more stable than you are. For a sensitive person, this will encourage that person to stabilize their own thinking and follow along with the social atmosphere generated by their friend or friends. If you don't know anybody who is more stable than you are, it is perhaps a good idea to begin frequenting places where people are trying to become better people and behave in a reasonably kind fashion towards each other. By this I mean houses of worship. There are also secular venues such as the Y, perhaps committees in the community which are seeking to better the life of others in the community – any group with a stated goal that is something other than serving their own egos or picking up people, is a place where you might make some friends.

As for myself, personally, I have to say that when I was manic I could be spectacularly manic (for example speaking nonstop for 96 hours in spite of medication) but the most I ever did against someone was to be sarcastic. Nonetheless, sarcasm can certainly be enough to make people not want to be with you; I had to work hard to get over my tendency to be sarcastic with, say, slow officials. Oftentimes it helps to tell myself I have nothing against the particular individual I am speaking to; my beef is with the inhumanity of the system and this one person talking to me did not engineer that system any more than I did.

If you really don't think you have a problem controlling your feelings or controlling your moods, try answering these questions, and since you do not have to show your answers to anyone, try being scrupulously honest.

A) How long ago was it that you last lost your temper with someone?
B) How long ago was it that you destroyed someone else's property?
C) How long ago was it that you physically attacked someone?
D) How long ago was it that you swore and/or raised your voice to someone?
E) How long ago was it that you felt like swearing or raising your voice to someone but you did not do so?
F) How long ago was it that you felt real resentment of someone?
G) How long ago was it that you felt like saying something cutting to someone, though you did not do so?
H) How long ago was it that you spread a vicious rumor about someone you dislike?
I) How long ago was it that you originated a vicious rumor against someone?
J) How long ago was it that you felt annoyed with someone, though perhaps you did not speak your annoyance nor act out in any way?

If the answers (and I do mean the candid, honest answers) about these questions are that the last time you expressed anger or annoyance in any way was many moons ago, (meaning at least six months) and you can't remember the details, then perhaps you don't need this chapter. If even the answer to question J) "How long ago was it that you felt annoyed with someone, though perhaps you did not speak your annoyance nor act out in any way?" is several weeks ago, then perhaps you do not need this chapter, but if any of the above questions had, candidly speaking, more recent examples in your past than that, then you do need to be a calmer, quieter, more satisfied and more happy person.

Now, how to do that? Well, first of all you need to become a good observer of yourself. Once you have gotten into the habit of keeping a watchful eye on how you feel, then the next step is to be able to question those feelings of annoyance or anger. One thing that is immensely helpful in this inquiry is to be a person who makes a habit of counting your blessings more than once a day. What are your blessings? One of them is that you are alive (you must be, or you couldn't be reading this book) and that therefore you do have some future in front of you – even if it's only a few choices about how you are going to leave this world, if you are on your way out.

I wrote a whole chapter on gratitude in my first book <u>My Money's on the Turtle</u>, and I'm not going to repeat the whole chapter here. But there are people the world over who do not have good health, do not know where their next meal is coming from, do not have clean air to breathe and clean water to drink and to cook in, do not apparently have a single friend etc. etc. etc. – so I'm going to leave it to you to fill in all the good things that you have in your life. Even if you don't like your work much, and you feel your boss and your co-workers are a pain, count having a job among your blessings. Would you be better off if you lost it? That is the procedure with anything you have. If you have a house which is small, dark, dank, cramped and ugly – would you be better off if you lost it? If the answer is no, you are better off at least for the time being to have it, then count it among your blessings.

Are you able to think, to talk, to walk, and to have your food digested and your metabolism proceed fairly normally? Anything like this is a blessing. Also blessings are the ability to see (again I presume that since you're reading this book) to hear (if someone is reading the book to you) to feel (in both the tactile and the emotional sense of that word). Do you have people in your life with whom you can regularly interact? Again the operative question here is would you be better off knowing no-one in the community where you are? If the answer is yes, then surely it is not too difficult to subtract yourself from whatever people you know. But do not despise lopsided or distorted caring – anyone is better off with someone in their life that cares about them than with no-one at all.

Now you have a list of your blessings. Try to put the best forward, (for example, say to yourself "I have a job, though I don't like the work very much.") How much better that is than to be saying to yourself "Well, anybody who is grateful for this job which is so awful and so low paid and with such terrible people is an idiot." The first statement, gratitude that you have a job, opens up possibilities of improving your lot, whereas the second statement opens up only more vistas of resentment and of being the kind of person that another employer (one with a nice job to offer, which pays better and which has better-tempered co-workers) would not want to hire. Nobody wants to invite a real grouch to be with them, so if you are a grouchy, negative kind of person, time to work on rethinking how you present yourself.

If you think of yourself as a person who has a lot of blessings, as well as things in your life you would like to improve, then it may not be difficult for you to question those few resentments or annoyances you do have. Don't forget the blessings of not being under immediate threat of bodily injury, not being under immediate threat of having your house repossessed, not being in a sticky divorce, or anything that you see around you from which you are free. This will help you to get yourself more free. For example, I think anyone who lives in the United States can count it as a blessing if they do not wake up in Afghanistan, Iraq, or Darfur or anywhere else with a great crisis of people shooting each other or a crisis brought about by a natural disaster. If you feel your co-workers are nasty, but your neighbors where you live are decent people, be sure to count the latter among your blessings. Or the reverse, if that is the case.

It is ironic, but it is my experience that the people who are grateful are those who are fighting for their lives or in some other great travail; whereas those who have a great many blessings and have had them for quite a while are caught in carping and griping. Try not to be one of the latter.

In the beginning of my moving away from surliness and annoyance to happiness, I had to identify my feelings and really chip away at the justification for those feelings. I would often come to the conclusion that I had no right to be surly or annoyed with the person in front of me, though my life itself was not very satisfying, and so I felt I had the right to be annoyed with Somebody for the way my life was turning out. As I got good at chipping away at the reasons for being disgruntled or moody in a particular situation, I found that I enjoyed feeling the absence of surliness or moodiness, and in the absence of surliness or moodiness or grouchiness, I could actually feel reasonably contented.

Then I began to see episodes of discontentedness as interruptions in my contentment, and to be able to decide that I didn't want my contentment interrupted, so I could just decide that I wouldn't let things get to me the way they used to. For instance, if you've ever had to call an insurance company, you know that the first person you speak to is never the right person, so you will have to speak to another person and another and another, until you do reach the right one. So I start with a whole page to write down phone numbers on and when I get to the third or fourth person I say "I do hope you can help me." This gets the third or fourth person ready to say "I'm so sorry, but this is the wrong department....", by which I mean they at least acknowledge they're sorry, and when I do finally reach someone who helps me, I think we both have a sense of mission accomplished and a sense of winning against the system. And when I see that I have to call an insurance company, I try and make the call in the morning since that is when I am most fresh. I just accept that a certain number of flat tires, lost keys, lost ID cards, need to call an insurance company, or whatever, is going to happen in life, and this is one of those times.

When I broke my arm, I needed surgery out of town (and out of network!) and endless calls to insurance. I just told myself that eventually the numbers of calls I had yet to make would die down, and there is no law that says I have to spend the time between contacts with insurance and patient billing department feeling bad. So I would get off the 'phone, do something to cheer myself up, and then get back on the phone for my next call.

This does not mean that I am perfect. I did raise my voice this morning (though my language was perfectly fine) to someone who refused to get me what I wanted for a reason I did not expect. So I still have to work on the unexpected demands of life. When the person I was talking to asked me to please not raise my voice against them, I did immediately apologize and the conversation was finished most cordially. But I have to remind myself that even in my sixties, I am not perfect and could do better.

If you know you have some contacts to make which you will not find pleasant, there is nothing wrong with scheduling one or two for Monday, one or two for Tuesday and one or two for Wednesday if you're not working against a deadline. If you are working against a deadline, remind yourself that after the deadline it will all be over, and plan something agreeable to do then. Note that by 'agreeable' I do not necessarily mean expensive – it could be a walk in the park in the sunshine. And when you do take that walk in the park, make sure you remind yourself that you are not undergoing anything unpleasant at that moment, that the unpleasantness you had recently is behind you, and that you have a pleasant morning tomorrow, without those telephone calls or other contacts, to look forward to.

In other words, you work to make the unpleasant time-limited, (it takes over a morning, it does not take over your whole life, and you still have the bowling club or your card playing group or your chess players which have nothing to do with the unpleasantness). Just put down these disagreeable things that occur in life as things that occur in everybody's life. They will be over when they are over, and hopefully going through them will not be so bad. Give yourself the goal of getting through all the conversations without raising your voice, if that is your difficulty, without saying anything sarcastic, or without saying or doing anything that is destructive to you own interest.

One of the most annoying things that can happen when you have started on your voyage of self-change is that you are changing but the people around you are not. It may be necessary to have a lot less to do with those particular people, especially if they are constantly carping and reminding you of how you used to be. As you respond less and less to their carping and you don't get into the old arguments, they will find making their remarks less satisfying because you don't reply, and the amount that they dish out to you may diminish substantially. If it does not, you may have to think of something more drastic. But in the meantime, the rest of your life – your work life, your life in the community, your social life, should be improving substantially so it may be that the carpers just become less and less important to you.

To sum up: to start changing your outlook in life, you have to want to. Your horizons become almost limitless when you do start to change yourself; I can say that from personal experience. The next thing is to become self-observant and to be aware when you begin to get annoyed or irritated or ticked off or wanting to say sarcastic things, let alone wanting to be destructive of property or to actually hit someone. When you are aware of these feelings, the next step is to start to argue with them. Who are you to think that you can call a bank, an insurance company, or some other such institution and get instantly the reply you seek, and have the content of that reply be what you want? While we are still on earth, we may expect a certain amount of frustration from such institutions (and I'm sure there are many others). When you do express anger or annoyance or irritation, or you do feel resentment or destructive urges, is there any other way you could interpret the situation? Are you absolutely obliged to feel annoyed or could you feel "Well, this person can't help me; maybe I can find someone else who can". Could you not say "Well, I didn't really expect to get the first person I spoke to tell me exactly what I wanted, so let's just move on to the next one"?

Then when you live mostly in contentment and are usually perfectly at peace with what's going on around you, you will get to a stage when you don't want anything or anyone to interrupt that contentment, and you will finally get to the point where you are not annoyed when something doesn't go your way, you just proceed down the line, to the next person, to another vendor and perhaps even (and this is for people and who want to really help change the world) you can make common cause with the person you are talking to and agree to perhaps tweak the system or make a note of something that will improve the system for the next user. Then you can have the satisfaction of making life better for someone else, the someone else being someone you don't know, but you can have a wonderful moment with the person you are talking to while you agree to improve things for this stranger.

Going to the Emergency Room

Let me first say that, if a person has been shot, is cut down from hanging themselves, has asphyxiated themselves and passed out, has cut themselves and bled enough so that their life is in danger (which I did twice) or has taken enough pills and passed into a coma (which I also did twice), let us hope and pray that they will be found alive and taken to an emergency room and cared for and given another chance to before they throw away their lives. I have said that my favorite assignment as a psychiatrist is to go welcome a recently suicidal person who is in intensive care back to the land of the living. I always have such a great sense of what a miracle that patient is (because we surely are God's miracles), and how marvelous it is that they have another chance to live, love, smile, laugh, cry in empathy, do something, connect with someone, and have a life. Emergency rooms do a great service in this way, and that is really what they're for.

What I'm going to discuss now is about going to an emergency room when a person is feeling bad, perhaps thinking of ending their lives, but hasn't done anything yet. In my own history, I would go along for days weeks or months not feeling too good, and declining the opportunity to think about self-destruction. I might then get to what seemed the point of no return, and go to an emergency room saying I was suicidal.

If perchance I happened upon someone who seemed to be willing to listen, I might cheer up because real listening is, I think, one of the rarest commodities on this planet. Sad to say it, but many therapists and many psychiatrists, psychologists etc. don't really listen, or at least not nearly all the time. And most of the professionals in an emergency room are geared for life-threatening situations which the patient never intended to get into, not ones they brought upon themselves. These professionals can be very bored and impatient (or scared) when they are in front of a person who is feeling self-destructive, but who is not bleeding, physically not hurt yet – not bleeding, cut down from hanging, nor comatose. They may feel "why is this person thinking about making me more work?"

The fact is, a patient, even the bad kind of professional patient (meaning someone who resists all attempts to change and presents the same way week after month after year after decade) is probably not as experienced in handling conversations about impulses to self-destruction as most mental health providers are. Patients may not be able to fall into a nice little pattern that we providers expect because the patients don't know their lines. Even a person with a history of previous actual self-harm may not see a pattern – those episodes were different because the patient was younger and/or there were different precipitating events. And, from my standpoint, I don't want to teach anyone their lines about suicidality, I want them to turn a page in their lives, and get a new take on their own presence here on earth, to turn away from ever thinking thoughts of destroying a life, theirs or anyone else's.

I once went feeling really badly to the emergency room, met someone who seemed willing to listen, started to feel better because that person had decided to listen for a few moments, and then was sent out of the emergency room as not needing immediate care; what I really needed was a few days' worth of being with people who would listen; I was brought back a day later in a coma.

You have to realize that there is one decision which is the overarching decision in any emergency room: to admit, or not to admit. If a person is deemed to be needing a psychiatric admission, then they will go up to the psychiatric ward or be sent to another hospital's psychiatric ward. If they don't need an admission, we may be in something of a quagmire. Because they may not have an appointment with their provider for several weeks, and it's Friday night, and we want to know whether they'll survive until Monday.

There are various ways around this. One is to ask the person, if they went home that night, what would they be doing tomorrow? If they can't come up with a single thing that they would do or a single friend they could call, that may be a danger signal.

Oddly enough, people who recite that they are going to go straight home and swallow twenty pills instead of ten and have it all very planned out, may often be just trying to press the physician into having an admission, because for some people a psychiatric admission, if they have nothing such as a job or a school or a family that would make them want to stay out of the hospital, may be entry to an elite social club whose members are other people who have experienced the same problems. (One sure way of having twenty to thirty other people around you with similar problems and plenty of help is to be in the hospital.) This can become very attractive for some chronically lonely people who have no reason to want to be outside of the hospital. They can also become very annoyed that their threats of self-destruction are not a guarantee for admission.

There were a number of people that I refused to admit when I was a resident that fell into this group. I never heard that any of them that I sent home actually did significantly hurt themselves. Usually I would say to them that I thought they were strong people with a good sense of taking care of number one (I thought that seemed true) and that they would make it through the night and probably the next day they would do what they usually did on a Saturday. I am fortunate in being able to say that I was never mistaken, at least as far as I know. I do know of one young lady in Philadelphia who insisted that she needed to be hospitalized (she had been hospitalized with a similar presentations fifty-three times in the preceding year and a half), and I heard that she took a late ferry to New Jersey and got herself hospitalized there, because of course, they did not know that she had been hospitalized fifty-three times with us.

The thing is, that patient was offered a placement in a group home after each hospitalization, which would doubtless have helped her, because she would have been surrounded by people who knew and understood what her problems were. But she always categorically refused, and insisted on returning to live on her own, which she was not able to do for more than a few days. Hence, we were stuck in this constant readmission/constant discharge. I knew this about her, and I felt that if she lived through a bad night or two, she would find out that she could live through them on her own, and she might learn that she had more survival capacity than she though she did. But she was angry with me for not letting her check into the local spa (the hospital) and so when I absolutely refused to admit her, she said "Well, I'll go somewhere where they understand what a sick person is." The other thing to say on my side of the argument is that she was in her middle thirties and she'd been doing this since she was about fifteen (that is, constantly threatening her to take her own life, and not doing anything else), and yet she never once had as much as a visit to intensive care. Somewhere underneath all her troubles, she had enough sense not to hurt herself.

I really did wish that I could refer her to a psycho-social club for mental patients, which do exist in some cities, but the Emergency Room when I was a resident did not list community resources other than shelters for homeless people. These are clubs in which are run by patients with only a few non-patient staff members, and they will ask a person how they are doing and listen to the answer, and they can call the police and have a person taken to a hospital if it seems to them a person is really in danger of taking their lives. I may add, as a person who has used such a club, that it is considered very bad manners to seriously threaten to the point where they have to call the police. If you're going to need the police, well then call them yourself. Or rather, don't call the police, call an ambulance. This is called self-rescue.

In other words, let's say a person has taken ten pills and is starting to feel rather groggy and then they suddenly realize they don't really want to die. The chic thing to do is to call the ambulance yourself. It would be considered very poor behavior to take the ten pills, walk to the social club, and dump the problem on their doorstep, as it were. And, most people do not want to be ill-thought of by their peers, which are the other members of the psycho-social club, other mental patients – they want their peers to respect them. As we all do.

It really worried me for a number of years that when I went to an emergency room, feeling suicidal, I would cheer up some when a person spoke to me and took an interest in me, and this would make people feel I didn't need to be admitted. There were other times when I knew I didn't need an admission, I just needed one night away from a toxic situation that I was living in. There was one time, when I was a student at the Catholic University of Louvain on the Brussels campus, that I managed to convince them to stay overnight in the emergency room for one night and that did me a power of good. I do have four suicide attempts in my record, all four requiring intensive care.

This was all some time ago, and I can confidently say that I am not going to be suicidal, because my whole take on what life is about has changed. I now think of life as an adventure, and expect bad times to alternate with good times. I also have the experience of hanging on through more than one bad time and finding that things turn good after it. If you have never experienced living through the long night of the soul, as it were, you won't believe the dawn will be coming.

Here is something as a suggestion for patients. I had the experience when I was in New Orleans of saying to a nice friend of mine who at the time did not know me very well but was a kindly person who was kindly disposed, "I'm feeling kind of bad, negative thoughts, not good things – could I come and spend the night on the couch?" and she was willing to let me spend a night with her. We watched TV, made some supper, and washed up the dishes. We didn't do anything spectacular, but I found out that as long as I didn't drag her through all the negatives in my life she was perfectly willing to be with me and be a sort of second reinforcer in my effort to stay away from those negatives. I just intimated what was going on in my head and didn't go into any yucky details, and she was able to be very helpful. At such times, at least for me, the main thing was not to be feeling very alone; having someone in the room meant that decent behavior was a social obligation, and I genuinely enjoyed her company.

Of course, as I say, things have changed for me, partly because I firmly believe I am sent here by my Lord, and it is true that I am never truly alone. All I have to do is say over one of my favorite Psalms or sing a hymn and the very real presence of God right there with me comes home to me. And I do feel God loves me, whatever I may do and however lacking or (at times) thoughtless I may be. I think most of my sins are not of commission, but of omission, that I just don't think about someone else because I get absorbed in my own little world. But then I think this is very common in Western culture. We do not feel obliged to think of others necessarily.

Having said what I said earlier about the wonderful job that emergency rooms do when the patient is very physically ill and truly in danger of death, I will say that people who have not put their lives at risk by self-harm, but who are thinking of doing so, will have a bad time in an emergency room. For one thing, the providers in an emergency room are far more invested in what they do best, which is to bring someone who is badly injured from the brink of death back to life. They are often very put out, annoyed, and I think a little scared and unsure of what to say, if they are confronted with (as they were in my case) a pretty, young, lively person who says she wants to kill herself. This seems illogical to them, and the atmosphere of an emergency room is not really conducive to assuming the patient's perspective.

For providers I would suggest the following: first of all, if it's very cold outside or very hot, take care of any patient's cold, thirst, or hunger first, before you ask anything, or do anything else. This will do more than volumes of perorations about how we at General Medical Center are focused on patient care. As I have said to students when I was senior resident, take that mission statement off the wall and just do it, you don't need to think what to say. I mean if it's hot, bring a cold drink, if it's cold, bring some blankets, if the patient has an obvious sore or sprain or cut work on that. That will do more to convince the patient that you care than any amount of speechifying.

Too, I always would go talk to a patient in an emergency room without pen and pad. I would talk to them the way you would talk to your neighbor about how life was treating you lately and listen to the story. Then at the end I would get details such as how they spell their name or what their birth date is or whatever else I needed. But rather than start out with "okay what's your name, where do you live, what's your social security number, what's your date of birth, I'd say "Hi, I'm Dr. Clark. What's happening with you?" and let them tell me. The question I would ask next depended on what they just said. It always seemed to me that if I couldn't hear one story as a story (told in a sequence different from the sequence we write it up in), and then rearrange the elements properly for the write-up, then I shouldn't be in psychiatry.

I would say an emergency room is not the best place to be, and I would tell patients you will have a harrowing time, even if you do get an admission, because an emergency room will not treat you well if you are not visibly injured. If you live in a city that's big enough to have a suicide prevention hotline, trained laypeople who will listen to you while you tell them whatever you need to say, call them.

If you can get involved in a local social club, so that you have some acquaintances and friends in your locality who know you and can say "Well now, come on, you survived last time, I mean, do you remember, you know you told us you went home and baked three chocolate cakes – would you like us to bake a chocolate cake for *you* this time?" There are people who can jolly you through your bad times, if you have some acquaintances who would understand what you're going through. Talk to them, certainly, and if you get to the point that you cannot think of anything except self-destruction, then you can go to the emergency room. But hopefully, you can avoid getting to that point.

This is a very serious subject, and I think I'm going to finish the chapter with a funny story. I was once interviewing a former professional athlete who was telling me he had no hope, he had been evicted, lost his boring job, and his girlfriend had left. Over the radio at the nurse's station came the news that his former team had won against the favorites, and were to be quarter finalists for the national championship. All of a sudden he beamed, jumped up and hugged a passing orderly (who did not take it amiss), and shook my hand saying he would be fine, he would be an idiot to leave this world, which was so full of wonderful surprises. He called a friend forthwith who agreed to take him in, we got him a cab voucher to go there, and he went on his way. The idea that his team had won was enough to blow away his fog of despond and thoughts of self-destruction.

CHAPTER 19

"GETTING STUCK"; PROFESSIONALISM FOR PATIENTS

I want to clue in the reader to something that sometimes happens in therapy and causes the patient and the provider a good bit of wear and tear and also can cause patient and provider to lose a lot of time, in the sense that time goes by and sessions go by but no progress happens. This phenomenon is getting stuck in a particular part of the patient's history or getting stuck when the patient for example attributes all their problems to their parents, or to a particular characteristic of theirs.

The "stuckness" reveals itself because the patient comes repeatedly back to the same old, same old explanation of their problems, and does not seem to be able to make any progress with a fresh view on anything, in the sense that if they start out on another subject in a few moments they are stuck again.

One technique that is used in such a situation is to break off and ask the patient to talk about how he has experienced his life over the last few days, without any reference to anything before then. This sometimes will get him past being stuck because he will be living in what psychologically is his present, talking of events not more than a few days old.

However, this frequently does not work. What is then recommended is to examine the stuckness itself. Why does everything in the patient's present seem to come back to his father's (or mother's) misdeeds? Why has he suddenly lost, essentially, the ability to consider himself an agent in his own life? For it is rarely that the patient is stuck over repeating the same story. The stuckness usually comes from the patient's desire to attribute all his present misfortunes to either someone else, or to a decision that he made a long time ago, for example in marrying the wrong woman. It may well be that his idea that he "married the wrong woman" is actually a way of covering up a whole group of feelings and decisions that were made, both his own and other peoples', which he has simplified in his own mind into one unfortunate decision in his past.

Sometimes it is a good idea to let the patient know that even our 'wrong' decisions are made as the best compromise we could think of at the time, and to talk about why, from the perspective of the moment the decision was taken, it seemed like a good thing to do. Perhaps the patient has changed since then, or perhaps they have become aware of other tendencies or desires or parts of themselves that they had not brought to their conscious minds at the time they took the decision they complain of. So it is sometimes a good idea to discuss what, in the patient's experience, led up to the event on which he is now stuck.

The above may seem a bit far-fetched for a book of this type. The reason I decided to point it out in this kind of a book is that I have known a good many patients to stay stuck for a long time, and I have also known therapists who accept that the patient is stuck and do not do anything to try to dislodge them from that situation and move on to be telling their story in a more fluid and varied manner.

Another attribute of stuckness is that even though it seems to the patient that they are telling the same story over and over, the patient feels the therapist will not understand, while the therapist is waiting for the patient to break out of it. Sometimes it is good to bring an entirely new element into the conversation such as "where would you like to be in five years?" This may have a psychological effect that is similar to bringing logs of wood and placing them under the front wheels of a car, in order to give those wheels something to grip onto while the driver is trying to get the back wheels to stop sinking ever further into sticky mud. My point is that in psychological treatment as in driving, our trying to get the car to move by turning the key and pumping may be as ineffective as it is to review the stuckness over and over and over.

I am trying to warn the patients of something that may occur in their treatment; perhaps they should start on a brand new tack and think more about how to connect their present to the future they want, than tell all over again all the sorry events that took place in their past. Sometimes it is as simple as saying something such as, "Every time you talk about the fact that you didn't go to graduate school after college, you start talking about your father's defects of character; why is that? Why should there a connection between your academic career and your father's character?"

Another trick that is sometimes used is to talk about something that makes the patient more lively – in other words get away from negative, slow, low-energy parts of the patient's history if they have dominated the discussion for a few sessions, and get him to talk about something about which he feels at least some enthusiasm. Above all, the main thing is to be aware when your sessions are boring, energy-sapping, and don't seem to be getting anywhere, and take action, rather than spend considerable money and time getting nowhere.

This may be less of a problem now when more people are going in for short term therapies whose content may be largely programmed into the conduct of the therapy, and people are doing a lot less psychoanalytically driven therapies. Or it can also be that the advent of a new therapist can open up new possibilities if the new therapist is determined to be having a lively session with the patient. I remember one patient I had when I was in training. She had been coming to the clinic for eleven years, and had a new therapist every year as the previous therapist graduated and was replaced by a new trainee. The graduating psychiatrist ahead of me just said to me "You can do nothing for her, just let her talk."

This casual dismissal of a human being made me angry, and the patient later related to me that she felt quite surprised that I wanted to understand every little thing she said. In her first session she said to me "Chris said this, and Tom said that, and Pat chimed in with this other thing" and she was quite taken aback when I asked her in detail who Chris, Tom and Pat were. The patient said she had become used to speaking aloud to a person whose face did not move no matter what she said, and who did not respond to her in any way.

She solved a number of important problems while she was my patient, and was a totally different human being when I passed on to her case to my successor. For example, from being a lady who was very much alone, she was dating a man who was very nice who lived across the street, and from being a lady who had always dreamt of having a certain little shop, she was applying to the Small Business Administration for a loan to start her own business. And these are not the only things about her life which she had changed.

Now I don't flatter myself that I "did" all this, because a readiness for real change had probably been building up in her for a decade, so that by the time she came to me she only needed a little bit of help to bring it about.

But I am making my point again – don't settle, as the patient, for being stuck. The most frequently applied idea is to analyze why you have gotten stuck in this particular place, and you can do it aloud by yourself if you have a therapist who is not very receptive. Stuckness is not necessarily a good reason to change therapists, because stuckness is part of the state of mind of the patient, and might not change with a new therapist – the patient might just take their being stuck with them.

You Choose Who You Really Are

The phrase "professionalism for patients" may seem a bit odd. It is perhaps more so when I explain that I would like to use this phrase in the opposite sense from the way in which it is usually used. Professional providers say that a person is a "professional patient" when that patient displays an uncanny ability to avoid growth, to sidestep change, to present always with the same pathology in spite of several providers' efforts. Thus it was with Mrs. Evans, a lady in her fifties who had told half a dozen people in the community the same tale of woe that she told me when I met her. Her problems had begun in childhood when an uncle molested her, continued in youth when her stepfather died (her own father had left the family before she was born, and she would bemoan the fact that she never knew her own father, but this loss was never very real to her precisely because she never knew the person she had lost). Her tale of misery went on with an impoverished young adulthood as she and her mother struggled to make ends meet in a small town full of nasty gossips, (and, apparently, little else). Mrs. Evans' mother was a member of a prominent colonial dame's family and disdained association with many of the people of Eastern European descent who populated the town.

Mrs. Evans had rather affected speech and one could imagine that though she might at one time have been strikingly pretty, she had never made many personal friends. Mrs. Evans was not stupid, and she went to a local business college, and learned to be a secretary. She deferred to her mother, deferred to her boss, deferred to anybody while at the same time expecting them to make a fuss over her and her pretty face. When someone did notice she was pretty, she was quick to rebuff them if their family had not been in the USA since the 1600's – so she had a perfect recipe for avoiding social success, she who laid claim to coming from one of the "first" families. Her notion of herself was extremely high, and yet she did not relate to many others in the community, so she remained isolated and was treated with little regard, a social position which she did not feel was congruent with her legitimate expectations, given her ancestry.

No one in the small city that we were working in had succeeded in getting her to ditch her preconceived notions and be open to opportunities around her, which, because she was pretty and quite intelligent, were fairly numerous.

So she settled into chronic complaining, never getting much better, and defeating the efforts of at least half a dozen practitioners. This lady was a good example of what the practitioners would call a "professional patient." She came to every session on time, and <u>said</u> she wanted her life to improve, but she would refuse to consider any suggestion of change in her attitude towards herself or towards others. At the time I knew her, her mother was still alive and was in her seventies. The daughter was so emotionally dependent on her mother that we all used to say that she might fall apart when her mother departed this life, which, in the normal course of events, was bound to happen.

What I want to talk about is a different use of the word "professionalism." What I want to talk about is the opposite of the intransigence and unwillingness to change, complete unwillingness to critique one's own behavior and find ways to improve it, that I have described in Mrs. Evans' case. By the way, Mrs. Evans had married in her late twenties but the marriage lasted such a short time that it never figured much in anybody's assessment of her life. Nevertheless, she remained "Mrs. Evans," using the title as an honorific.

With respect to the concept of professionalism for patients, I want to use it in the following fashion. I want to say that a professional patient is someone who is interested in engaging in changing themselves so as to become more open to possibility, more able to free themselves of their own past (able to say for example that something happened and note a reaction without getting all tangled up in the emotional reaction to the happening), able to take on a new initiative in life and look at probabilities of succeeding squarely, able to, as Kipling says, treat good fortune and disaster both as "imposters" and not get caught up in self-adulation or self-deprecation in either instance.

We usually have scripted our lives so that the idea that we could have reacted differently, we could have made wiser choices, things could have progressed other than how they did, is very painful. We are not necessarily responsible for what happens in our lives (my father, for example, was warned about continuing to eat things like chocolate fudge sundaes, but he continued to do it, and I am not responsible for that decision and I am in no way responsible for the fact that he had a third heart attack close upon the second one, from which he died). But the interpretation, the color that I give to these events is my choice, and I can choose differently as time gives me distance and perspective on events.

There are a number of situations in which a person can either freeze into constant complaining of the difficulty they are having, or, after some genuine suffering and some complaining, move forward to attain a new level of success in life. Many people, when they are at one of these moments, say to themselves "Well, most people would not be able to move beyond this," or "I don't think I know anybody who could move beyond this" and take it as a given that they have to have the limitations that perhaps most (a majority) of people might have. Yet if they were disposed to see themselves as people of almost limitless potential (which I am thoroughly convinced, after more than twenty years of practice, that we all are) and proceed in a fashion which is courageous and yet practical, they might attain a result which is far better than what "most people" can get to.

I am frequently struck by the way in which people cling to their sorrows and their grief and say "Doctor, you don't understand, I have a <u>right</u> to feel the way I feel!" As long as a person is trying to justify negative feelings (of resentment, anger, envy, jealousy etc.) which make a better future impossible, they are not going to get that better future. A better stance would be "Well, I felt pretty bad when it happened, as you can well understand that I might, but now I have taken a new look at my life and I understand that I need to be more self-driven, I need to be kinder to people around me, I need to appreciate other peoples' efforts more etc. – in other words I used to have a dysfunctional attitude, but I have come to see that I need to change my response to this set of circumstances." In psychiatry we're always looking for a new perspective which will be more loving, more accepting, more looking for and seeing possibility rather than being despairing or resentful or stuck in any entrenched negative perception.

I'd like to close with the idea that there is being a patient and then there is being a patient. I myself have been a patient for nearly forty years. In the beginning of my career as a mentally ill person, I was full of complaint, very lacking in self-assurance, and needing the approbation of my provider or providers before I engaged upon any course of action. I saw providers frequently and my self-perceptions went up and down like a barometer, and I had apparently as little control of my own viewpoint as any of us have over the weather.

Nowadays I see my psychiatrist maybe three or four times a year, (unless I'm changing my medications) have my blood work done twice a year which is the minimum (I'm not entirely responsible for this, it's because all the parameters which need to be regularly checked are quite stable which is my current good fortune) and I see my therapist once in 6 weeks, as required by the clinic to keep seeing my psychiatrist. I do not have to wait to get professional approbation for embarking on a new endeavor in my life. I do tell the doctor and the therapist, but I tell them when I next see them – I do not feel I need to consult them to get their approval of what I am doing. So I am a patient, but I am quite able to decide things for myself. This is a huge change from what was going on when I was a young person.

I don't remember when the change came about exactly. It was a progression. Big in my life was forgiving my mother for all sorts of things, some of which were probably not her fault anyway. And if something is completely forgiven, it is no longer in the forefront of the mind, so I don't have any old issues that are continuing to present themselves, even though I have quite a history.

The last part of my effort has been over the last few years, to be able to get over my own history – in other words, my own past is not what I come forward and speak about at a social gathering with new people. My past has been useful in that I recognize a commonality of experience with many of my patients' stories, which I think made me a better psychiatrist. Not that I think our experiences were ever identical, because of course we're different people with different life histories and different gifts– but by my having something in common with many of my patients, the patients and I can reach a better understanding of whatever situation the patient is in. When you want to help someone, it's good to have walked in their shoes.

I think a little word about identity is in order here. If you ask people who they are, they will often give their name or their profession or where they come from as the first part of their identity, but all of these actually represent circumstances, not a part of who you fundamentally are. And by making ourselves identified with a certain social position, a certain kind of work or a certain expectation of wealth, we place ourselves as hostages to these circumstances. Meaning that if we were deprived of our ethnic identity, our work, our standard of living, we would feel that something essential to us has been taken away, and would open ourselves to years or even decades of feeling terrible.

It is important to cultivate an identity which is "I am who I am" which has to do with qualities of soul rather than external circumstances, because it is these qualities that will carry you through even the loss of those particular circumstances. Ask yourself how you would describe yourself. Are you adventurous, innovative, dependable, a risk taker, a person with a gift for making comfort and coziness and home,? Because these qualities will be good to have if you are deprived of your professional standing (you lose your job) or deprived of your belonging to a particular group (if for example you have to go to another country where that group is a tiny minority) or deprived of your comfortable house (the recent collapse of the mortgage system or a number of natural disasters could operate here). Are you a person who gravitates towards new people, appreciates the gifts of others, likes to try something new with other people? You can understand that these qualities would be useful anywhere except on a deserted island.

I'd like to suggest that you close this book now, take a piece of paper, and write down all the qualities that you have that are not dependent on a particular life circumstance, things that are a part of <u>you</u>. Your day to day <u>experiences</u> are perhaps part of you, but your standing is a circumstance. Make the list, and review it every few months and ask yourself if you are changing. This is your personal journey, a most vital part of who you are.

Now I am going to talk about my own personal experiences of stuckness. After I left the hospital of my second hospitalization, the one in which the doctor thought I had a conversion disorder when in fact I had a severe scopolamine intoxication superimposed on my bipolar disorder, I lived in a residential hotel in New York City, eked out a living as a temporary secretary in various assignments in Manhattan, and seemed to spend my time with the doctor complaining about my mother, first, and second, refusing to give up on my dream of ever becoming a physician.

As to the complaints about my mother, I literally did not remember much of her abuse; that memory came back to me when I was forty years old and living in New Orleans. So I could not give an accurate history, had I wanted to, and the good doctor took no interest in trying to find out if there were any additional facts that he had not been told.

I left the hospital at the end of November. The rest of that year was fairly uneventful, although I remember one of the loneliest Christmases I ever had in my life. I spent Christmas Day serving Christmas dinner to homeless people, which was okay, but I felt a little uncomfortably close to being homeless myself, and so was not able to bring as much joy and good cheer to it as I would have liked.

The following May was when my boss at the Congress of Racial Equality (C.O.R.E.) raped me. I have already in this book described what profound pain this event brought to my life. As I said, before I was raped I was a virgin, and I felt most cruelly violated.

But when I got to see the doctor again, I simply could not tell him. He by this time had evolved from a somewhat distant person who stared at me blankly without showing anything on his face no matter what I was talking about, to being someone I was certain was not listening to me. Later, when he decided not to continue seeing me because, I was, in his words "boring", he told me that I had been so "boring" that during our sessions he had been fantasizing about building himself a boat – in other words, he had not even tried to listen.

Let me say to all providers that a complete disconnection from the patient as evidenced by the provider's is not even attempting to listen to what the patient is saying, is one of the most damaging things that a provider could do. I had a sense that he wasn't really listening, but I did not know that he had made a decision to absent himself from our sessions and to daydream of being elsewhere doing something else.

I have often regretted that I did not have someone sympathetic to me to listen to me so that I dared speak of the rape, and have also chided myself for my lack of honesty, which is quite unlike me. I have also deeply regretted that when I did get to a good psychiatric service in Belgium, I was offered an opportunity to talk about my romantic history (or lack of it), but the idea of mentioning my sexuality to anyone out loud was so difficult that I did not take advantage of this opportunity. This was the one time in my whole history I did not explain whatever I was asked to explain, and I regret it to this day. I would ask the reader seriously to take heed of my statement that if you have something that is painful or humiliating or difficult to talk about, that is what you should talk about.

The real problem for me, I think, is that my mother formed the idea when I was a little girl that my twisted body, crossed-eyes, and pronounced limp made me profoundly unappealing, and even as I changed over the years she did not fail to remind me that according to her I rated minus something on the attractiveness scale. She kept telling me when I was growing up that I would never have a boyfriend, never marry etc. etc. – and though I have had a few romantic flings here and there, I wish I could feel that her prediction did not come true. Something that starts when you're a toddler is awfully hard to shake, and I do admire those of my patients who can change their opinion of themselves later in life, when the disparagement and negativity started when they were very small.

So you can see, dear reader, that acceptance by therapist and patient of a block or of being stuck, if you will, may totally arrest the therapy. My doctor wouldn't listen, and I felt I couldn't talk to him, so each of us for different reasons were participating in not talking about what we should have talked about. To providers I would say, always remain curious about your patient and never ever fantasize that you are elsewhere doing something else. If you find yourself consistently tempted to engage in daydreaming while seeing patients, then by all means stop seeing patients and go wherever your daydream takes you, but do not impose upon a patient the experience of having a provider who sits a few feet away and who is not paying attention.

For patients, I would say the pain or discomfort of talking about something which is negative about yourself is far less than the pain and discomfort of living with this same problem for decades henceforward. Pluck up your courage, and say what needs to be said.

CHAPTER 20

RESPONSIBILITY IN MENTAL ILLNESS

Obviously, whether a person is the only one in the family to have a particular mental illness, whether they are one of a number of affected individuals in an illness that "runs in the family", or whether they have an illness which is definitely known to be genetically inherited, no-one is responsible for getting a mental illness in the first place.

But the main point of this chapter, is that people who get mental illnesses are indeed responsible for the way they handle the illness. When it is that a person comes to attention to be diagnosed depends upon a) the natural history of the illness and its usual age of onset (schizophrenia usually has its onset in the mid- to late teen years or in the early twenties or, on occasion in the thirties but rarely after that); b) how disruptive the illness makes the patient become in such a way that they would draw attention to themselves as acting abnormally and so get someone to take them for professional help; and c) how easy or difficult it is to diagnose the condition and get an effective treatment for it. But after that, staying on the treatment or not staying on the treatment, having or not having more episodes of acute illness, is for the most part up to the individual.

Outside of hospitals, there are a few facilities in which someone is responsible for seeing to it that a mentally ill individual takes their medication on time. And then, there are patients who have become adept at elaborate ruses to avoid taking medication. Now, some of this is countered by using medications which are given by a parenteral route (i.e. not by mouth) but even in these situations, even with case managers to take the patients to the nurse to get their injection, patients can cooperate or not. For example, they can be "unfindable" on the morning they are supposed to go to the nurse for the injection. Also, in some states like New York, patients who are not dangerous have the right to refuse medication. The only problem for them is that they may postpone their discharge from the hospital by their refusal.

There are some individuals who spend years avoiding proper treatment in this fashion. And they have their own reward, because they may never be able to sit calmly and quietly and enjoy a sunny spring morning, for example, the way the rest of us would. They undoubtedly feel some sort of sense of triumph in being able to stymie the efforts of clinic employees to give them the medication they need. Some of them end up doing untoward things and end up in jail, which is a lot less forgiving. Such people do not in general have any sense of responsibility to the common welfare. By "such people" I mean the people who avoid taking the medication which would help them have a basic sense of what is appropriate behavior and what will keep them out of trouble with the legal system.

I am not condoning the way the legal system handles the mentally ill. The situation is that people when on medication behave reasonably rationally, and then, if they are given the opportunity to go off the medication and they do so, they earn themselves incarceration where only about 10% of the incarcerated individuals who need mental health services get them, and so 90% do not, and they become extremely ill while in jail. They may then become too ill to be competent to appear in court, and so they are sent back to the hospital to get well enough to go to a court, they are then returned to the jail and the process recommences. This is a horrendous state of affairs for which really there is no excuse except to say that the system is broken.

But that is not the situation I am trying to discuss now. I am trying to discuss the situation in which a person who is acutely mentally ill is taken to a psychiatric facility, treated, returned to some approximation of his former self, and released to live perhaps in a group home in the community. But this individual has no sense of his own responsibility to take his medication and treat his brain well, rather than subjecting it to many repeated flare-ups of his illness. As I have said before, such flare-ups will cost the patient IQ points.

So, having no sense of responsibility, he has further episodes of illness due to not taking his medication as a primary factor (though certainly not the only one) and the patient needs to go with some regularity to the hospital again to be treated again, set right, only to be released from the hospital and to start the process over again.

Anybody is entitled to their first episode of illness without criticism; the first episode hits one perhaps like an express train – (it is so unexpected, so hard to describe, so totally baffling). But at some point in that hospitalization it should be borne in upon the patient that his further success as an independent human being depends very much upon his taking personal responsibility for accepting his treatment.

Now I know this is unpalatable for some people, but although we have some inklings as to what might be done to prevent, say, schizophrenia or bipolar disorder, we still are a long, long way away from being able to <u>cure</u> a new case so that episodes will not return even if the patient is off medication. It is therefore of paramount importance that the patient understand that his future depends upon being able to take medication and being able to articulate as well as he can any particularly objectionable side effects. We do fairly well now for those who can be persuaded to follow doctor's recommendations; as time goes on and our choices for medications become more and more sophisticated, a wise psychiatrist is more and more adept at choosing the best medication available.

There are now some bona fide schizophrenics who hold good jobs and keep their schizophrenia in good enough control so that they can take their place in the work world; ditto with people with bipolar disorder. As this continues and more such cases are evident, one would hope that the dismissal of patients by their providers by saying "Oh he'll never amount to anything" will become less common.

But it is the responsibility of the patient to take his own illness, as President FDR said, "by the scruff of the neck and the seat of the pants and shake a result out of it." It should be said that if schizophrenic or bipolar people are not responsible for having gotten the illness in the first place, that they <u>are</u>, at least in part, responsible for recurring episodes of the same illness. To take the view that the patient has no responsibility to ensure his own sanity robs the individual of their dignity as a human being and I, for one, do not think of that as a kind or good service. Patients are also ultimately responsible for treating whatever other issues (such as substance use) may have cropped up along the way. As I said, about half of bipolar patients have substance use disorders, and about half of those with substance use disorders are bipolar. This makes the picture more complicated, but the patient is still responsible for dealing with the illness as best he can, or he will find himself dealing in a very real and concrete way with the consequences of his own irresponsibility.

This shows in many ways. I have tackled patients who had been screaming in the dayroom, once they have calmed down, and said "Why did you choose to scream?" They often bridle at the use of the word "choose." Then I say, "Oh well then, so your advice is, the next weekday I wake up and don't feel like coming to work, I should just stay home?" If they are telling me they have absolutely no control over their own behavior, they're telling me they have no choices, and it is my contention that every human being has a choice, from moment to moment. Perhaps not in all the details of the circumstances in which we find ourselves, (other people make choices too and strange things happen) but certainly in our interpretation of our circumstances. And in taking responsibility for our own choices lies all our dignity and all our real freedom. It is in doing "whatever we damn well please" that we cancel our own dignity and our own freedom; if we do whatever seems to take our fancy, changing direction with every passing moment, then in a quest for freedom we become slaves to our own unpredictability.

I have also gently chided staff members who fall into the assumption that if Joe or Susan or Jerry or Margery's behavior is habitually out of control, they never will be in control in the future. The ultimate staff putdown is to say "He or she (the patient) is always out of control." And, just as, if people will predict, foster, and endorse significant change, they will see change, if they predict and endorse saneness they will see saneness. The best way to bring about real change is to expect it.

In my work in state hospitals, I was continually surprised to notice that although there are periodic meetings to discuss the progress of each patient, and the patient may well be present at such meetings, the patient is the only one in the room who does not understand the limiting factors in his or her behavior which mean that he or she cannot be discharged at that moment. Usually, the list of absolute contraindications for discharge for a patient comes down to one or two things. Perhaps the patient wets the bed every night (and community residences cannot cope with an endless number of wet sheets). I'm not talking about senile people who belong in a nursing home, I'm talking about much younger physically healthy adults. Perhaps the difficulty is that the patient gets angry easily, and gets into fights with his peers over such things as who was first in line for the shower. We cannot discharge someone who may be physically dangerous. Perhaps the person just doesn't get up in the morning, and so is not seen as fit for a community residence in which people have to get up, get breakfast, make their beds, and get dressed fairly expeditiously every day.

But the sad fact of the matter is, the individual patients in state hospitals are often clueless as to what the limiting factor for them is. What I do (which has resulted in dozens of successful and long-lasting discharges) is to ask the patient if he would ever like to get out to the outside world. Most say that they would like to, very much. I did once in my career come across a man who said he was "instootionalized" and who would sabotage his own discharge because he just didn't want any change. But that is rare. Then, when I have the patient's interest because he is interested in leaving, I asked him why he is still being kept in the hospital? The most frequent answer is "I dunno." If I then tell him the one or two behaviors which are a limiting factor for him, and which keep him locked up in the state hospital, many patients really make an effort to eliminate those particular behaviors.

This means that they may not appear totally 'normal' when they leave the hospital, but for a patient who's going to a community residence for the mentally ill, that's OK. My point is, that I have found most mental patients (out of several hundred in chronic wards in hospitals that I have known, there have been perhaps twenty that could not be discharged under any circumstance that I could foresee) most are perfectly capable of moving out into the community. And surely, that is what a hospital, in the public or private sector, is for – the patient goes to the hospital when they or people around them can't cope anymore, and we work with them on getting them better so that they can return to the community. An admission to a state hospital should <u>not</u> be treated as a lifetime sentence. Of course, most state hospitals are paid a certain amount per patient living there. The lazy way for the staff is to make admissions and discharges few in number and continue endlessly with the patients who are already there. It takes a lot of work to discharge a patient.

Further, if a person will take no responsibility for their conduct when they are ill, no-one is going to give them any credit for improvement when they get better. Whereas, if a person is willing to say something such as "I feel really unstable today, but I'm going to make it a good day anyway, and do everything I can to damp down my mood fluctuations" then, when they succeed, other people will realize that this was came from some effort on their part.

I first had a "nervous breakdown" at the age of twenty-two, after six months of my first attempt at the hundred hour work week which was then required in this country of medical students, interns and residents. There are some places in which laws have been written against this requirement, and I know some attending physicians are feeling the strain of having to do some of the work which used to be done by senior medical students, interns and residents. But a) the enforcement of these laws is highly variable and b) if they choose to, attending physicians can make themselves into people who are so scary that the house officer (as interns and residents are called collectively) are terrified and would sooner die than call the attending – at least if it's about having too much work and too little time. I do not mean that people are generally frightened to call an attending for some extremely difficult procedure – but no one would dare call an attending for scut work, at least not in any hospital I ever worked in.

From the patient's point of view "scut work" may be absolutely vital. It includes things like inserting IV's for lifesaving medication, inserting catheters for procedures to take place the next day, drawing blood if in this particular institution this is done by physicians rather than phlebotomists who may become extremely busy. A classic example of "scut work" which can be lifesaving is an exchange transfusion performed for a premature newborn, whose immature liver cannot handle all the fetal hemoglobin that is broken down a few hours after birth. Exchange transfusions involve having a three-way stopcock system such that you can alternately withdraw a few cc's of blood with a syringe, then inject some blood that is to replace it, then go back to withdrawing a few cc's, and so alternate withdrawing and replacing, withdrawing and replacing, sometimes for many hours. If this is not done in a timely manner, the newborn baby may develop kernicterus, which is a severe, lifelong, and untreatable condition which occurs when the unmetabolized fetal hemoglobin, having reached an unacceptably high level, begins to bind permanently to the baby's nervous system.

This is called scut work because you put blood in, record that, then blood out, record that, and repeat the process over and over and over and over for hours on end. It probably will one day be done by a machine, but for now no robot has been devised that is completely reliable. A written record is kept of the time of each injection and withdrawal, so that you don't "lose your place" so to speak, and withdraw twice in a row or replace twice in a row, because the sheer monotony of it can be a danger. But work is work. Whether fascinating or monotonous scut work, it is important to the patient, and part of a doctor's responsibility.

Let me say immediately that I do not share the perspective implied by the phrase 'scut work' on the different parts of a physician's job. I wrote part of a chapter in my first book, My Money's on the Turtle concerning spending a whole night doing an exchange transfusion on a tiny little baby named Elizabeth Clark and the wonderful effect it had on me. I think I can say without bragging that it was also good for her, because no one will argue with the fact that I saved the life of another human being that night. I'm not saying no one else could have done it – anyone else could have done it, but I was the one who was willing. Dr. Rachel Naomi Remen has written a wonderful passage about the difference between wanting to "help" people who may be patients, and wanting to "serve." For me the difference between the two words can be summed up as follows: that "help;" means doing something constructive whereas "service" means getting the job done. I may help an old man across the street and then just leave him on the other side. If I wish to be of service I will ask him if he wants to tell me where he is going and help him get all the way there. A person is being helpful if, seeing someone collapse on the street without getting up, they call 911. They are being of service if they see the person collapse on the street and ask someone else to call 911, do CPR themselves, and tell the paramedics when they get there whatever they know about that person in terms of what might have been the problem just before he collapsed. "Help" can expect notice, thanks, a pat on the head where "service" does not. Therefore "help" can sometimes create more of a problem than it solves, whereas service is always putting the needs of the other person first. Sometimes a person might say it would be helpful if someone would get them an alcoholic drink. Real service to that person may mean ensuring their safety in sobriety.

I'm going to tell the story here of how I managed to get to my polling place to vote the first time that I was old enough to vote, even though I was locked up in a mental hospital, and did not have the right to leave the hospital building by myself. This, it seems to me, is a good story of how satisfying it can be to fulfill one's obligations to our society as a grown-up, how satisfying it can be to be responsible. It seems to me that our democracy is suffering greatly from the autocratic selfishness of some of the folks who have been in political power in recent years. But surely, if the response of the public at large is total indifference, so that they don't even bother to go to the polls, then our beautiful dream of a participative democracy in this country is indeed dead.

I remember the first time that I was old enough to vote. I turned twenty-one in July, 1971, but the voting age had been lowered to eighteen a few months earlier. This took a little from my anticipation of what being able to vote would mean, but only a little. So, when I was hospitalized on October 26, 1972, I was very determined that I would vote in the Presidential election in early November, 1972. I asked the social worker the day after my admission to get me an absentee ballot, and she did not say anything, but she nodded.

Election Day was, I believe, the seventh of November and I remember wondering if absentee ballots were still available, but the social worker seemed to be nodding agreement that she would take care of it, and I believed her. In any case, I was too manic at the time to realize that she said nothing.

About a week later I asked her if she had received the absentee ballots, and she said they were no longer available. I then said I would have to get to the polls. The problem was, that though I knew exactly how to walk to my polling place, I was not yet allowed out of the hospital on a pass by myself. So I needed to find someone who would accompany me.

I thought of asking my mother, but I wanted so much to get to the polls under my own steam. Then I thought of asking the hospital volunteer department whether they had someone who would take me to my polling place on Election Day. I was pretty sure I could get an accompanied pass, since I had by this time been out several times with a group of other patients and a couple of staff members, and everything went well.

The volunteer department said they had no one they could spare on Election Day, and then I faced a dilemma. How was I going to get someone to accompany me? All my adult friends were my mother's friends, and my medical school classmates were people to whom I did not want to admit that I was in a locked psych. ward, so I was a bit at a loss.

Then something occurred to me: I had already spoken to the family solicitor about suing the hospital for admitting me and depriving me of the one telephone call I was entitled to, and I had told him to hold off. I knew I was ill, though the hospital's approach to the matter seemed way off base.

I called back the family solicitor and asked, would I have grounds to sue the hospital if they deprived me of the civil right to vote? He said yes, I told him the situation, and he told me to call him back on Wednesday morning if I had not managed to vote on Tuesday. He wished me good luck, and we rang off.

I then called the Chairman of the Board of the hospital, getting past the secretary by telling her that I needed to speak to her boss to avoid an impending lawsuit for him. I was put through quite quickly. I then explained to the Chairman of the Board how he could avoid a big headache (the lawsuit) with a two minute 'phone call, if he would call the volunteer department and tell them they had no choice but to find someone who would accompany me to the polls on Election Day. I said to him, "This is a no-brainer for you – a two minute 'phone call now, or you will find yourself with a big headache, because I come from a Mayflower family (this is true) my father was a multimillionaire, we live on Park Avenue and I have already spoken to our family solicitor about suing you, and he told me the case would be a slam dunk in our favor (all also true). So, you make the 'phone call to the volunteer department now, or you face one of the biggest headaches of your career."

He did make the 'phone call, although he did not tell me he was going to, nor that he found someone. (I had to call the volunteer department back myself). I did also have to make sure that my pass was valid for all day. I had two hours, to start whenever the person accompanying me got there, and to finish two hours later.

On Election Day, the volunteer did come. She was, I would guess, in her sixties, and she told me that as a young girl she too had wanted to become a physician. But then somebody made a dirty joke concerning her, and she gave up on the instant any idea of joining the medical profession. Privately, I thought that such a wimpy person did not belong in medicine, but then I had to remember that the world had changed much in the preceding forty years. My strongest reaction was that I wanted to stay away from anybody who told a story of wanting to be a doctor but who was defeated. She made no bones about it – she told me several times that I would be defeated too. I can only think how small-souled she must have been to want to predict for somebody else a repeat of her own failure. But, I reflected, there are people like that, and I said nothing.

We went up to my dorm room in Columbia on West 168th Street on the subway, got my voter registration card (so I would have ID) and then went to my polling place. I don't remember the process of actually voting very well. I do remember being glad that it was the middle of the day and the lines were not long so I was able to make it back to the hospital before my pass expired. Since then, I have asked other people if they wanted to vote when I was the ward attending, and I could have arranged it for them. Unfortunately, I never got any takers on my offer, which I think is very sad.

I heard later that my mother came to vote later in the afternoon than I did, and she had tears in her eyes when she saw that I had already voted. She said she had a great regard for me for my courage and persistence, to get to the polls in spite of being on a locked ward in the hospital. And I did feel a sense of pride.

I do think the patient benefits whenever they discharge a civic or social responsibility as they should. I think it helps their self-esteem. Therefore, I would ask anyone who is hospitalized to think of asking to register as a voter and to get an absentee ballot, or get accompaniment to the polls, if they have any means of doing so. And I would like to ask my colleagues to think in terms of arranging to have their patients vote. We're talking civil rights here.

CHAPTER 21

ATTITUDES OF PROVIDERS

Being a professional has in practice come to mean refusing to allow personal bias to intrude upon one's performance of one's duties. It does also cover some behaviors which an untrained person might indulge in but which hopefully are no longer of interest to a trained staff member, such as gossiping.

That's the theory. Unfortunately, what does happen is that a whole team can decide as a group that a certain patient is not likeable or is never going to get better. Let me tell the story of a man I will call "Patrick" who was hospitalized in the ward for people with severe and persistent mental illnesses as well as physical illnesses in a state hospital in the State of New York where I worked a few years ago. Patrick was a man of about forty who had been in the state hospital for approximately fifteen years, since his mid-twenties.

In a team meeting on one occasion, the staff was discussing why it was that Patrick had such difficulty getting dressed in the morning. One of the morning staff piped up and said, "I remind Patrick to comb his hair or put on his socks and shoes (the staff there had learned to say "socks and shoes," mentioning socks first, so that no patient would get the notion that you were supposed to put on your shoes and then put on your socks).

Then another staff member said that she too would remind Patrick to do "whatever he hadn't done already."

An idea began to form in my mind of some possible confusion for Patrick. So, I made a note to see him after the staff meeting. Then we got to the principal reason why Patrick could not be placed in the community. He wet the bed "every night or almost every night." Then, I was told, Patrick would pull up his wet sheets in the morning and pretend he had not wet the bed. (I could imagine anybody of an adult age might feel ashamed of bedwetting and might want to conceal it.) It is true that supplies of dry sheets were readily available, and Patrick knew where to get them. But he would have to take the wet sheets off and carry them down two long corridors to put them in the laundry hamper. And of course, everybody along those two long corridors would know why he was changing his sheets.

Then in the meeting we came to the summary of Patrick's behavior over the preceding six months. At this point, I had been working at this facility only a couple of weeks, so I really didn't know much about Patrick's past behavior.

The treatment plan summary was a most ungrammatical and bureaucratic statement that Patrick was still "failing to conform to social norms" in that he wet the bed. I don't have the actual sentence construction as it was, but it seemed obvious that several people had edited this sentence over a period of time, and no one had gone back to the beginning of the sentence to make sure it all made sense (I have quoted the part that did make some sense.) It went on to say that poor Patrick "consistently failed to master his ADL." (ADL stands for Activities of Daily Living and covers things that everybody has to do every day such as wash, get dressed, go to the bathroom, make their bed, put their dirty clothes in the laundry hamper, etc. In any setting other than the state hospital where meals are provided by the kitchen, ADL might include basic budgeting, food buying, food preparation, putting out the trash and so forth – whatever are the basic things that everybody has to have covered before they can go to school, take on a job, or be a parent, for example.)

Patrick's treatment summary, as it was, suggested a complete failure, and there was no suggestion in the summary of any strategy that might be used to improve matters. I also noticed that it was always Patrick who had failed. There was never any "the staff has failed to teach Patrick to…;" it was always "Patrick has failed to…." And since the only asset listed was good physical health (Patrick's heart condition, which got him on this ward of patients with both physical <u>and</u> mental health problems, was much improved with medication) there was nothing to build a better treatment plan on.

I went to see Patrick after the meeting. To figure out what the problem really was about his getting dressed in the morning, I asked him why, with everyone trying to help him, nothing was happening. I asked him in the way of saying, not, "why have you failed?" but rather "how have we as staff members failed you?"

The picture I got was suddenly understandable. Patrick said, "Well, I'm standing in my room minding my own business, putting a clean sock on, when a nurse comes by and says, 'Patrick, comb your hair.' So I put down my other sock and go to combing my hair and the next staff member comes by and says 'Patrick, finish putting your socks on and then put on your shoes.'" Patrick got very flustered and actually burst into tears of frustration and pounded my desk gently as he said "I'm trying! I'm trying! But none of you gives me time to do what the last person said before you interrupt with another instruction!"

I calmed poor Patrick down and said now I understood what the problem was. I then gave him a piece of paper, asked him to sit in a little alcove outside my office so he wouldn't feel my eye was upon him, and asked him to take his time and write down in proper sequence how he got dressed in the morning from the moment he woke up dressed in pajamas until the moment he was ready to walk off the ward to the treatment mall. I said he could take his time and just do his best.

What he brought me in a few moments was not bad. He had left out putting on deodorant and combing his hair, but otherwise he had gotten everything down. He had also not mentioned what to do with wet sheets.

I didn't manage to finish with Patrick that day because I had to go to another meeting. A few days later when we had another team meeting, I suggested that perhaps someone such as one of the aides could take the information I had and provide Patrick with a complete list in short phrases of what to do in the morning which he would then use as a guide until he had learned it. No one wanted to do this, and so a few days later I did it myself.

I saw Patrick again and asked him about the bedwetting. In answer to a question of mine, he said that he did indeed feel it when his bladder was full, but it was a long distance down the hall to the bathroom and sometimes he "just didn't feel like getting up and walking all that way." I then asked him if he wanted to get out of the institution and live in the community. "Oh, yes," he said with interest and intensity, "Yes, I do want to get out." I then told him that if he wanted to leave the institution, being in control of his bladder was extremely important. The reason, I explained to him, is that a state hospital has a big laundry with an almost limitless capacity to wash urine-soaked sheets. No accommodations in the community, be it a group home, a supported apartment, or family care (this is an arrangement by which a mentally ill person is taken into a family's home and treated like a family member, it's like foster care for adults) – no community setup would be able to accommodate a change of sheets every night or nearly every night. I said that when he woke up in the middle of the night with a full bladder, he should think about his future, and if he wanted to have a future in the community, he'd have to get up and go to the bathroom.

This had never been made clear to him before, and he told me he would change. Then I tackled the question of his ability to get dressed. There was nothing in the sequence of dressing that he was unable to do, which is an important thing to check. Some people do not cooperate with staff about something because they have a disability, a dyslexia, or some other kind of problem. The patient will very often not speak up and say they cannot do what is asked of them – they just don't do it, and don't say anything.

All I had to do was to insert 'use deodorant' and 'comb your hair' in the right places and add at the end, "check to see if sheets are wet or dry; if wet, remove wet sheets and put them in the laundry hamper, get dry sheets and put them on the bed and make the bed; if the sheets are dry, pull up the bed and make it," and we were all set.

I wrote this out in very simple language (for example, item number one was "get up," item number two was "go to the bathroom," item number three was "wash" etc. When I got to socks I said "put on socks, one foot, and then the other" because people who are mentally ill will often put on one and forget about the other one. I told him to put this in his bedside drawer and consult it every morning – meaning, when it says "number one get up, number two go to the bathroom" when he's finished going to the bathroom, he should come back and look at the list and see that it says "number three, wash," do that, come back, and look at the list again and do as it says until he had done the whole list. Each time, undertake one thing, do that, and then check the list again.

About two months later when he had another three month review, everyone said he had vastly improved and his wetting the bed had dwindled to about once a month. The staff was not very certain as to what had brought this about, and they didn't seem to take it as a real change, even though they noticed it. Sometimes staff members will say "oh well he's just doing well for the time being but give it a month or two and he'll slide back into his old ways."

Unfortunately, I was not able to impress the staff with the idea that he was trying very hard to choose to be a capable person who would be qualified to live in the community. They were not convinced, but they heard it and I kept on saying for several more months until I left there. I also revised the treatment plan summary to read "Patrick White". I always put the last name, I do not think we should patronize adults by calling them by their first name only in an official document. I think if the document is signed by Shana Clark MD and so-and-so LCSW (which stands for licensed clinical social worker) so-and-so RN etc. that we should at least call somebody Patrick White (not his name) not "Pat" or some other nickname. In the treatment plan we should say Mr. White. This to my mind is consistent with respecting the dignity of the individual. I know I am in the minority on this; staff feel that if they have known a patient a long time, they are entitled to use the first name as a nickname, such as 'Joey' or 'Susie' or 'Andy'. Yet the physician stays "Dr. Johnson" and the nurse is "Patricia Reveley, RN."

Getting back to what I was saying a moment ago; I changed the summary to read: "Mr. White still has occasional difficulty deciding to get up in the middle of the night. He does feel bladder fullness, but he is not always able to convince himself that a good future lies in keeping the sheets dry and bothering to walk down the hallway to go to the bathroom.

He has improved greatly in his ability to dress himself, with the aid of a very simple sequential list kept in his bedside table."

I remember very clearly Patrick saying that the staff confused him terribly because he would be trying to do one thing and someone would happen by and tell him to do something else so he'd try and do the something else and then a second person would come by and tell him to do a third thing. But I realized that many people don't seem to be able to put themselves in the situation of a person who can be easily confused.

While I couldn't say anything bad about the professionalism of the people in that group, I regret once again that professional concern does not for many people mean kindness or consideration or empathy. It usually means only such things as avoiding taking the patient's expressions of anger personally or putting up with abnormal behavior without obvious judgment. Staff often seems to think that all they have to do when a patient behaves badly is keep their mouths shut. They don't seem to understand that body language and what they're thinking and feeling can cast just as much judgment on the patient as if they were actually saying insulting things. While I very well know that it is hard to put up with patients who can be very nasty, I think it is unfortunate that more staff people don't see the need and the sorrow and the pain underneath the nastiness and think about the suffering human being inside that carapace of negativity.

I think I should at this point mention that I have seen some nurses in my travels – I have to say nurses because the other doctors that are working will see patients on their own (just as I saw my patients on my own) so I don't often see other doctors in action. I run my ward my way and another doctor runs his or her ward his or her way and we might never get to see each other as we are working. But I have seen nurses who have a gift and a kindness and a generosity of spirit that makes my heart sing. I remember in particular one of the nurses in a state hospital in New York where I was once a patient. I am thinking about how this nurse reacted when another patient walked across the day room with lumps of fecal material dropping on the floor behind her. The patient had been severely traumatized – raped by several members of her family when she was young – and had had some bad luck with boyfriends as well. The result was that the patient lived in an almost continual state of dissociation.

Dissociation is a state in which a person's body is in one place, but their mind and soul are somewhere else. Most people are familiar with this because most of us have driven past a destination, forgotten a familiar turn or failed to get off the bus at the right stop, even though we well knew when we were supposed to do so. At such times the body is in our car or on the bus but the mind and soul were somewhere else, perhaps in a daydream, perhaps in a worry, such that they did not come back to the present in time to make the proper turn or get off the bus. Some people have described a state of being in a daze before an accident happens, in explanation of, for example, why they ran a red light.

Our usual explanation for this is that we were "distracted" but there is a difference certainly of degree between distraction and dissociation. Distraction would be a very temporary preoccupation with something else which is somewhere else, whereas dissociation can be a profound absence from one's own body or a profound fracturing of the personality into host and alters (see the description of Dissociative Identity Disorder in Chapter 4).which can last for years or even a lifetime. The young lady who walked across the dayroom with regal gestures dropping feces as she did so was hardly ever present in herself.

I remember a time when I was a patient in that hospital when dinner did not arrive for over an hour. Apparently, there was a failure of the electrical appliances such that frozen food could not be warmed up. Eventually, staff figured out that they could make us all sandwiches, and then they got the appliances functional the next day before lunch. But as we sat in the dining room waiting for something to come up from the kitchen, most of us had our stomachs growling. This young lady's stomach growled just as much as anybody else's did, but she was far away from any idea of feeling hunger – because she simply wasn't connecting to being in this world at this time.

My admiration for the nurse came because as the nurse got out the janitor's bucket to pick up the feces and mop the floor she spoke to the young lady in such a loving, kind way. She invited her to join us, and be with us, to be present where she was, as if inviting her soul and her mind to come back and inhabit her body. I was so much moved by this that I said to the nurse that she had a remarkable gift, and the nurse laughed and said something like "Oh, yeah, that's why I'm mopping shit off the floor." But I said to the nurse that she should not be so self-disparaging because she had a gift of being so kind and wonderful and nearly angelic to this patient. I saw that nurse operate on other occasions, and to me the difference in the way she handled things vs. what others did was very moving.

I'd like to discuss the matter of using the word "care" as in the phrase "I care about you." While what we do as clinicians is routinely referred to as patient care, there is a strict feeling that we should avoid saying that we care to the patient. We should say, trainees are told, that we are "concerned" about the patient.

I am a renegade about this. Since my student days, if a patient asks me "do you care about me?" I say "Yes of course I do – just as I care about all my patients."

The danger of the verb "care," as opposed to the noun, is that apparently if one says to someone "I care about you" the patient may be inclined to take this as a signal of romantic inclination on the provider's part, or, alternatively, that a romantic involvement coming from the patient towards the provider would be welcome.

I find it very unkind of people when asked, "Do you care what happens to me, Doctor?" to say "Well, I am concerned for you." This to me sounds like pushing someone away. But including "I care about you" in a phrase which finishes "as I care about all my patients" says that the patient belongs to a very privileged group, the people who are this provider's patients. It seems to answer people's need to be cared about, without opening the door to an unintended and wholly inappropriate attachment. All I can say is, that by saying it in this way, I know my patients do feel cared about, but I have never had a patient mistake my meaning. In a hospital ward, for example, there may be twenty or twenty-four or thirty patients, and if a patient feels cared about in the same way as twenty-nine other people are, then he or she is not very likely to think that the doctor is falling in love with him or her. At the same time I have not backed away from saying that I care about someone, an avoidance which could be very bruising for our patients.

I'm going to say one more thing under the heading of professionalism. I think we professionals as a group think far too much of ourselves. Some of us have the idea that we are in service to others (please note I say "service," not "help"). Others of us are very proud of our professional attainments and seem to have an idea in our heads that we are in some way more important or more valuable or of greater interest than our charges.

From my point of view, I keep in my head the scripture which says "Whatever you do to the least of these so you do to Me", and I keep in mind that all human beings are children of God and that all of God's children are equally precious. I sometimes have had students, and I have said to them that they must remember that any patient is worth just as much in the eyes of the Almighty as they are. They may be a little uncomfortable with this. I remember one time I was talking to a very smart third year medical student who was destined, he said, for a career as a cardio-thoracic surgeon. He could see nothing of worth in psychiatry. We had just seen a patient who was in her late sixties. She was obese, diabetic, slovenly, spoke poorly and had lost many teeth. I said to the young man that he should remember that she is as precious to Almighty God as he was himself, and he looked at me in horror. I confess I was trying to shake him out of his complacency and out of his dismissal of psychiatry as irrelevant and silly.

I have often said to medical students that whereas I can be certain that I will never be practicing cardio-thoracic surgery, pediatric neurosurgery, or some other subspecialty, everybody in medicine practices psychiatry in one way or another because the patient comes with their "stuff" and the provider comes with his or her "stuff" and either does well with the patient or does badly. The question is, is the cardiac surgeon or the orthopedic surgeon or the pediatric neurosurgeon practicing good psychiatry, or bad?

How well a patient functions depends upon the context they are seen in. I can remember for myself several instances of being hospitalized in a fairly bad state, and rising to being one of the most functional of the patients present. When I was hospitalized for the first time, in 1972, a hospitalization which lasted twenty-five days, I was not permitted for a walk out of the building on about day eight, but by day twelve I was elected to be one of the officers of the patients' council, and by day fifteen I was ordering the supplies for the kitchen, secretary of the patients' council, organizing trips to various places (meaning, talking with social workers and art therapists about having excursions to those places, and asking who among the patients might be able to go). Admittedly, this was in the day when a patients' council brokered a lot of decisions about life on the ward, because patients generally stayed long enough so that people could get to know them, and therefore peer pressure could be used as a tool to get the patients going about improving such things as personal grooming, etc. It also was a time when an enterprising patient could be doing quite a bit.

But then, when I got discharged, instead of having several people wanting to talk to me, I would be living by myself, and usually my level of function took a nosedive for a while until I adjusted to this new condition of living.

The era of the therapeutic community had a lot to recommend it, not the least of which was that a considerable amount of day-to-day decision making could be done by the patients if their decisions were reasonable. This gave the patients a feeling of being respected.

That era is gone, I think forever, because of the continued shortening of average length of stay. A place where a person is admitted, diagnosed, treated, and discharged within a week or at the very most two weeks cannot sustain a therapeutic community because there's too much turnover in the patients.

Furthermore, a lot of the treatment becomes "one size fits all" and, the therapeutic groups can degenerate into things like lists of things to do when you feel blue or lists of strategies for anger control. It can be good to engage people by having the members start with making a list, but the list should not be the group's destination. The treatment needs to be much more individualized if an individual patient is going to benefit from it.

Let's take the case of Richard. Richard was admitted to a hospital at the age of nineteen, having been diagnosed with schizophrenia at the age of sixteen. He was admitted to the hospital, because he was psychotic and had anger management problems as well. Because of his psychosis, his family did not know how to react to his anger.

Richard had a history of throwing things when he got mad. He would pick up whatever was handy, be it a stuffed animal belonging to a younger sibling that would not suffer any damage when thrown, to his grandmother's most treasured heirloom china; whatever came to hand, Richard threw it. His internal emotional temperature went up slowly at the beginning, and then reached a critical point, where, if no intervention were made, he would be throwing whatever was near his hand.

The standard list of things to do when you get angry, which includes such things as take a walk, throw a basketball, or talk to a friend, did not work well for Richard. What he needed was a) help in recognizing that he was becoming angry early on in his escalation and b) help in talking about what was upsetting him. He needed to learn how to say "I don't like the idea that we are not going to go to Grandma's tomorrow!" or "I feel that you are being very disrespectful in telling me that I cannot do x, y, and z until I have had a shower!" because in Richard's family they tried to handle his reluctance to shower by simply saying "If you don't get under the showerhead with running water within two minutes, you're grounded and you won't go Grandma's." No one ever discussed things with him when he <u>wasn't</u> angry.

Richard was rather alienated from his contemporaries because of the schizophrenia, but he and his grandmother shared a wonderful bond. In Richard's case, what we had to do was sit down with his family and arrange more reasonable consequences, explain to Richard many many times why showering was so important for his functioning in society, and encourage him to use words rather than throw things.

The list of alternate activities was not useful, because by the time he picked up something and threw it, he was much too angry to be able to remember a list. And at the time when he needed to deescalate his mounting negative feelings, he needed to use words rather than, say, going out of the house and taking a walk. We tried having him take a walk when he was really angry and, when cooled down, come <u>back</u> to speak about what he was angry about, but this did not work for him.

Also, his family needed to have explained to them how to respond when he was uncooperative. They also needed a lot of work to teach them to <u>expect</u> he would cooperate rather than saying things like "Of course a loser like you won't do this, but just for the record I'll say you need to shave" and to teach him that there is great dignity in doing what you should be doing. Also, his family needed to learn that they had to be consistent with the application of any consequences or penalties, which should be well known in advance. Consequences to behavior should be known, not a capricious spur-of-the moment decision on the part of exasperated family members.

A lot of people who teach anger management may say that all of this may be part of anger management. I do know that. I said that in some places (not all, thank goodness) anger management has degenerated into lists, because the emphasis of the institution is on admissions, very hasty therapy and medication adjustment, and very rapid discharge. Some places have a high rate of what we in the trade call "bounce backs" which are people who come back into the hospital immediately after they have been discharged. Usually, this is operationalized to be a readmission somewhere (the same hospital or a different one) less than thirty days after a discharge. Before I consider working at a place, I will ask how many bounce backs they have. Of course, the high ups in a badly run place may not be aware of their proportion of bounce backs, so the people who have a job on offer may not be able to give accurate information. But this is certainly something that patients and families can be aware of when they are inquiring as to the quality of care at a given institution. Note that a readmission a year or two or three later may add up to many admissions in a lifetime, but the person has <u>lived</u> in the community between admissions.

I have said many times in this book that we as families, or providers, or the general public, allow ourselves much too much entrenched negativity about mental patients. A patient who is not expected to get better by anyone has to have an enormous amount of energy to achieve progress in spite of all those negative expectations. I know; I've been there, and I was one who had enough energy to counter all the negativity that surrounded me, (mostly because I felt that the providers did not know me or understand me). On the other hand, that does not mean we should fail to tell a person what is really going on.

Here I will tell a personal story of what happened to me when I was a patient in an NY State Hospital in 1987. I was nearing discharge and had secured the job that paid me $8 an hour (minimum wage was under $6 an hour at that time) calling the chiefs of various computer programs around the country, and asking them a series of marketing questions which our client wanted answered. I was paid more than the others because I could get hold of the head honcho of some very prestigious university's computer science department himself, and did not have to settle for the opinion of an assistant or a secretary. The idea was that I would save up enough money for my key money and my first month's rent on an apartment, and a little money for food, and then I would leave the hospital.

The hospital had set up meal times so that each nursing shift would have to deal with serving one meal. This meant that breakfast was served towards the end of the night shift. The rule was that everybody had to go to breakfast, if they went, in street clothes, so that one had to get dressed and be in the dining room by 6:30 a.m. Then one was supposed to come back to the room, undress for morning showers if one wished to take a shower in the morning, and then dress again for the day. Patients were not allowed to go to the dining room in their sleeping clothes with a bathrobe on because many patients had holes in their clothes and would have been exposing themselves to appear in public so dressed. Hence the rule that one went to the dining room in street clothes only.

You can understand that having dressed for breakfast, most people did not want to get undressed for a shower in the morning only to get dressed again. Therefore most people showered in the evening.

I always showered in the morning, because the showers were almost empty at that time and I found it much easier to be dealing with undressing and soap and water and all those things when there was not a racket around me. I was at that time already somewhat unsteady on my feet, and so dropping the soap and having to pick it up was a major effort, not to fall over. So I would have to think very carefully about where I put things, to avoid dropping them.

The showers in the morning were supposed to open at seven-thirty a.m. But they were never opened on time. At that time, the nursing staff were all in the nurses' station discussing the patients for the change from night shift to day shift.

I would wait until seven-thirty five (I always give people five minutes) and knock on the nurses' station door and ask to have the showers opened. Since the ward schedule included opening the showers at that time, nobody could refuse me. There was a young nurse's aide who was detailed to go with me and sit just outside the shower. (Showers are supposed to be supervised in case somebody falls or faints or has a medical problem when they are in the shower). This young lady came with me every morning and opened up the shower and let me in, and sat outside the shower until I came out again. She was supposed to mark down on a sheet that I had showered, but I found to my ruing that she did not bother to do this.

Sometime after I began working to save the money to have my key money and rent money and food money for when I would leave the hospital, it came up to almost ten days that this young lady had not marked down that I had showered. The ward psychologist noticed this, and concluded that I refused to shower. So she wrote in the chart her opinion that I was having difficulty with commercial employment and was expressing my difficulty by acting out (refusing to shower), and further wrote that she planned to cancel my pass had I not showered before a certain date.

Then, one night, there was a real fire somewhere in the building. It may not have been more than flames in a wastebasket, for example, but it was a real fire, so we had to get to the lobby downstairs. This occurred in the middle of the night, so it was not hard for the patients to understand that it was a real fire, not a drill, and they needed to hurry up. But the patients, instead of focusing on lining up and getting downstairs, panicked, or at least many of them did.

I sympathized with the nurses (there were only two of them for twenty-eight very ill patients) and so I started getting people to focus and get lined up, to calm down and realize that a fire in the wastebasket on another floor was really no danger to us, it was just policy that we get downstairs.

The next night, the night nurse told me that because she appreciated my help from the night before, she was going to be nice and give me a heads up that I either had to take a shower that night or all my privileges to leave the floor (and go to my job) would be cancelled the following morning.

I asked her if she was uncomfortable being near me. "Because" I said to her, "this is midsummer and if I hadn't showered in ten days, your nose would tell you. I just want you to realize you're not uncomfortable being near me, so my story that I shower in the mornings, which is verifiable by checking with the day shift head nurse, must be valid."

The night nurse replied that I could run the risk if I liked, but since the matter was only of taking one shower that evening which would save me the problem, why not just take a shower? So I did.

What I would like to focus on is that the psychologist, instead of asking me was there a problem with my job, instead of telling me she had noticed there was no record of my showering and was wondering if I were expressing something by refusing to shower, never approached me. She asked me nothing, and set it up so that my privileges would be revoked the following day without telling me.

There was a man whose privileges had been revoked the week before. He told all the patients all about it, but didn't speak to any of the professionals responsible.

I always find as a physician, that the first thing to do when I have indications that all is not well with a particular patient, is to get my facts straight. This involves talking to other professionals; it also involves speaking to the patient, and giving the patient a chance to present a different view of the story. At least half the time, in my experience, the details of the facts are in the patient's favor. I have encountered very few patients in my career in a hospital who attempt to lie to me, at least not about a dispute with another patient or with staff.

Outpatients are a different story, because people who come in from the outside world who will be in the patient's role for an hour, realize that you can't check up on them, and substance abusing outpatients are notorious for the stories they will tell. It still is the provider's business to get to the bottom of the story, but it can be quite a bit more difficult.

I would like my colleagues to take note of this story, because there were dozens like it that happened to patients of mine where a staff member presumed that something is the case which is not true, just like the psychologist presumed that I had not showered because the nurse's aide had not done her duty and made a record of my showering. I remained indebted to the night nurse who let me in on what was going on and gave me an opportunity, by taking a shower the night after the fire, to thwart the plans of the psychologist to take away my privileges.

I would like to suggest that something as draconian as taking away all off-ward privileges should not be done without warning. We, the providers, should stop playing 'cat and mouse' with our patients.

Now I'm going to tell the story of a patient that was my patient when I was the attending, a story that turned out rather differently. The patient, Clifford, was in the chronic ward of a state hospital in Pennsylvania when I was working there. Cliff had a sort of sallow complexion, I thought he might be of southern Mediterranean ancestry in spite of his German surname. He was one of the worst people to refuse to shower. If you could get him to go under the shower heads he would allow only a few drops to drip on him, and then, without ever really getting wet, he would pronounce that he had finished his shower and insist on going to get dressed.

I remember a team meeting with him in which he said he was fed up because he had been in a state hospital for twenty years, and he just wanted to get out of the hospital and go home. I asked him if he knew why we all thought he wasn't ready to go home? He answered, he was not sure.

So I said, "It's summertime in Pennsylvania, Cliff, and since you don't really shower when you're in the shower, you stink. I can smell you from here," which was from across a large meeting table. "Until you can keep your body clean, you are not going anywhere."

Cliff replied that it was very unfair that he had been "locked up" for twenty years. He suggested that he didn't think that showering was all that important, but I interrupted and said, "If you will agree to shower -- which means really get wet, sopping wet, then lathering up with soap, scrub-scrub-scrubbing with the soap and then washing all the suds and dirt off every day, you can be discharged. Come back in a month having showered every single day between now and then, and we're talking discharge."

So Cliff agreed to it.

The following month he came back and he was several skin shades lighter. His skin color was the pale pink-and-white of the northern German ancestry his last name suggested. He told me he had showered every day, I asked for the shower roster to check that, and then I said "Fine. We're talking discharge."

Unfortunately for him, Pennsylvania had just shut down their state hospital in Harrisburg, and the remaining Harrisburg clients, all four hundred of them, had been sent to homes and hospitals all over the state, so that, when I had this talk with Cliff, the system was rather full up. Therefore, I did not get to discharge him before my assignment ended.

But I did use a real consequence (namely telling him that people do not like people who smell bad) to get him to change his behavior sufficiently that his appearance became several skin tones lighter. Sometimes, it's best to really tell it like it is. We do not do favors by refusing to be candid. Cliff had not been told this in so many words before, though people had done all sorts of things to try and get him to shower, without having him understand why it was important. Once he understood that it was important enough to cancel his discharge possibilities, he decided to cooperate and become dischargeable.

Please realize that when I told Cliff he stank and that I could smell him from across the table, I said it in a pleasant, matter-of-fact tone, as if I were saying we needed to make lemonade, or that the temperature outside was 88° F. There was no disrespect in my voice or body language, no exasperated self-righteousness. I provided him with some factual information (about his malodorousness), the ongoing consequence this had on confirming the team's decision that he was not a candidate for discharge, and the possibility of a different consequence which would follow changed behavior on his part. I gave him a clear choice -- to shower, really shower, daily, or to fail to do so, during a set timeframe of 30 days. I explained simply and straightforwardly and left him to choose.

Some mentally ill people may continue to choose badly for a long time. But how often do we put them in front of a clear choice? We often say "you don't do it right!" without explaining why it is so important they do differently, and exactly <u>how</u> to do what we want them to do. After two or three attempts, we allow ourselves to be sarcastic and exasperated, and to give ourselves airs of superiority.

No-one, be he a homeless, toothless, hallucinating street man, or the CEO or professor, or artist of great eminence, will make effortful changes in behavior unless they see themselves as choosing a preferable consequence. As professionals, we need to provide information so patients can make a thoughtful choice, and, if need be, we need to motivate our patients.

But a fictitious superiority, sarcasm, or mockery have NO PLACE in our professional toolbox. If we model for families how to treat patients properly, the families may learn more constructive ways of communicating with their mentally ill members. I do wish we could get beyond petty egotistical attitudes in our dealings with patients. It is in that spirit, in that hope, that I tell the following story.

Shortly after I took over as attending on one of the chronic wards of the Binghamton Health Center in Binghamton, New York (it is a state hospital) I was accosted by one of the patients as follows: "You goddamn motherfuckin' cunt whore bitch!"

According to my training, any obviously deliberately targeted use of foul language such as the above should be met with "How dare you address a physician in such a fashion? I am going to cancel your grounds privileges" (the patient's right to go out on the grounds of the mental hospital by himself) "for a week!"

Please note that a person who does this has no idea why the patient addressed them thus – what is going on in the mind of the patient. I would submit that a better answer would be "Oh, Mr. Jones – you're upset. Come into my office and talk to me." The Mr. Jones in question (of course that is not his real name) told me that his mother had sent him three pair of briefs, as he said, "brand new and really clean" for Christmas. He had worn them and washed them in the ward washing machine, but when he went to take his load out of the dryer, they were missing. Mr. Jones concluded "Someone took my mother's Christmas present and I'm holding you personally responsible, Dr. Clark."

I did tell the patient that I am not personally responsible for everything that everyone else decides to do, but I did also tell him that I would have the staff quietly look for his briefs. I took down some information about the size, the brand, the appearance of the waistband etc., and told my staff to slowly go through all the other rooms during the day. I also told Mr. Jones not to mention their disappearance to anyone.

At around mid-afternoon they were found, in the room of a man who had been sent to us after having spent three days in intensive care because he was brought into an acute care hospital unresponsive, in a very bad state, with his electrolytes (salts in the blood) quite abnormal. During his stay in intensive care, it was determined that he was a psychiatric patient and arrangements were made to send him to our facility.

I gave Mr. Jones back his clean briefs, and told him again that he should not be speaking to anyone about the fact of their disappearance. I simply said to him "You got your property back, and there's an end to it. I don't want to hear anything more about it." I then made an announcement to the patients to the effect that when they put their wet clean laundry into the dryer, they should make a note of the time, and since the dryer ran for one hour, return to the dryer in a little less than an hour so that clean laundry did not spend any time unattended in a non-moving machine.

As for Mr. Jones, two conversations and ten days later, he came to me one morning and said "Good morning. Excuse me, Dr. Clark, could I have a word with you sometime today? I just need a few moments of your time, but I really do have a problem I need to talk about with you." Notice that he had gone all the way from a string of expletives to "Good morning" and "excuse me" in a matter of ten days.

I will also add that this patient had been sent to me by another ward as "incorrigible". I did ask Mr. Jones about why he had been furious with me initially, and he said in effect that he assumed that we were going to be indifferent to his plight as the institution had been indifferent to his loss of clean new clothing a number of times previously.

The contrast between my chronic ward and the other chronic ward became so marked that people took to assuming that I had all the "easy" patients whereas in point of fact if a patient was ungovernable on another ward, they were sometimes sent to me.

The main idea that I would like my colleagues to take away from the above story is that if we are interested in why the patient is so upset as to be using filthy language to us, more than protecting our own delicate egos against unprintable language, we might get a good bit further towards helping our patients. If I had merely said the "how dare you…." and taken away his grounds privileges, I would have made Mr. Jones transit from a frustrated patient to a frustrated patient who feels like he is being treated like a caged animal, and he might then have begun to harbor fantasies, at least, of hurting me or other staff.

This is something I saw handled the wrong way over and over and over in my career as a patient, which I will remind you preceded but to some extent overlapped my career as a doctor. One does far better to take a tirade as indicating the patient's level of upset than as indicating a personal insult to the physician. The irony is that I have heard some of my colleagues react strongly to bad language and then half an hour later in a staff meeting use the identical bad language to describe their feeling toward, shall we say, a car mechanic who overcharged them; yet in that instance the physician does not lose any "grounds privileges" or anything similar for merely expressing frustration and would be astounded if a loss of privileges were suggested.

I found repeatedly in many different institutions in different states that treating patients as if I empathized with their upset, but yet expected them to return to decent behavior and printable language in short order because they were grown men and women who were able to be reasonable, got me the result that I asked for.

This is a big chunk of the difference that I made on several different chronic wards in several different institutions, turning them from the most violent wards in the hospital to a place where everyone would say good morning with a smile. I never directly said anything to criticize a patient's use of language, with the result that not infrequently, they would apologize to me the next time they saw me, and the apology was sincere. I also think that my colleagues could think about what it means to a patient if a one minute release of frustration with no threats or dangerous moves, means that the patient cannot walk freely on the grounds for a whole week. I'll leave that for others to think about.

I remember on the first day I arrived at a particular hospital I saw a package on top of a filing cabinet. The package was at about shoulder height, so it wasn't as if it were way too high to be something that other people could notice, given that I am 5'5". The package was addressed to one of the patients and it was sent express mail which is the post office's overnight mail, which meant that it was quite expensive to send.

I asked the nurse in charge whether there was any particular reason why the patient could not have it, noting that the postmark on it was December 18 and we were now in early February. It looked to me as though a family member or friend were trying to be sure, by sending it express mail, that the patient would get it before Christmas. And we were, as I said, already in February. I was told there was no reason she could not get it, so I handed it to the charge nurse and asked her to deliver it to the patient, since I had just arrived and didn't know who was who yet.

The next day I noted that it was still there on top of the file cabinet. I asked again that the nurse deliver it that day, and thought no more about it. On the third day, noting that it was still undelivered, I told the nurse to deliver it. I also said that if she did not deliver it right then and there that I would write her up to the nursing supervisor for insubordination because I had asked her the first day and the second day to deliver it and she had not done so. I do not fathom why the nurse would be reluctant or unwilling to give a patient a Christmas present; it would seem to me that any staff should be delighted to bring a patient a gift, since that would probably brighten the patient's day and the patient might be grateful to that staff member.

The gift was finally delivered and it turned out to be a beautiful sweater from the patient's father, which he had spent a lot of money to try and make sure she received before Christmas, as I had suspected. That left me wondering why in the space between December and February no one had actually given it to the patient. The best explanation I could come up with was that it was in no one's job description and this was a state hospital so people were very often reluctant to do something that could be said to be even a little beyond the scope of their usual duties.

You can understand that patients often think of staff as totally indifferent. Failure to deliver a Christmas gift for over a month is a perfect example.

I remember once when I was hospitalized in a place which had a countertop around the nurses' station and then bulletproof glass up to the ceiling except for a little mouse hole where the patient standing in front of the nurses' station could talk to the people inside. I saw a letter addressed to me in my sister's handwriting propped up against the inside of the glass, so I asked the clerk who sat right next to it to give it to me. She told me that this was not an appropriate time, and so I came back two hours later. Again, she refused to deliver me my letter. So I waited until after the shift change at three o'clock, hoping the afternoon clerk would be a little more reasonable. At three-forty five I approached the afternoon clerk, and she similarly told me it was not a good time, so I asked again at five o'clock and was about to be refused again and I said in a very level tone, sounding not in the least upset, "I have been trying to get someone to hand me that letter since nine o'clock this morning. What I need you to do is reach forward, pick up the letter, and then move your hand about four inches to the mouse hole and hand it to me. Couldn't you just give it to me instead of having another conversation to tell me that this is the wrong time to ask? I have been very patient all day waiting for someone to give me my letter." At that point, I was finally handed the letter.

I see a pattern here. While staff pay attention to institutional requirements, what a clerk is required to do, what a nurse is required to do, they are not paying attention to patient preferences even when such paying attention takes seconds (as for example in reaching for the letter and handing it to me). This makes me feel very sad that many if not most of hospital staff need an attitude adjustment.

Patients are people; they want the gift from a family member or a letter as much as staff does. Why are so many staff who are well-trained and good at their jobs otherwise, so totally indifferent to the humanity of their patients? There are some exceptions of course, and encounters with those stand out in my mind. But the vast majority of staff behave as if the wellbeing and happiness of the patient were the least of their concern. Getting them their medications on time is important because that's one of their assigned duties, but being polite, being understanding, being nice are nowhere in the list of things they aspire to be, and I just don't get it.

Another thing which I have noticed about staff is that they have absolutely no tolerance of letting a patient express frustration. For example, they may tell a patient that his family, who arranged three weeks earlier to come and visit him, is not coming today. When the patient says, softly, not in a disruptive way, "Damn!" and very softly taps the edge of the desk, causing no harm to anything or anyone, the staff immediately thinks that the patient needs restraint or needs an emergency shot of extra medication.

This is not good for the patient. Everybody has to learn how to cope with frustrations and contretemps and upsets and things not going your way. What surprises me is that each one of these staff members in their private lives could appreciate that saying damn once under your breath and tapping the edge of the desk very gently (in other words, the patient is not screaming, threatening, or doing anything really disruptive) can be done by themselves or by friends and no one suggests restraints or medication.

Now, I can understand that if we are dealing with a patient who has a history of going from being frustrated and swearing under his breath to violence in two minutes, the staff would be concerned. But most patients, like most people, are not like that, and why it is necessary to impose upon the patient that they must behave as if they had reached Nirvana and nothing at all frustrates them then I don't understand.

I often refused to medicate or restrain someone if they said one swear word, if when I talked with the patient he said he was feeling "bummed" out or some other negative but he wasn't threatening anybody. I know this is different from other doctors, some of whom order medication over the 'phone without even asking what the patient has done that is out of line.

It is a much better learning experience for the patient to learn to cope without the crutch of more medicine or restraints, and since these are often situations in which a) it is very understandable the patient would be frustrated and b) the patient's reaction was not disruptive in terms of a scream, a threat or some other behavior which is unacceptable on a mental ward, I would ask staff members who may read this to consider carefully how they behave. I don't think staff need to be as nasty or as thoughtless as they often are.

I'm talking about usual times, not when they are under pressure trying to take care of someone who is dying or in some other particular difficulty for them. I'm talking about the normal, day in and day out work attitude. The professions have an awful lot to work on here.

I suppose I am in a particularly unusual spot, because I've seen this sort of thing from both sides: the patient's side <u>and</u> the provider's side. We are always telling our patients that they must change their behavior; I believe we the staff must change our behavior as well.

I do wish many doctors would realize how arrogant and indifferent they seem, when for a little more effort on their part they could be seen as caring. I know from experience that the idea that the doctor cares is critical for a patient's well-being, and I keep thinking how these arrogant doctors eliminate the possibility of seeing many patients get well, by their own attitude. I suppose this may get better with time, but I wonder if the doctors could think a little more, and try to see the world from the point of view of their patient a bit more. That would go a long way for better results for the patient, and better job satisfaction for the doctors.

I do not think I would be behaving as I should if I did not broach another subject about some of my colleagues' attitude and behaviors. Some people are so negative about their patients' prospects that one wonders if they are just lazy. I know there was one physician who lost his staff position at another State Hospital in New York because he had made a generic progress note and had put that same note, word for word, in several patients' charts for many months running. Apparently, nothing, not even an episode of lithium toxicity that the patient experienced, could induce him to write a progress note which was actually about what was going on with the patient. I find this very sad, and totally unacceptable. I will say that I found it was standard procedure to copy electronically a patient's note from last month (these were long-term chronic patients and only one note per month was absolutely required), "tweak it" a little bit (which meant often rearrange a sentence or two without really putting in any new information) and thus the state requirement of a progress note per month was satisfied.

Shana Wibberley Clark, M.D., Dr. P.H.

I will say that when I worked in state hospitals (and I did work in five of them, spread out over three states) that I never once in my entire professional career did that. Every one of my monthly notes was written from scratch. I never copied anything electronically and so never found myself making errors such as not changing information and so perpetuating (for instance) that a particular incident occurred two months ago when in fact it was three four and five months since the event took place. From my point of view, this ensured that I would actually have to <u>think</u> when I did each patient's note about how they were doing in the past month, rather than mechanically reproducing old (and possibly out-of-date) information.

But what I'm getting at is something more fundamental. Personally, I have no doubt that I have treated some of the sickest people in this country. I have encountered only a handful of people who could not learn and could not improve their behavior if they had a clear incentive to do so – if it were clear to the patient, in other words, that what we considered an improvement in behavior would result in a consequence that the patient found desirable.

Considering that patients are shunted around between doctors to suit the doctors, or the administration, and that most state hospital doctors don't try to connect with their patients, the idea of being more esteemed by the doctor is a very poor motivator. But there are usually quite a few things such as more grounds privileges or more time in the gym etc. which patients are willing to work for. My impression is that they have such a low self-esteem that praise from a doctor who sees them at long intervals has no effect on them, so praise from a savvy nurse who sees them every day or nearly every day might be much more important.

I've often wondered why my colleagues are so negative. I regarded the sicker patients that I had charge of as simply those that were more challenging to me, though I noticed that it seems the kind of person who is willing to become a state employee is not looking for challenge or interest or something new on the job, and tends to regard every lapse in patient behavior as a headache for the staff which is to be stamped on as soon as possible, not as a learning opportunity for the patient.

There have been many prominent people who have let it be known over the last few years that they've had at least one episode of significant mental illness. There is a famous psychiatrist who is schizophrenic, who worked in California, there is a psychologist who is a brilliant researcher who has written a book about being bipolar, and there are eminent parents as well who have written about what it is like to have a schizophrenic child. But although we do have examples of such good control over years that the person can be considered to be functionally cured (even though they continued to take medication and to see the prescriber of that medication), it seems that the profession which should be in the vanguard of advocacy for these people, namely the psychiatrist, is often bringing up the rear.

It is fifteen years since I myself had a significant mood episode. I did hospitalize myself shortly after 9/11/01 because I felt very unsafe (though I am not alone in this). I was hospitalized for five days, and the time away from work was merely taken out of my vacation time. I've had incredible ups and downs over the last fifteen years; my success against my mood disorder is not because my life is very quiet and without incident.

My point here is that my good result in terms of controlling my psychiatric symptoms has not been because I've had a very easy time of it. My good result comes from having developed an ability to cope with whatever adversity comes my way, which is what I used to invite my patients to do.

In no other field of medicine are the practitioners down on their patients for being patients. Surgeons don't despise their patients for getting sick. Neither do internists look down on their patients for having illnesses. Why do we in psychiatry have such a negative take on our charges instead of thinking of the sicker among them as needing more work and more time and being more challenging to our skill, but being people nonetheless? I've never met a patient, even people who have not said a sentence that made sense in thirty years, who wasn't a human being. Why can't we all realize this?

CHAPTER 22

HOW TO MAKE A GEOGRAPHIC MOVE WITHOUT RUNNING OUT OF YOUR MEDS

First, when I say "making a geographic move" what I mean is, making the kind of move such that you will have to change your providers <u>and</u> change your insurance. There are a lot of good reasons to move, such as going to live with someone you care about (and who cares about you also), moving to a better job, moving to a better climate for you (I say better climate for you, because if you are an avid skier you will want to be in a place with lots of snow and winter – different people have different ideas about what is a wonderful climate to live in.) Other reasons to move include going to school, moving somewhere where you may be able to engage in your favorite hobby (I knew one man who moved from New York City to the Finger Lakes district of New York State because he was an avid sailor and he could have a boat up on Keuka Lake without having to spend huge sums of money on marina fees).

Whatever your reason, let's say you are facing that move. About changing providers: if you have known your providers a while and they have served you well, the idea of leaving them may fill you with dismay. Take comfort in the notion that whatever you have learned, be it how to clean a room, how to organize your day, how to avoid getting stuck in memories of events long gone, how to cope with your other symptoms, or wisdom about life – whatever you have actually learned, you will take with you. You will start at your new place with your new providers from a new baseline. They may not understand how bad it used to be (assuming you have made some progress since the beginning), but they also will not be able to look down on you because you once were in a sorry state. They will treat you as the healthier person that you are, and might even see you as having more potential than your present providers do.

If, on the other hand, you have never fit in very well with your present group of providers, then an iron-clad need to change – because you have to move – might not be a bad thing. Life is an adventure; try always to remember that you are a <u>person</u> with a diagnosis or with particular symptoms or with particular difficult experiences; you are a great deal more than a mental health diagnosis. To run your life according to your psychiatric patient status is indeed to let the tail wag the dog.

Now, as to choosing a new provider: look over what I said about choosing a provider in the beginning of the book. Realize that you should always go for someone that you would like to be talking to even if you did not have your mental health problems. If you have no clue as to how to find a good provider for yourself, but yet you have moved to your new place and have met a decent primary care provider, ask him or her where he or she would send a spouse or a close family member for treatment, and see if you can go there.

If you will be going to a public clinic, realize that you probably will first meet an intake worker who will take down some essentials such as your name, telephone number, address, age, and next of kin, and a general description of the problem, and then you will be assigned to a provider and put on the schedule. This may cause a delay in actually seeing your new provider.

This is what happened to me when I came back from six and a half years in Belgium in 1981. I could hardly call transatlantically to set up appointments in New York City, and I knew perfectly well that I would not go forward with my medical career until July 1 of that year. So I had a period from late January to July to fill in. I got myself a temporary job as a secretary, and then looked up a public clinic in the city which would serve my needs for getting my medication. Seeing the intake worker was not difficult; I was given an appointment during my 'phone call. But I did not realize when I walked into her office that she would not give me an appointment with the prescriber until seven weeks later.

This is because there is a regulation on the books that all patients discharged from a hospital in New York City must be seen by a prescriber within the week. Add to these people just exiting from the hospital those patients that the prescribers have who have been out of the hospital for some time, and the prescriber's calendar is filled quickly. A new patient coming from the outside world (that is, not coming from a hospital discharge) is the last in order of priorities for the prescriber to see. This is why a new outpatient gets a long wait before they see the doctor. This is what will happen to you too if you wait until your move is made before you make your appointment.

This is why my suggestion to you is if you know that you will reach New City on the first of June, call in April and make an appointment to see the intake worker for June 10th and to see the doctor shortly after that. If you can give a New City address (your plans to stay with your friend or your choice of a residential hotel have crystallized) and you give your 'cell phone number or your telephone contact, making an appointment will be easy to do.

But I, coming back from Belgium did not know any of this, since I had always gone to clinics after a hospital discharge, and those patients are first priority in the clinic's schedule. When the intake worker told me I would have to wait seven weeks to see the prescriber, I asked what I should do since I had been living abroad and had no prescriptions for the intervening seven weeks. I actually had about ten days' medications left but, as I explained, I thought I would be seeing the prescriber very soon. So the intake worker suggested I have "tide over" prescriptions until I see my new provider. Fortunately the bottle that I had from Belgium each mentioned the generic name of the medicine, which is international, in addition to the French language brand name, which is not the same as English. So the doctor in that clinic knew what medication I was on. When I got the medication I left the clinic immediately. I had had to wait two hours to get the "tide over" prescriptions, and I was very anxious to leave that very noisy environment.

That's where I made my mistake. The physician who wrote the prescriptions for me had written half the dose per pill of one of my medications than I was used to. So, to keep taking my usual doses, I had to use up the pills twice as fast. The doctor had been very reluctant to give me a thirty day supply with one refill (necessary to have enough medication for seven weeks) and when I went back to the clinic showing him the bottle from Belgium and the prescriptions he wrote, it took almost two more hours to straighten things out.

This is why I tell my patients to a) accumulate a supply in the ways that are detailed in this chapter before they make a move and b) if they are going to a public clinic, call the clinic and make an appointment with the intake worker and the prescriber long before they actually make the move.

I would also say to anyone that before you leave the clinic (or more precisely before you leave the prescriber's presence) you review all your medications to make sure you have the right number of milligrams per pill, the right number of pills to be taken every day, and therefore the right total number of pills to be given to you. If you are not good at doing mental arithmetic, I would suggest you write this out in advance so you can compare what the doctor wrote very quickly with your list. After all, better do that which might take ten or fifteen minutes than have the doctor make a mistake and have to go back to the clinic in which you saw the doctor, explain your situation to half a dozen people and wait for that doctor or a colleague of his or hers to give you a fresh prescription. Physicians as a rule do not like to admit they made a mistake, and they are always very busy, so to interrupt them, get their attention and get the mistake corrected is a major undertaking. Also, if the clinic keeps a list of the medications you are on, make sure that that list is accurate and stays accurate. Otherwise, people will simply point to their list and tell you that your notions are faulty.

Now about building up a supply of your medication before making a move. If you fill your prescriptions every thirty days, you are probably allowed to fill them after the twenty-second day, in other words you may fill them on day twenty-three, twenty-four, twenty-five, twenty-six, twenty-seven, twenty-eight, twenty-nine or thirty at no additional charge. If you know for some time that you are likely to be moving (even if you are not sure where you will be moving to) then start filling your prescriptions on day twenty-three several months before you go. Also, find out if your insurance of the place that you are leaving allows you to have what is called a "vacation override". A vacation override is a once-a-year permission to get sixty days' worth of medication at one time, because the person is going to be on vacation and out of their usual area when their medication is due to be refilled. It is wise to inquire about this some time before you are actually going to be leaving, because some form filling may be needed. Also, you must do it in advance so that you are covered by insurance in Old City for the full sixty days from the day your prescriptions are filled. That may be up to 75 days if you have to mail the script in. Don't forget to allow extra time if there is a holiday in those 14 or 15 days that you are allowing for the script to get there and the time to get it filled and sent back to you. If you know you will be moving, go ahead and order your vacation override 3-4 months before the move. (The vacation override is sent to your present (pre-move) address.)

Do not think of this as necessarily to be used only for vacation. The 'vacation' designation is to explain to the insurance company why once a year they will provide sixty days' worth of meds at once. It allows a person to be out of their home area one time out of twelve. If you are planning to move, by all means get your vacation override and leave town with an extra supply of medications. Also, if you have at the same time been filling your prescriptions twenty-three days after you last filled them (see above) you will accumulate a week's worth of medication for every month in which you fill in advance in that fashion. As soon as you know you're going to be moving, or even if you know that there is some likelihood that you may not be staying (though your moving plans may not have crystallized yet), start doing this. You don't have to explain or apologize to anyone and it may get you those extra few weeks of meds before you can find a new provider in your new location.

If you are a person who fills your medications through a ninety day supply house (which would mean you have been taking the same medications for some time, because this arrangement is meant for people who must take their medications chronically, not for people who are going to be having their medication changed with some frequency), you may usually fill your medications any time during the third month. An exception is new medications which are still under patent which can be horrendously expensive. These, your insurance will probably not want to let you have a month before you run out If the medication is fairly new, you may be able to get some samples from your provider's office, or there may be a patient assistance program such that the manufacturer will give you free meds.

Patient assistance programs are means-tested (they won't play if your income is above a certain amount, which may be different for different medications). They may require you to have a form filled out by your present provider (i.e. the provider of the place you're leaving) and they may also require an explanation as to why older medications which are off patent are not advisable in your case. For example, for anti-depressants, it is often required that three medications be listed that the patient has already taken which were a) ineffective or b) not tolerated – that means they caused a reaction such that the patient couldn't keep taking them, for example the patient had an all-over-the-body rash or other severe allergic reaction or was very sleepy when they took this medication. (The latter is a little harder to prove.) This is where having a little list of what medications you've been on and what happened when you took them with the dates and the dosages can be invaluable because you can simply trot this out any time your doctor has to fill a form and have the information ready to hand. It is not a good thing to be saying "Oh, I think I've taken that, but I'm not sure what happened with it" – because that won't convince anybody that you cannot take it again. See the description of how to keep a medication history in Chapter One.

I cannot say too strongly to my colleague providers that the kind of expectations we have for our patients is mirrored by the kind of results we get. If a patient is treated as if they are childish, lazy, irresponsible, negative, etc. it takes an ENORMOUS amount of energy on the patient's part to countermand that and to succeed in spite of us. We would have so much better outcomes if we assumed that a good outcome is not only possible, but probable, and that the beginning of constructive change will be evident fairly soon. Any successful businessman or professional succeeds in part because they think they are going to succeed. A surgeon does not pick up the scalpel thinking to himself "I can't possibly do this". A teacher does not say "My class will never pay attention, or write their papers, or take the final exam." A policeman does not pursue the suspect thinking "I'll never catch him, and if I do ever catch him, I couldn't possibly arrest him, and if I did arrest him I couldn't possibly read him his rights." Whole books are written on the subject of staying positive. Yet we surround mental patients with a negativistic atmosphere day in day out. And then of course when they fail, when they show no interest in a program, when they don't make any effort to come and see us, we say, "You see? They're lazy, or they don't understand even though they've been told that they have to take care of their illness, and there's nothing we can do." And we go through the motions, convinced in advance of failure.

Now about getting appointments in a new place: when you know when you're going to move and where exactly you are moving to, it is not a bad idea, unless you're going to be paying for private sector care, to call the county mental health clinic. You can find out which county your new town is in on the internet, and, armed with that information, you look up the telephone number for the "Cayuga County Mental Health Department," or some such.

My point is, if you know you're moving to New City on the first of June, you call the county mental health center in April and say that you would like an appointment with the intake worker for June 10, (having checked that it is a weekday). Give the address of the friend you will stay with, or the residential hotel you plan to stay in for the first few days in June, and your cell phone. Then you don't have to have a two month wait to see the intake worker when you get to New City. You give yourself ten days after arrival because you don't want to be having to dash out to the mental health clinic the very day after you've arrived, but you're not wasting time on a waiting list, using up your carefully accumulated supply of medications, and running out of medications before you even get to see that intake worker.

Now, some clinics will have a prescriber appointed to give "tide over" prescriptions to anyone the intake worker sees that day who needs medication. These "tide over" prescriptions would be for more of of what you can prove was prescribed before the move. This is generally something you have a prescription for, or something you have the bottles for that say what medication it is, how many milligrams per pill, and how many pills you take when during the day.

There is an advantage for having gotten to the point of stability and being able to use a ninety day supply. One is that you get ninety days of pills for one copay, rather than thirty days of pills three times for three copays, so you do save some money. The other is that these supply houses will generally send the pills to anywhere within the forty-eight continental states, if you have refills left and if you are still covered by your old insurance on the day the supply house is asked to send you a refill of the prescriptions.

You may not realize it, but your prescriber in your old city has the ability to write prescriptions which can be filled only in states in which that particular prescriber is licensed. The only exception to this is, if that prescription is either sent over the internet, faxed, telephoned by the doctor's office, or sent by postal mail to these supply houses. I personally worked for fifteen years in many different states east of the Mississippi, having medications sent to me based on prescriptions written in New York State by my New York State provider. If I were in Wisconsin and he sent me a prescription, and I in turn sent it to the supply house (which I believe was headquartered in Texas, with another office in Ohio), then the supply house would send me the medications to wherever I happened to by anywhere in the lower 48. All I had to do was call up the supplier and let them know my current address. So I did not have to worry when my work took me to another state that I didn't have a prescriber for (a Wisconsin prescriber for Wisconsin, or a Maine prescriber for Maine, or an Alabama prescriber for Alabama etc.) Most retail pharmacies that you walk into are still limited to filling prescriptions written by a prescriber licensed in that state.

Occasionally a national chain can oblige you, if you walk into a national chain pharmacy in one state and they communicate with your pharmacy in your home state and the home pharmacist says, yes, indeed, this person does take this medication, and the last fill was on such a date, you can then get the national chain to give it to you where you are, but they are doing you a favor. (This does not work for controlled substances such as opioid pain killers, benzodiazepines and stimulants used in ADHD.) Sometimes people want to be helpful, and sometimes they're not in such a positive frame of mind, so I prefer to work with the system where the system thinks it's perfectly normal to send my New York doctor's prescriptions to anywhere in any of the lower forty-eight states. I have not gone into what would happen if I were to go to Alaska or to Hawaii for an extended period of time, but if I were going to do that I would make inquiries by calling the customer service department of the supply house that sends me my meds. I would get an individual's name before I go, so that I know whom to call when I get there.

The one thing you have to keep in mind is, that with the exception of using the supply houses for existing refills of medications you take continuously, your provider in the old city may not be able to send you a prescription or to arrange for medication under his authority to be sent to another state, and your provider may very well not want to do it in the same state, after you have left that provider and are no long his or her patient. In other words, if (shall we say) you move from Buffalo in Western New York to New York City and you run out of medications in New York City before you get to a New York City prescriber, it will not do you much good to call your provider in Buffalo. Certainly, providers in a public clinic do not want to give medications to someone they are not going to see. And if you go to another state where your provider is not licensed, then except for the supply houses of medications that are taken continuously as described above, there's nothing your provider in the old city <u>can</u> do.

I remember I had a family of patients (meaning the mother, the father and two of the children were all in treatment) who suddenly decided that they were going to leave Mansfield, Pennsylvania and go to Tennessee. Maybe they took a long time to make the decision; I don't know. But they certainly did not say anything until a few days before they moved to either me or their social worker therapist or the personnel in the front office who schedule appointments, about thinking about moving to Tennessee.

I got a distress call one day saying that the children had run out of their medications. But the family had no connection to a supply house, and I told them that even if I sent them a prescription, it would not be valid in Tennessee. I told them I was licensed in seven states, but Tennessee did not happen to be one of them.

Now I will add that the last two appointments I had with this family (the last only two weeks before they left), I did tell them that if they were thinking of moving they should orchestrate this beforehand. I suggested they make an appointment in Tennessee before they left Pennsylvania since it's a few days' drive away. (That's what I suggested above about calling in April or May and making an appointment with the intake worker for the tenth of June if you think you're going to arrive in your new town on June first.) But they were not willing to have any planfulness, and so there was nothing I could do to help them.

I am trying to make my reader a savvy consumer. It is a royal headache to have to do all this, but if you do it and just get it done it's like other headaches in life – paying your taxes, sorting through a distant relative's possessions when they die, whatever – it's just one of those things that has to get done. You can do what you need to, or refuse to do it and pay the consequences. And for some, if they run out of medications they may well end up in a mental hospital.

I don't like to think what would have happened to that family if all four of them had run out of their medications and they were in a state of total disarray unable to cope with much of anything. I tried and tried to interest them in planning their move. They did have the idea that they had to move out at the end of "a month" (when I said earlier that they did not say they had decided to move to Tennessee, it was because they said "Well we may go at the end of some month or other," and did not specify when. They knew they had to move out at the end of the month because they didn't want to be paying rent in Pennsylvania for the next month. And they knew that they had to put all their possessions in boxes and suitcases and get them carted out of their premises. But there was nothing I could do to convince them that they also had to plan their move from the point of view of psychiatric providers and medications. I have wondered many times since then whatever happened to those people. They must have been in a terrible mess.

CHAPTER 23

HOW TO TALK TO A MENTALLY ILL FAMILY MEMBER

Greeting

When you see your family member, be sure to greet her, if possible, with the same enthusiasm and level of informality that you are mutually used to. In other words, if in the outside world your usual is "Hi, Susie! How are you doing?" said with an all-enveloping hug, try to do something similar when Susie is in the hospital. It is a tremendous downer for the patient if the aunt who used to greet her as described now says in a subdued voice "Well hello, Susan," with no hug. I don't mean force yourself to do something that is not genuine, but consider what effect a big change will have on poor Susan/Susie who is struggling against a major problem thinking, behaving, etc. and who may have been counting on your greeting to keep her going for that day. In other words, give the greeting some thought; if you are feeling uncomfortable seeing her in the mental hospital, you can say "It feels uncomfortable to see you in the hospital. I'm longing to see you out of here." Better admit it's the surroundings, than have Susie think it is <u>she</u> who makes you so uncomfortable.

When I was first hospitalized in Belgium, because I went to see a French-speaking doctor an hour early by mistake, a Dutch-speaking doctor came into the waiting room and talked to me, and when I said that I would go and register myself for the June exam session, he said, "You are not going anywhere," and punched me with a right uppercut to my jaw, knocking me over backwards. This same Dutch-speaking doctor took me to his hospital and I was there from April to August 1975. During those four months, my sister visited me I think four times, but my mother only came once. My sister did hug me; my mother did not. In fact, my mother had to be persuaded to speak to me. This caused a permanent deterioration in our relationship. My mother did negotiate when later that year I wound up in a French-speaking hospital, to get me Professor Herbert Guillemot as my attending, by waiting in his waiting room for a whole day and most of the next day, until he would see her. She also negotiated, a few years later, that the United States Embassy sent a letter to the Belgium insurance saying that the United States government would take umbrage if I were essentially kicked out of Belgium for spending too much money in their health care system, given that my father had given so much of his time to the establishment of the Common Market.

My mother knew how to do extraordinary things in times of genuine crisis, but she just couldn't cope with ordinary problems. Also, she wanted always to be the center of attention and when a member of the family is in a mental hospital, at least when you are visiting them, they should be the center of attention, not you.

Please be understanding if the patient does not meet your expectations as far as his or her appearance when you get to the hospital. If you have a pass to take Susie off the grounds, I suggest you do some soul-searching if you find yourself wanting to say "Do you have to wear checkered pants and a flowered print blouse?" At any rate, do say hello and show some warmth and some affection before you come up with any comments on your family member's appearance. You, as a well family member, have no idea what your family member who is the patient, is going through, and you have no idea how much effort has gone into getting ready to see you. So if the patient is clean but oddly dressed, or well-dressed but perhaps not so clean, cut them some slack and don't protest much. If you really need to say that they stink, the way to say it might be "My goodness, you must have worked hard this morning and sweated quite a bit. I do appreciate your being on time to see me, but perhaps it would be a good idea if you took the time to get washed up before we leave. You are a bit smelly." If you can't hug your relative who has some body odor, I pity you. I know I put that strongly, but as I say, you have no idea what the person is going through. If they had two broken legs or pneumonia and they coughed up into an emesis basin something that looks and smells pretty awful, you wouldn't take it out on them, so please don't take the evidence you see of their mental illness out on them.

I have seen patients plan for a week before their family member arrives what they're going to wear, what they're going to say, how they're going to look, everything – trying to please the family member. So realize they may have put a great deal of effort into their appearance for you, even if that appearance to you seems to be not that good. Give them some credit. And don't be so shallow as to cancel their off grounds visit because they look a bit odd.

After all, supposing your family member has been in a bad car wreck. We all know that we don't walk into the hospital and see somebody with lots of bandages and tubes and immediately blurt out "Oh my God, it's awful to see you looking like this." Well, the same etiquette applies to mental health. The appropriate greeting to someone who is daring to come out of the hospital with you and spend some time with you is not "Oh my God, you look awful." And yet how often have I heard patients who go out with their family for the first time return and say that is exactly the greeting they got.

How you behave when the patient is ill will have a great deal to do with whether they get better, and how fast they get better. If you can teach yourself to look beyond the superficial of the shirt that is untucked or the chin that is not clean-shaven, or the reds that don't match, or whatever it is, and tell yourself "This is my beloved child; I have to help him in this time which must be so difficult for him" and realize that the patient is sick, not willfully endeavoring to distress you, the sooner your family member is likely to get well. Remember how much you love him or her, and don't stress out on the superficial qualities of whether he or she looks pale or whether he or she has had his hair cut to your satisfaction, etc.

One important point is this: try not to be using your visits with your family member to be working out your own feelings and reactions to his or her being ill. It may be that you need some talk therapy yourself to handle the disappointment, the grief, the loss, the shock, the sheer rapidity of the change that many families go through when a close family member quite suddenly seems to become ill and strangely beyond their reach while still sitting in front of them. But you need to work on this for yourself, and not take your frustration or your perplexity or your sorrow or whatever it may be out on your family member.

Where to Go On a Visit

Visiting a hospitalized family member may be a tricky endeavor, depending on your recent relationship with that family member. If the hospitalized patient is nervous about going out with you, then perhaps a visit on the grounds or in the visiting room (where there are usually several tables and the person sees the family member at a table, and the whole room is supervised by staff) might be a good idea. Don't be afraid to ask staff how they think your family member is doing, and whether they think your family member is ready for an off-grounds visit yet (as well as, do they have a doctor's order to go off the grounds with you?). Realize this has much to do with whether your family member is adjusted to his medications and can walk and sit without dizziness and would not be in danger walking in traffic with other pedestrians. An important consideration also is that drivers would not necessarily realize he takes psychotropic medication and might expect a faster reaction time than your family member exhibits today. This is as important as whether or not they get along well with you.

Also ask the patient what they would like. If the patient seems to have no particular reaction and no particular preferences, don't assume they won't go to the places they used to enjoy, or that they want to avoid those places. Short direct questions such as, "Would you like to go to the corner café?" "Would you like to go to (name of restaurant)?" or "Would you like to go to the park?" are in order here. Ask each one as a separate question, and be willing to be a little patient for an answer. Tell the patient that he has a lot of control over where you go, that you want to make the outing as pleasant as possible, so the choice of destination is his.

Sometimes, if your relationship with the patient has been stormy lately, it might be of some interest to take the patient somewhere where the two of you are unlikely to get into long recriminations about your recent encounters. Be sure to ask the patient whether they want to go to any of their old hangouts or not. Sometimes patients will be delighted to return to places they know well, which make them feel more normal and more like themselves; other times that's the last place they want to go, because it will make them think of the contrast between when they used to go there (when they were well) and now going there as a psychiatric patient, how far they have fallen since.

I remember vividly one young woman who had been admitted to the hospital five or six days earlier and had finally arrived at having the right to be taken out on a pass by her parents, but no one told the parents. (This occurred when I was a patient). When the parents came they were determined to see the young girl in the visiting room, and would not listen to her statement that she had the right to go out on a pass with them. They kept telling her not to lie. If your family member tells you they have a pass, and no one from the staff has spoken to you, go verify what the situation is. If the patient has a particular request, such as to go to a café or someplace which they know well, consider that. Probably the safest off-ground pass with family is one in which the patient does not get out of the car, but it is perhaps kinder to say, "Let's try driving around a little bit, and then if things go well we may go to the café."

The above situation is one in which the patient is eager to go out, and the family is not sure she is up to it. There is also the opposite situation, in which the family is bent on taking the patient to one of her old haunts, but the patient, who used to find this particular place fun and exciting, now finds it overcrowded, noisy, and difficult to navigate. Patients, particularly those with schizophrenia, are not good at articulating the problem they may have with being in a particular place. I have known patients who did not want to disappoint their family spend two hours in a place which from their point of view was hellish, and arrive back at the mental hospital saying that they wanted to spend the rest of the afternoon in their room alone. What is easy to you as a family member may be overwhelming to the patient, even if the patient had been dreaming of going to just exactly that place when they got locked up in the hospital. It may be a significant disappointment to the patient to realize that an environment which they used to consider fun might now be overwhelming – and what we would ideally ask a visiting family is to be flexible. Don't have your heart set on going to the café or driving around or whatever it might be. Don't have your heart set on taking your son to the football game, particularly if you don't give him a lot of leeway in terms of how he manages to follow all the ins and outs of the game – mental illness affects one's ability to think, and he may not respond in the way he used to. Let that go. Have your heart set on giving the patient a nice family visit with possibly an outing.

If you have significant issues that you want to discuss with the patient (such as why they behaved in an odd and even anti-social manner when they were first hospitalized) these are better saved for a meeting between the patient, you as a family member, and the patient's treatment team. The treatment team may be able to help interpret what the patient is actually feeling, while to you the patient just seems stonily silent and indifferent to your complaints.

One other situation seems worth mentioning here. That is, supposing you are to be going out with your mentally ill family member, but you dread appearing in a café which all the family and your friends, and, it seems, the whole town knows well, with a son who is disheveled, perhaps somewhat malodorous, pallid, a boy whose clothes don't seem to fit on his bones, who is also stonily silent and uncommunicative, he who used to be so witty and intelligent and the life of the party. If you can't stand the idea of critical glances from friends, tell your family member you don't want to go there. But I hope you care most where your family member would like to go.

Cleanliness

Many people who are significantly mentally ill do not wash as consistently and as thoroughly as the rest of us do. They therefore may have a certain degree of body odor. Now, your relative may have tried especially hard to take care of "grooming" issues, but if they have failed, try to let it go, at least initially. If you are getting along well and things seem to be going smoothly you may mention this later. I suggested above a way to excuse the patient's odor by suggesting they "must have worked hard this morning" and that they should shower before the two of you go out. It may help to point out that they should lather themselves up with soap, and scrub, and then rinse it all off in the shower. Similarly, if faced with a young woman who is wearing a checkered skirt or slacks and a floral print blouse, you might say something like "Why don't you put on the lovely white silk blouse I gave you on your last birthday? I think it's hanging in your closet, and it looks really nice on you." But be ready to concede something to the fact that your family member is not well and should not be held to the standard of someone who is 100% well. Whatever you say, phrase it carefully so as to save the self-esteem and the dignity of your family member.

Are you avoiding going to the familiar café to save your own feelings or to save your family member (the patient's) imagined feelings? If it is to save your family member's imagined feelings you can simply check with him by saying "Would you like to go to the café?" and seeing what he has to say. If he is overmedicated or drooling or totally out of it, then perhaps you had better not take him to a place where he might feel completely overwhelmed (see above). If on the other hand he says "Oh yeah, sure" with an air of indifference, then I would assume he <u>does</u> want to go. After all, you asked him if he wanted to go and he said "Sure".

If you have any place that <u>you</u> don't want to go to, for fear that the patient will look or act oddly or embarrass you, there is a tactful way to say that. You can say "We can go to X but if we do, please understand that I'd like you to behave in a conventional way." Or, if you are very unsure, you can suggest aiming to go there next time.

If you meet someone you know when you're off the grounds with your mentally ill family member, be sure and introduce him or her in a way that respects their dignity. People close to the family will probably know something about Junior's recent hospitalization, and people who are not close to the family hardly matter anyway. If the patient's appearance is such as to excite mockery from other people, be sure to know whose side you are on – you should be on the side of family, not the stranger. Besides, one should never be on the side of making fun of someone else. If the patient looks very odd, then the relative stranger may be dimly aware that something is going on, and may be reluctant to talk to either one of you. But if the relationship with the person in the community is distant, then you do not owe them any explanation. If you do try to explain something to someone, make sure that you do it in such a way that your patient family member feels that you handled the situation sensitively. After all what is more important to you – to seem normal for someone you hardly know, or to seem kind and considerate to someone who is family? Perhaps one facet of choosing where you go, would be the relative likelihood of running into someone you know only slightly; if you feel embarrassed to be seen with a mentally ill person, I would suggest you not bringing up to the family member the possibility of going off grounds with them.

I remember vividly being in London in the 1970's. I had been put on a medium dose of haloperidol, which actually is contraindicated for me because of the brain damage I was born with, which includes having a somewhat spastic left side. Haloperidol increases spasticity, and so would get me, as I put it, "twisted up like a pretzel" which was only a mild exaggeration. Nowadays, I tell a new psychiatrist on my case never to give me haloperidol.

My mother and sister and I were getting ready to go walking in central London. It was morning and I took the dose of haloperidol which was precisely what had been prescribed for me. It had the predictable effect of making me somewhat dizzy, bent over sideways, and speaking like R2D2, although of course R2D2 had not been invented at that time. My mother took one horrified look at me about forty-five minutes after I took the medication, and said that she would not allow me to come out on the street with her.

I spent the whole morning in the hotel room, penalized because I was compliant with my medication. With effort, I could appear nearly normal to a person who did not know me well, and who would ascribe some of my difficulties to my neurological injury rather than to the medication. Therefore, my mother's statement that people would 'recognize me as crazy from far off' was quite unfair. And she preferred to refuse to be with me rather than risk being seen with what she called a 'crazy person'. It was very painful to me to see where her priorities lay, and this was from my point of view one of the contributing factors which led to an impaired relationship with her.

I mentioned before that if there is an activity that you and your patient family member have enjoyed in years past such as watching the football game, by all means you should give the patient the opportunity to do that, but do not expect them, as a person who is not well, to be able to follow all the details and the ins and outs of it as he would if he were in the pink.

When I was in the hospital, I once had a visit from a half-brother who brought me a selection of magic tricks, showed me how to do each one once, and then expected me to do all ten of them in succession perfectly correctly. I was not well, but he didn't seem to realize this so I unintentionally, half on purpose, turned my dinner tray over on his lap. Well, he was a very fastidious individual, and my dinner spilled in his lap got him going in a hurry. I did not see him again during the course of that hospitalization, but he and I have made up since. He actually did apologize to me for his expectation that I should be able to learn new magic tricks (and it wasn't as if magic had ever been "my thing") when I had just been admitted to the hospital with a serious diagnosis.

How you behave will be remembered by your mentally ill family member for years, if not decades, if not the rest of his life. So try not to come at the patient with a huge list of expectations which they must meet in order to be on good terms with you. Would you do that to the family member who had been in a car wreck? Good grief no.

Last point: please realize that you may well be not the only one grieving the fact that your mentally ill family member has to spend graduation day in the hospital, or has had to forego his driving test, or has missed out on some other event that was important to him, because of his illness. He may be all too aware of how he's slipping away and is trying desperately to cope. That is how it seems in the beginning anyway; the abyss of mental illness may be opening up in front of him or her, and he or she is plunging further and further into it. Do everything you can to make it clear to him or her that a) you still love him or her; b) you always will; and c) you will have patience in expecting improvement. Mental illnesses can take decades or a lifetime to recover from.

The more you recognize that you still love your family member, but that family member has a problem which might make their thinking, their speaking, their behavior difficult for them and for you, but that all their misthinking or misbehaving is not intentional and is not invented for the sole and unique purpose of frustrating you, the better off you will be. Take it easy.

If you're part of a large and loving family, then the mentally ill family member is still a member of that family, and can be expected to take part in every family event, even though he may not be very active, at least in the beginning. If there are things that the patient has said or done which have embarrassed you in front of other family members or have embarrassed your family with respect to the community – things such as urinating in public, trampling all over the neighbor's prized petunias, spray painting someone's property, then the thing to do is bring this up to the patient's treatment team. Tell the team what your beef is about; we are committed (at least the treatment teams which I have worked on have been) to making patients aware of the consequences of their past actions, and if there is any possibility of doing so, having the patient make amends or apologize or pay for a broken window or whatever it may be.

Set yourself back to the parent or family member you once were of a seven, eight, nine, or ten year-old child and ask yourself what you would have done if your son had trampled all over the neighbor's prize petunias or waded into a fountain naked or done something which is not a felony, but which is generally considered not a good thing. Would you not have made your child apologize, acknowledging the wrong and make him make at least an attempt to clean up the mess? It is no different with a mentally ill family member. The only thing is, if you would have had a tendency to just yell at your kid and say "I hate this, this is bad, you're a bad boy," then I will tell you that berating and bullying the mentally ill has no place. We have to bring up their mistakes to them with patience and love and with a constant invitation and open arms to welcome them back into the human family of responsible individuals.

The author of the book "Crazy", who works on the New York Times, points out that these days many mentally ill people end up in the judicial system where they truly do not belong. I could not agree more with this idea, and if you can keep a mentally ill person out of jail for minor infractions, that is a very good thing. But whether you are in court or whether you are just trying to broker an understanding between your neighbor whose property has been damaged or vandalized and your family member, keep in mind that some wrong has been done and the first thing for the mentally ill family member to get around to, is to admit to it.

If however you feel so hurt and exasperated and angry that your beloved child or family member could have done such a terrible thing, I would suggest you get some therapy for yourself to help you take the strain of having this problem of mental illness brought into your life, and I would also suggest that you take the question of how to correct the mentally ill family member to the treatment team. Do not venture on doing it yourself, unless you are sure that you are not going to start yelling at the patient. He can be very puzzled by having everyone look at him very oddly, quite apparently aware that he is so ill that he is barely recognizable, while at the same time coming at him with the same standards of behavior as if he were class valedictorian. Also, joining a NAMI group of other families of mentally ill people might be an excellent idea. You can look up contact information for local offices of NAMI at NAMI.org on the internet.

Communication Style

It has been shown that families who do have high expressed emotion are more difficult for mentally ill people to navigate than families which do not have high expressed emotion. By that I mean if something does not happen as it is expected to, do the members react with expressions such as "Oh my God, what's going to happen??" or "Good lord, this is a disaster!" or "Oh my goodness, what next?" If the response is likely to be surprise, consternation, shock, or other very marked emotional reaction, this is much harder for a severely ill mental patient to manage than a family in which they say, "You lost your job? Oh well, I suppose you'll find another soon enough", or "The prize flowers froze? What a pity, guess we'll have to plant more next year." In other words, families which normalize unexpected happenings are much easier for a mental patient to live in.

This has been studied, and has been fairly conclusively shown to be true. What I have noticed, though I don't think this has been researched, is another point. In some families, a lot of inherently unanswerable questions are asked. There's a lot of "Well, I never, what comes next?" or "What would grandma have to say about that?" or "Well, that's one way of putting away fresh fruit" when the hapless patient accidently upended a bag of cherries into the garbage. Some of these are rhetorical questions, some are sarcastic, and some are fairly indirect ways of trying to manipulate behavior.

The double bind is a classic. R.D. Laing described this and gave some examples such as the following: a mother gives two gifts to her child, let's say two ties. The next day, when he's going to be seeing her, he puts on one of his new ties. She then says "Oh, don't you like the other one?" – which is a double bind because he couldn't very well put on both, and whichever one he chooses, he's damned if he chooses that one and damned if he chooses the other one

What I mean about indirectness is saying things like "Do you want to come in to dinner or do you want to stay out there forever in the backyard looking at the stars?" Now, a patient's reaction might be to be thinking, no he doesn't want to come in to dinner right now, but he doesn't want to stay out there forever either, so this puts him in a quandary. It would be a lot simpler for patients if people could learn to say "Dinner is ready. Please come in." This follows the general pattern of, "The situation is x. Please y." Unfortunately some people seem to be almost natural born smartasses and they don't know how to change their communication style when someone in the family develops a severe mental illness. Another example: "Well, if you're going to help with the dishes, I guess about now might be the time." How about "Now it's time to wash dishes"? I will close with a little story of an interaction I saw once when I was working in a hospital in Maine. The patient was a forty-eight year old bipolar (that means the same as manic-depressive) man, who, though he was not nearly as manic as he had been when admitted ten days earlier, was by no means having normal thought speed. (What happens in mania is that thoughts can accelerate greatly, and what can happen to a person who is having manic thoughts (which can go around the world in a very few seconds, skipping from subject to subject,) is that it can become very difficult for them to hear anything in their surroundings, because their thoughts occupy all their attention.)

It was at mealtime. One of the nurses was trying to get this patient, who was new to the step-down unit where I was working, to come get his tray and sit down and have lunch. She said to him: "Oh Mr. Smith, why don't you stop jabbering like a magpie and be a reasonable fellow and come over here and get your tray and sit down and have lunch – you must be hungry."

Mr. Smith registered when he was called, but a glazed look came over him at the cascade of syllables which followed. He made not a move to come any closer to the nurse, the tray, or his meal.

I said quietly to the other nurse, "Here, let me try." I then said "Mr. Smith," beckoning him with my finger, "come." He came to within a few feet of me. I then pulled out a chair and motioned that he should sit down. I said "Sit." He did so. I then got his tray and put the tray in front of him and said "Eat." Mr. Smith was doing well and could cope with a hospital tray without assistance, and so he ate his lunch. Please notice all I said was three one syllable words: "Come, sit, eat."

I will add for completeness' sake that it is not necessary to ask a person what they want in their coffee, or whether they want salad dressing, or whether they want extra salt or pepper on their meat, etc. All that you need to do is put these things in front of them; if they want it they'll use it, if they don't they won't. But, speaking as a formerly manic person, I can say that being constantly asked to verbalize more decisions can seem like an interrogation and be very hard to deal with. Most people know what they like and will look for it, and when they see it, will use it – and there's an end to it.

So the final message for this chapter is that one part of communicating is to say what you mean and mean what you say (as Lewis Carroll, who wrote the <u>Alice in Wonderland</u> books, had it) and not go in for a whole lot of unnecessary verbiage. Sarcasm has no place. If you want to make a comment about wearing dress black shoes with old jeans you could say, "Are you sure you want to wear your dress shoes? Why not put on your sneakers?"

It is very puzzling for the families of mentally ill patients to know what they should say and what they should not say. I would have people express themselves tenderly, openly, and honestly about what they're thinking if and only if what they're thinking at that moment is of major importance. But I would not have people consciously stifling themselves not to say anything about the appearance of the mentally ill family member or their behavior if the family thinks it is truly way out of line.

What needs to change is not so much what is expressed, as the manner in which it is expressed. For example, think of a young woman who dresses in very flamboyant colors and seems to have an enormous amount of make-up on. The proper way to approach this situation is to say first and foremost "See here, you are my daughter and I love you no matter what. But you have to realize that many people who see you today, if they see you the way you are now, will be staring at you, because according to our view of things, you have much too much make-up on. Would you like me to help you change?" This approach puts firmly in the forefront, a bond of love that exists in a family as much more important than mere physical appearance. If there is a family out there (and I'm sure there are) who would feel uncomfortable expressing love first, then maybe the so-called healthy members of the family should get into treatment as to why they don't have their priorities straight.

A child, dressed, undressed, hungry or sated, in very proper attire or in very wild attire or in minimal attire should be more important as a human being to their family than the fact that their appearance may deviate from social norms. The ill family member should be gently encouraged to conform to these norms, so as not to excite negative attention in the form of stares or nasty comments. But, push comes to shove, the mentally ill family member should be allowed to go out and be seen, provided they are sufficiently clad not to excite police attention for indecency. Mentally ill people learn as normal people do, and an experience of being stared at and having whispered comments behind hands may straighten out a young girl more than comments of her mother or someone of the mother's generation which is obviously a generation older than she and therefore perhaps classified in her mind (at least in matters of fashionable attire) as "fuddy duddy". Reality is a great teacher, whether a person is mentally ill or perfectly sane.

Again if it is the mother who is feeling embarrassed because of the stares and the behind-the-hand-comments, then perhaps the mother needs some therapeutic support for the difficulty she is experiencing which does go above and beyond the difficulty of an average mom who is raising an average daughter. As a quick one-minute image, I might suggest to such a mom envisioning her daughter going out dressed in a bizarre and over-made-up fashion versus her daughter committing suicide and being carried as a bloody corpse down the stairs where she lives. Any reasonable mom will see the pain of escorting and oddly dressed daughter as much less than the pain of going to their daughter's funeral, so that may help put things into perspective. Because mothers who have gotten extremely angry with their zanily dressed daughters have on occasion been known to lower the daughter's self-esteem so much that she contemplates suicide. Schizophrenic people who communicate little are particularly vulnerable in this way.

At the same time, making no comment at all as a mother is not a good thing, because the daughter may have lost her ability to look at herself critically and see the bizarreness of her appearance. If this is the case, having a mother who agrees to some of it but says that she definitely needs less eye make-up, for example, is being helpful.

My mother and sister, whenever they visited me, would flatten my collar, straighten out my belt, even up my sleeves on my coat etc. etc. and then greet me. May I make a very firm suggestion that this is the wrong way to proceed. The greeting, the hug, should definitely precede any comments about appearance or straightening, and a person over twenty-one may well feel insulted if you straighten out their clothes instead of suggesting that they might straighten them. Treating the family member as if they are not alive, not a human being but some sort of dressed up doll for you to fiddle with is definitely not the way to go. My family was very consistent about this behavior, I complained about it consistently, and it sometimes started a family quarrel as soon as we met. I would suggest that if there is anything that predictably starts a family quarrel between you and the patient, could you not find a different way of approaching the matter, if it needs to be talked about?

I recently met a woman who was the mother of a young man in his late twenties who had had a major psychiatric illness since his teens. She said that her son was very disciplined about taking his medication because "he doesn't like to be dull." Yes, she said, he had worked extremely hard when the supermarket where he was employed in was taken over by a larger supermarket company in April. He had worked ten or twelve days straight, and had sometimes worked ten or twelve hours a day.

In late summer, he started to deteriorate in terms of his mental status. He began to feel that the police were after him, that 'planes that flew overhead were looking down on him, and when his mother asked him, "What would the police be after you about?" he said, "Oh, I made a nasty face in the car six weeks ago when I was frustrated about not being able to go to the movies that day."

His mother would then say to him, "You know perfectly well it is okay to make a wry face, that is not illegal nor is it something that would interest the police."

He would then say, "Oh, I guess I knew that."

The issue that this lady brought to the fore was that her son was losing his ability to leave the house alone. He retained quite a few good friends from the people he grew up with. (That is a blessing – for many people with a mental illness, the hardest thing of all is to make strangers into new friends. Patients are far more comfortable with people who already know them and appreciate them. Willingness to go into an unfamiliar environment and encounter a lot of strangers is an index of social health, for so-called healthy people and mental patients alike).

What this mother was worried about was that he was beginning to lose faith in his ability to go out of the house alone, or to leave the car and go get something alone.

I warned her, as I would the family of any patient, not to fall into thinking that because he was nervous or uncomfortable, he could not do something. After all, all of us in life have to face situations which may make us nervous or uncomfortable. We may have to present a talk in front of a group, we have to start a new job, we have to move house and change our neighbors, change our church affiliation, etc. It is not a kindness to tell people who have mental illness that because they are uncomfortable with something that we would find easy, that they should not struggle to do what they find difficult. Everybody should be involved in some effortful endeavor.

I told this mother that she should not allow her son's temporary discomfiture with going out alone or leaving the car alone to overtake his life.

I warned her that a person may get a completely frozen shoulder if, in response to an injury, they put their arm in a sling, don't use the shoulder at all for a period of weeks, and then find that when the sling is removed the shoulder is "frozen" – meaning that they are not able to move it at all, or can move it in a limited way, with pain. By analogy the same "frozen" state can occur with respect to emotional movements. Social skills are very fluid and if a person gets in the habit of saying "I can't go to the corner store alone" or thinking that they can't get out of the car by themselves, or any particular thing, it will settle on them and become reality, and that is one way in which people with mental illnesses can deteriorate over time. We do not do people with mental illnesses a favor when we say "Never mind, you don't have to do that" and so create a dependency on other members of the family or other members of the community.

I told that mother that the best thing to do would be to say "Of course you can," if her son expressed doubts about being able to leave the car or go to the mailbox or get out of the car and buy something simple like some milk or some coffee or whatever at the store. I even told her she might engineer needing him to do some errands for her by not buying something, driving by the store and saying to him, handing him a ten dollar bill, "Go in and get me some coffee. You know the kind we usually drink," I told her not to let his psychological "shoulder" become frozen.

In my professional life I am often struck by the idea that the treatment team for chronic patients often establishes no real plan or goals. Treatment plans are written in a perfunctory way to suit the demands of the bureaucracy. People sitting around the table will say "He'll never get any better – he wets his bed almost every night." To which I reply "What are we doing to help him stop wetting the bed?" Sometimes, for this particular problem, medication is used, sometimes simple maneuvers (like not drinking water after supper and making sure to void before going to bed) are sufficient. Sometimes, a patient has to be awakened in the middle of the night to use the toilet, so that they will have dry sheets in the morning. Sometimes, discussing with them how important that problem is in terms of the terribly detrimental effect it will have on their future can make a big difference.

One of the most discouraging things about being a physician in state hospitals today is that people will say for instance "He will never get out of here – he wets the bed almost every night" to which I have said "Well, in preparation for today's meeting I looked up the records and per the records he has wet the bed twice in the past five weeks. That's two nights out of thirty-five, which is less than ten percent of the time, which means that over ninety percent of the time his sheets are dry in the morning." Sometimes you can get people to get on the bandwagon of making patients better, and sometimes you have to work for many months before people begin to see change. In my experience, even the toughest case can change substantially in six to eight months, but it may take that long and it may take effort such that those that are in the vanguard of the effort feel they are drilling through concrete.

However, an "onward and upward" attitude is what we need as professionals. The time has come and gone when a person with a chronic mental illness could be considered to be doomed to be chronic institutionalization. We may not be able to teach people all the skills and flexibility they would need to live independently, but they don't need to be hospitalized indefinitely, either.

There are professionals who have schizophrenia, professionals who have bipolar disorder, and we should not be settling for an elitist approach about this, that mental patients should be hospitalized for life.

Of course old attitudes die hard; people don't like change; they just want to collect their paycheck and retire. But the negativistic attitude (hopefully not the staff member) must die. If we can't influence the attitudes of those in our working environment, why should we be trusted to be in charge of changing the lives of our patients?

We all need to get on the side of life, liberty, and the pursuit of happiness for everybody. Making lists of what John or Susan will never be able to do is not part of that picture.

I will close with what the devastating effect hearing such remarks had on me when I was in my early twenties and first entered the world of being a mental patient. Many, many people said I would never get back to medical school, and would essentially never do anything with my life because "now you have a mental illness." This reminded me of what people used to say to me when I was a little girl when I was the cripple in school and my classmates, and sometimes even my teachers, would make fun of me. I would go somewhere where I could be alone and I might cry for a moment or two and feel devastated. After all, if a doctor or the charge nurses who are supposed to be helping you get well are telling you you will never do anything with your life, how is any result to be achieved?

I was very lucky in having a wonderful man for a father, who, though he died when I was only ten, instilled in me a terrific "never say die" spirit. So, I have now achieved being a psychiatrist, a music student soon

(I hope!), to become a composer, and a writer. Yes, I made it through the horrendous sleep deprivation that we demanded then of our young physicians. It nearly did me in, but as my father and I used to say together, "'almost' doesn't count."

The first thing that I would suggest to families and patients who are mentally ill is, don't give up, don't <u>ever</u> give up. As my father taught me when I would come home and complain of the way other students in class laughed at me while the teacher either said nothing, or even, in one or two cases, joined in the fun, "Just because someone else doesn't understand you, doesn't mean you have to accept what they say as truth." He taught me that verse in the Bible which says get the beam (big log) out of your own eye before you fuss about the mote (little fragment) in your brother's eye and said "Shana, you have an eye problem – but nobody else can see straight. They don't know you, they don't understand you, so don't take their statements or their evaluations as gospel. Ever. You are who you know you are."

I remember a particularly poignant part of my own story. When I lost my pediatric internship, which occurred because after six months of the hundred-hour work week I just could not continue, (I had not done anything harmful to a patient nor failed to do what was needful, but it was obvious that the strain on my cognitive faculties was considerable, and I needed to stop for a while.) Sleep deprivation is just terrible for a person with bipolar disorder in the first place. I did not have an admission to the hospital at that time – I was just told to go home and take a rest and call in on Monday about what would come next.

A very kindly director of an institution for children with brain damage that was bad enough that they were not verbal and were way behind in their motor development, was good enough to offer to take me under his wing and drive me every day for a month to his hospital and let me examine patients with him. These children had severe brain damage, and at first I had an eerie feeling that this was one of the places that the doctors who examined me when I was little were referring to, when they told my parents that I should be taken to an institution and placed there. These doctors told my parents that they should forget about me, but the attending for this particular hospital certainly did not forget any of his patients. Some showed very little reaction to the doctor, others cooed pleasantly when he came by, and yet others seemed to enjoy playing little games with him to show off the motor coordination that they had learned. I remember one little boy who was five and a half who had finally learned to take a small block and transfer it from his left hand to his right hand and back and when the doctor came he would pick up the block and transfer it at a great rate of speed, smiling as if to say "Ooh look at me! Look at me!", though in fact he was completely nonverbal.

This was clearly a place where one had to drop any preconceived notions about what a five year old should be like or how much a four year old should be talking – drop all the "should" and just enjoy whatever you could from these children. The doctor assured me that they had therapists for at least a couple of hours a day to try and help them advance as much as they could. The doctor also said that he thought I needed a little kindness away from the critical eye of the director of the pediatric training program, for whom anyone who could not hold to <u>his</u> standards of working under great pressure, when exhausted, had no worth as a physician or even as a human being.

After thirty days with this man, the training program came up with the idea that I should work in the pediatric emergency room for about ten hours a day five days a week. I also had some twelve hour shifts on weekends to do. I worked under the tutelage of a very clever and very devoted man.

As the end of June of 1982 approached, I went to sit down with the pediatric emergency room attending, and discuss with him what possibilities I had for my future. He said to me that I knew pediatrics well, that I had a terrific ability to communicate with sick children, and that I was very good at explaining to parents the decisions they had to make, the attitude to take etc. and was also good at explaining to third parties such as schools or the police, who had an interest and a stake in decisions concerning the children.

"But," he said, "if you cannot tolerate the sleep deprivation which is required for getting through a residency I don't see what future you could possibly have in medicine."

I felt wonderful when he gave me all those fulsome praises. But when he said "if you can't tolerate the sleep deprivation, I don't see any future for you in medicine," I felt absolutely crushed. I had worked as hard as

I was able for six months with a man who at the start was very reluctant to take me since I was in a sense the residency failure, and I had watched him warm to me and realize that I function very well with patients, with parents, with third parties, and never came up short on my knowledge of pediatrics. If this same man said that my one problem would mean that I had no future in medicine, what was I to do?

I went home for a weekend off duty, and I began to think more closely about what he had said. He said that if I had the limitations which I had to admit I did have, that he could see no future for me in medicine. Maybe the problem was just that – he could not see what my future would be. Maybe there was a future for me somewhere in medicine, but it was only that he was blind to that future.

I did not give up at that time, and I did pray about it although I did not have then nearly as secure a connection to prayer as I have had since. The connection was forged from having taken risks for other people, saying in my prayers that I was counting on God's help, and having received that help.

And what I imagined did come to pass. I still have the letter that the director of the pediatrics training program sent me when I sent him a letter saying I was finishing up a residency in psychiatry. He was most congratulatory and most complimentary and then he said what a fine physician I was, which he had known from the beginning – it was only that I needed to overcome certain obstacles. I have forgiven him that he did not really help me to overcome the obstacles, it was rather he who put the obstacles firmly in front of me and said that I was a failure because I could not do what most people do. But it was wonderful nonetheless, to have his attitude change from pessimism and guarded restraint (not paying me anything at beginning of my six months of working fifty hours a week, then paying me half a salary, then refusing to give me any residency credit at all for that work), to a much more accepting and congratulatory point of view.

I would then say to my readers, that if someone tells you no you cannot go into their program, then that will obviously not be your way of making progress. But if they tell you (in this extraordinary world of wide possibility) that because they cannot help you or will not try, that there is nothing that can be done, don't take that as gospel. Take that rather as the limit of their vision, the boundary of their understanding. We are all human beings, we are not perfect, and sometimes we are very negative and most unwonderful. Pray to find out where you should go, and work to find the place that the Lord has made for you.

Some parents and siblings of young people struck by a mental illness may go overboard in an attempt to be kind and considerate. Schizophrenia is an illness that has its highest likelihood of onset in the mid-teen, late teen, and early adult years. This has several consequences, not the least of which is the fact that the schizophrenic patient may not have arrived at full maturity in terms of being able to make stable choices, to choose wisely among different options, to have a good sense of what is important, and to be reliable as the adult world expects a person to be reliable. The patient may go on to their mid-twenties thirties or forties, and still not have developed an adult work ethic. This may not be because they are lazy – it may be that when they first became ill at the age of fifteen, they had a teenager's perspective on the importance of work, which because of illness, did not mature.

Parents, siblings, or providers who have no positive expectations of the patient, including that he or she should learn an adult work ethic, are not doing the patient any favors. I'm not speaking of times when the patient is obviously floridly psychotic, hallucinating, doing bizarre things. I am assuming the patient has had enough medication aboard and enough therapy that they can behave quite acceptably. The family has an immense impact here. Perhaps they should not expect a person with a major mental illness to keep even with their contemporaries in terms of speed at which they learn, but there should be some positive expectation that they will learn and that they will get to understand what constitutes adult behavior.

Teaching people by showing them consequences is what I think is best. I tell my schizophrenic patients point blank that every episode of schizophrenia (I mean an acute episode in which they are hallucinating, behaving wildly, etc.) will cost them a few IQ points because an acute episode of illness seems to be toxic to the brain. I tell them that after several such episodes they will begin to lose some of their intelligence. If they are in an in-patient service, or if they have been in an in-patient service in the past, I remind them that they may have seen some old codgers who were not very bright who had the burnt-out kind of schizophrenia. I explain that that's what happens to people when they don't pay attention to their medication regimen, and repeatedly have breakthrough acute episodes of psychosis. I then emphasize to the patient that the way to avoid being old before their time is to a) take their medication and b) complain constructively about any side effects they may experience to their provider.

My point here is that a good life may come for those who put in the effort. Doing nothing when you wake up in the morning never got anybody anything interesting in life. This is something that sometimes affluent or wealthy people do not understand. They think that if they don't need to make more money, then they should be partying and relaxing continually, that it is fine to spend their entire lives in vacation mode. In my view, such people miss out, because they never have the deep satisfaction of making a contribution to the world.

Everyone living in the community can do at least part of taking care of the basics that we all have to do just to go on living which are called "Activities of Daily Living" – keeping your body and clothes clean, getting and preparing food to eat, and cleaning up. Anybody living in the community should be expected to do that, or to learn to do that. If a person fell ill at the age of fifteen, they may have been in a rebellious frame of mind when they didn't do their own laundry and they didn't clean up their own room. However, this is not an excuse to be perpetually dependent on someone else to do the things for them. They can learn to clean up after themselves just like other people can. At least, I think that is the attitude to take. If the attitude of those around them is that they cannot learn and they will never do anything meaningful, this is stifling to any hopes they may have of making a contribution and having a life with meaning.

Parents who go to their children's apartments and clean them up FOR them are not really doing a good thing for their offspring. What they should do is clean the place up WITH them, so that the younger generation learns how to do it for themselves, and then have them clean up with progressively less supervision, until they can do it all by themselves without assistance.

I know this can be extremely difficult and exasperating. I also am aware that the parent may still be grieving over the fact that their wonderful and much loved son or daughter now has a major mental illness. But to hasten to do everything for the patient so as to be able to forget that the patient needed help, is not a good thing. Show the young person how to do it, and tell them that you will be showing them so that they will learn. Build into your activity the idea that you are not going to be doing this forever.

It is often a question when a person develops schizophrenia (or for that matter bipolar disorder or major depression) what kind of help they should receive and what should be expected of them. What I am encouraging people to expect is a learning curve, even though it may not be as steep as it would for a young person who has no illness. Also, if it is at all possible, I like to see young people who have had a nervous breakdown in the middle of a course of study, (be that high school, a community college, a four year college or graduate school), resume their studies, if at a slower pace. There is no question that it is much harder to go to class, take notes, write papers, take examinations, and so forth if you have a major mental illness than if you do not. But there ought to be an attempt to find something between going back to school at the same pace as people who do not have a mental illness, and giving up school altogether. It makes a person sad to have to slow down their curriculum and therefore be unable to graduate with the rest of their class, that is true. But there is a special feeling of wondrous achievement when the person who has had to slow down does complete their degree requirements and take their degree. To have been affected by the mental illness is hardly surprising; what I am advocating is that being affected does not mean giving up.

I personally lost many years in pursuing my professional goal of becoming a physician because of my mental illness. I was originally slated to graduate in May 1974; I graduated from medical school overseas in January 1981. Because I had great difficulty dealing with the hundred-hour work week killer schedule that we in the United States seem to find necessary for young doctors, it was not until January 1997, sixteen years later, that I had finished my psychiatry residency.

Along the way I got two other masters degrees and another doctorate, an applied doctorate in public health. So I was still working on climbing that mountain, it's just that I had to take a very roundabout route climbing very slowly, but I did reach the end of clinical training and the ability to work in clinical psychiatry as a physician.

As I have said before, we tend to give up on ourselves and on others much too easily if we are not able to complete a course of study or training in standard fashion. Yet if we persist, a way may be found so that goals can be reached.

There were many times during my training when I felt I just couldn't do what I had in front of me in terms of, say, four examinations in two days or something like that. I prayed hard and dove straight into the next task. As a good friend of mine says, "Just do the next thing" – meaning don't think about whether you can or you can't, just get started and keep going on whatever it is you know you must do.

I am very glad that I did finish what I set out to do. I didn't set out to become specifically a psychiatrist, psychiatry found me as it were by happy accident. I know I will never again be able to do what I call with only a little exaggeration the "forty hour shift" again. This is waking up and starting, shall we say, on a Monday morning at seven a.m., going through all day Monday, all night Monday night, all day Tuesday, and finishing Tuesday evening perhaps eight or nine o'clock at night. I could not do that again, and I'm very glad that I no longer have to; it nearly killed me. It is very difficult to hang on when you have a mental illness and you are horrendously sleep deprived. I would not recommend it to anyone else. But at the time, the Horsemen of the Apocalypse themselves could not have dissuaded me from the course I had set myself, and I did feel a kind of eerie elation when I had finished it all. It was eerie, because so many of the people who told me that I could never achieve what I wanted to achieve were dead and buried. It was spooky too, because very few people that I knew had known me long enough to realize that this was the achievement of my number one lifelong dream.

Everyone should be encouraged to do whatever they can to contribute to the world.

Pass Orders

Now I want to say something about the way a pass order should be written. A pass order will be in your family member patient's orders, and it may say the patient has an off grounds pass with (and here you as a family member are identified) on Saturday (date) between two and four p.m. This is the bad way to have a pass order written. I will explain to you why this is not a good pass order.

Suppose you as a family member have to come from some distance, and life being what it is you do not arrive at two p.m. as originally planned, you get to the hospital at two-thirty. Then suppose the nurses are busy with another patient when you get there, and so you don't get signed out (that is, the patient signs a piece of paper stating that they are aware they are to be back by four p.m., and you as a family member may or may not have to sign a paper saying you take responsibility for the patient during the pass time). You definitely will have to sign such a paper if the patient is a minor; you may not have to if the patient is an adult, depending on the state, the nature of their commitment, and the policies of the institution. But the nurses don't get to giving you the papers to sign out until 2:40.

Your two hour visit has been cut to one hour and twenty minutes before you set out. This may in practical terms make the itinerary you planned impossible or very doubtful, or you may be under great time pressure to be back in time, which is not very conducive to having a relaxed, happy time together.

The way the pass order should be written is that the patient has a two hour pass in the company of (and here you will be identified) between the hours of one o'clock (this is the time that lunch is over) and half past five (this is the time that dinner is served). This means you could leave any time after one o'clock and return two hours later, provided that you are back by half past five. Therefore, you could leave at 2:40 and return at 4:40 and be perfectly within the limits of your pass.

In other words, the pass time should specify the number of hours you can be away, but it should be any period of time of that length within a much larger period of time, which allows for your difficulty getting there and the nurses' unavailability at the precise moment you want to sign out. Of course, it does not allow for difficulty (such as traffic) getting back unless you are wise enough not to plan an itinerary that will take absolutely all the time. And you as the responsible party have to plan when you are going to start to head back. Again, I would suggest you do not expect perfect traffic and road conditions on the way back – you should allow extra time.

In any case, if you are going to be back late, it is <u>extremely important</u> to call before your pass expires and let the ward staff know that you are going to be late, when you think you're going to get back, and the reason for your lateness. In other words, continuing with our example if you left at 2:40 and are to be back at 4:40, if at 4:15 you are still thirty miles away, and you are traveling at about forty miles an hour, you might want to let the staff know that you will be about twenty minutes late.

Theoretically the attending doctor has the right to send the police out after a patient as soon as he or she is late returning from his or her pass, and if that happens, the patient may be confined involuntarily – they may lose their voluntary status. This would mean that patient cannot have another pass for some time to come.

I remember one case of a young man who had been in the hospital a long time which both he and his mother bitterly resented. He was given the right to a four hour pass in the afternoon, and was expected back in time for supper, but did not come back. This was a patient who had a considerable history of dangerous suicide attempts when he had been living with his mother some years before. Therefore, after two and a half hours of his not coming back on time, the police were sent out after him.

The patient was found at his mother's house, and was brought back that night, safe and sound. But, because of the legal liability that giving him passes to his mother's house represented, he lost his voluntary status and was not permitted off the grounds in the company of anyone for some time. I hate to say this, but putting the hospital in a state of medico-legal risk is a very poor move, and it is much wiser to come back on time. Call if you need to (which I would advise if you're not quite clearly going to be a little early – that is before your pass expires – when you come back).

What I am advocating is that you behave like a responsible person. If a short pass is negotiated successfully, then you are likely to get another pass, which might be for longer, soon after. This will also figure well in the patient's efforts to get discharged and be allowed to live in the community once again, because he or she will have shown him or herself to be a responsible individual. For the same reason, it is very important that the patient take his or her medication on time when he or she is out on a pass, if there are any medications to be taken.

Usually, the first passes are given between medication times so that neither the patient nor the family member have medications to remember when they are out on a pass. Giving them pass times which encompasses medication taking is something that will follow later if they negotiate simply being out of the hospital and coming back on time first. But in my mind, speaking both as a patient and as a provider, there is absolutely no excuse for failure to contact the ward if the patient is going to come back from a pass even as much as five minutes late.

Wards vary in whether they will offer you the number for the ward when you leave for a pass, so if you are going to take a family member out of the hospital for some period of time, make sure you have the right number to call from the outside so that there is no difficulty reaching the right ward. Also, there is no dishonor in coming back from a pass early if the patient gets tired or if things aren't going well. Of course if you come back <u>very</u> early it will be judged that it was inappropriate to give you the pass in the first place, whereas if you come back only fifteen or twenty minutes early there will be no such adverse conclusion.

While you are out on the pass, try and avoid contentious subjects and be glad that your mentally ill family member is well enough to have a pass, that you have good weather if you do, and try and spend some pleasant time together. Don't forget to say good-bye, until the next visit as warmly and caringly as you know how. Like your greeting, your leave-taking will stay very much in the mind of your mentally ill family member.

CHAPTER 24

PARTICULAR SITUATIONS

Part I: Co-Managing Mental Illness and Pregnancy

As I was finishing my psychiatric residency almost 20 years ago now, I became aware that a number of the leading medical centers in this country had started a department which is a hybrid of obstetrics on the one hand and psychiatry on the other, for the management of pregnancy in women who are known to have a psychiatric disorder, usually a mood disorder. These centers had actually started ten years earlier, so the departments exist from as long as thirty years ago.

The fact is, simply taking a woman off all her psychotropic meds because she is pregnant has been recognized as unwise. Some women may be able to tolerate prolonged periods without psychotropic meds, but many would see a return of their affective disorder with a vengeance and, after all, if the mother-to-be completes suicide because she is depressed (for example), then her baby dies with her.

It should perhaps be explained that most medications that are used in psychiatry today are not without risk to a fetus. But the risk may be that the odds are much higher that a pregnant lady's baby will have a malformation which does occur among those who do <u>not</u> take psychotropics, albeit at a lower rate than among those who do. Let me give an example of what I mean.

The risk to the general population of prospective mothers under forty of having a baby who has Down's syndrome (which is a genetic fault of having an extra chromosome twenty-one), is perhaps one in a hundred thousand live births. In other words for a woman under forty the risk is very small, though it is not unknown that a mother under forty gives birth to a baby with Down's syndrome. The risk to a mother over forty of giving birth to a baby with Down's syndrome may be as high as one in ten. This means there is a ten thousand fold increase in risk for the older mothers vs. younger mothers. Down's syndrome is a serious condition because it is associated with mild to moderate intellectual disability and an increased risk of a number of illnesses throughout the child's life.

But please notice that if the risk to a mother over forty is one in ten, that means she has a ninety percent chance that her baby will <u>not</u> have Down's syndrome. So while the increase in risk is very large, the likelihood that a mother over forty will have a normal baby (as far as Down's syndrome is concerned) is still ninety percent.

So it is with women who take psychotropics (psychiatric medications) vs. women who do not take them. The risk of malformation increases for the women who take psychotropics, but it is not a foregone conclusion that a malformation will necessarily exist in the baby, or that if it did, it was due to the medication.

Now, I just mentioned that simply taking the mother off all her psychotropics for the period of her pregnancy is not a good idea, because many women with affective disorders cannot go untreated for so long.

But it is now known at what point in the pregnancy many medications exert their malformative effect. Thus, a medication which causes cardiac malformation is exerting its ill effect from week two to about week eight in the pregnancy. Therefore, this is the high toxicity period for that particular drug. Other drugs have different windows of time when they exert their malformative effects, and so, with this information, IF the pregnancy's gestational age is well-known, the mother can be off that particular medication at the critical time.

Notice that I mentioned a cardiac malformative effect beginning as early as week two in the pregnancy. This means this strategy will work with a planned pregnancy, in which the mother takes advantage of the fact that a woman's core body temperature rises by a fraction of a degree and is higher for the first two or three days after her ovulation (in other words, in the time conception must take place for a pregnancy to occur in that cycle) and she must know with some degree of precision the gestational age of the pregnancy – otherwise, all the information in the world about the timing of teratogenicity (the likelihood of causing malformation in the fetus) is worthless. Putting it succinctly, if we know during which weeks a teratogen (potentially damaging drug) works to cause malformation AND we know when the pregnancy approaches that time for a particular case, then we can avoid giving that drug during that time period. It should be clear from the above that knowing the gestational age of the pregnancy with some exactitude is absolutely essential, and under most circumstances the only way to be sure is if the pregnancy was planned.

There are a number of situations in which, if a specific drug is particularly dangerous, another medication which is either structurally similar or at least has a functional similarity with regard to the mother's mental health, can be put in its place, at least in the early part of the pregnancy when a baby's organs are most vulnerable.

This would require several things: first, the prospective mother should get in touch with the combined psychiatric/obstetric services before she gets pregnant. I know such departments exist at Harvard and at the University of Pittsburgh. I have contacted both of those services when I was working in the boonies and got some guidance for a patient of mine, and I would encourage other practitioners to do the same; next, have a pregnancy which was planned so that the gestational age of the fetus (down to the day on which conception occurred) is known. If the mother knows that she ovulated sometime during a particular day because her core temperature was low the day before and had risen by half a degree by the next morning, and she had sex with the prospective father of her child that day, and she becomes pregnant, she knows when conception must have occurred. She will therefore know the gestational age of the pregnancy very precisely.

It is important that before she becomes pregnant she is registered as a patient at the obstetric/psychiatric clinic and preferably has met the expert in the management of psychotropic medications and pregnancy already. The mother must be in a condition of life such that she is able, not only to comply with her medication regimen, but to tolerate changes in that regimen throughout the pregnancy; and, the mother should be within easy distance of the hospital at which the birth is to take place, which of course would be whatever hospital the obstetric/psychiatric doctor works at.

I have known people move house temporarily in order to make sure their baby is born healthy. They don't want to be far away from their obstetrician if an emergency comes up and they need to be seen on an urgent basis. This strikes me as wise, if it is doable.

Under these circumstances their obstetrician is also the expert in psychotropic medications, and would be able to order the resumption of full psychotropic dosing after the birth of the child when it is desirable. This is important, because I have known of a case in which a woman gave birth after much effort on many peoples' part to a normal baby, but she had her baby on Wednesday and was not given any psychotropics until she left the hospital on Saturday. By Monday morning she was psychotic and killed her newborn son when the child's father was out of the house. The enormous drop in female hormones which occurs very rapidly after birth is something that women with affective disorders have great difficulty tolerating; the drop makes it hard to maintain a normal mental outlook. Some women who have not been diagnosed ahead of time as having a mental illness become psychotic and do destructive things to their children anyway; the risk to a woman who already has an affective illness is that much greater.

I heard it said in a lecture that a woman should be put back on her psychotropic medication within four hours of the birth of the baby, not as in the tragic case I mentioned above, several days later. The problem is twofold – number one, it is not usual to write orders "give medication X, so many milligrams, within four hours after the birth." Nurses are used to having medications ordered for clock time so the obstetrician has to be vigilant, be paged at the time of the birth and, when that time is known, write a medication order to be given, say, two hours later. Obstetricians who are not psychotropic experts may forget to order psychotropic meds, because they're not thinking about the mother's state of mind postpartum.

At the time of the birth, the mother involved in the tragic instance cited above seemed perfectly normal, because it is only after the birth that female hormones drop precipitously and it is that precipitous drop that causes women with affective disorders to get into psychological trouble. The psychiatrist was blameless in that instance, because she emailed the obstetrician what the mother should be given and when, and the obstetrician answered the email with a reply thanking her for the information. But the obstetrician said in the malpractice trial that he simply had not remembered to write the order after the birth that the medication be given, and so the tragedy happened, as I have said.

To sum up: if a woman has an affective disorder, she would be wise to plan her pregnancy so that she knows the gestational age of the pregnancy with some exactitude, and then take advantage of doctors' ability to remove the offending drug at the critical time, and substitute other drugs with a similar function or even coast for a few weeks without medication if the condition is such that the mother can take a gap in her treatment. Close proximity between the obstetrician/psychiatrist during the pregnancy is highly advisable as the woman may not react entirely well to this change in her medication, and may need extra support or further dosage or regimen adjustments. The possibility exists, however, for women with affective disorders to have perfectly normal children, and this is something that was not possible when this writer was in her twenties.

Usually the best way to contact the department is to call the administrator of psychiatry and ask them do they have anyone who has combined expertise as a psychiatrist and as an obstetrician. Much teragenicity occurs very early in the pregnancy, and so it does need to be planned.

Part II: Management of Mental Illness Before and After Elective Surgery

This is one of the areas in which communication among physicians could majorly improve the health of our patients. I have had a number of patients who tell me a week in advance that they're going to have elective surgery, even though they knew it a couple of months before, but the patient had no idea that <u>all</u> their post-op orders are written by the surgeon, and the surgeon needs to be well-informed about the medication that the patient is taking.

The attitude of many surgeons is simply to take the patient off all psychotropics as soon as they come onto the surgical service, which sometimes has disastrous results. I have been called a number of times to a surgical floor because Mr. X is taking out other people's catheters, refusing to stay in bed, throwing food implements, or engaging in some other unacceptable behavior. I have sometimes been very hard on my surgical colleagues who took the patient off their psychotropic meds without a second thought and without asking for a consult before the surgery so as to know how to control the situation. A little bit of proactivity does wonders in a situation like this. Particularly, people who have been on anti-psychotics for decades, living in a home in which their medications are given to them, should not be taken off their medications without a second thought. It is also important for the patient to be able to <u>taper</u> off their medications rather than stopping very abruptly, because the abrupt stoppage adds, to the lack of medicine in the bloodstream, whatever withdrawal syndrome exists for that particular medication.

This is made more complicated by the fact that sometimes the patient's reaction to having their medication stopped may not become objectively visible for two to six days after the medication is stopped – so the staff think the patient is doing perfectly well, and then on day three, say, his behavior goes haywire, which the staff does not attribute to the medication stoppage, since the patient acted perfectly normally on the first few days after the medication was stopped.

As soon as I find out that a patient is going to have elective surgery I write a letter to the surgeon, advising him as how to handle the psychotropics and, if there is time, telling him that he can turn the page over on which I have written my letter and write anything that he would like to say back to me. I give this to the patient if at all possible, because most of my patients will get it to the surgeon, and it won't come in a pile of other mail and so be filed away unseen, or forgotten by a surgeon who sees the information when he is not seeing the patient to whom it applies. I tell the patient to hand the letter to the surgeon saying "This is for you from my psychiatrist."

This may be the first time the surgeon finds out the person <u>has</u> a psychiatrist. I don't know how many times I have told people "Look you only have one head, one heart, one stomach, etc., so everybody who prescribes for you or operates on you or does anything to your mind or your body should know about everybody else who is working to help you." We have a lot to do in this area yet.

Shana Wibberley Clark, M.D., Dr. P.H.

There is one special case I would like to mention here. This is for the medication called clozapine which is commercialized under the name Clozaril^R as well as some other names. It is the only medication to date whose name, both generic and proprietary, begins with the letters "CLOZ" and so I'm hoping it will stick in my readers' minds. Clozaril^R is an anti-psychotic which has existed since about 1949 and which can be extraordinary in bringing people who had been thought irredeemably crazy to come back to our consensual world of sanity. All of a sudden, they are able to speak coherently, to mention their preferences, to react in a way that we can understand.

But clozapine has some inconveniences. Chief among them is that if it is stopped for more than twenty-four hours, it must be restarted at starter doses, that is, 25 milligrams twice a day, to be increased only every four or five days and then by 25 milligrams, just as if the person had never taken it before. Many patients, before the operation, were taking 600 to 1,000 milligrams per day, divided into two doses, morning and evening. In other words, stopping the medication for more than twenty-four hours will mean the patient has to start as if they were a Clozaril^R novice and will take a long time to get up to their pre-surgery doses, which is what they'll need. The other inconvenience with clozapine is that the United States has decided to create a national Clozaril^R registry and has agreed to take a CBC, with a differential, with a view to noticing sudden drops in white blood cell counts which may be caused by the medication. Pharmacies are not allowed to dispense Clozaril^R to someone who has no CBC drawn within the last week for a person who has been taking Clozaril^R for less than six months, within the past two weeks for a person who has been taking it for longer. There are now some people who can go four weeks without a CBC, but these are in a small minority. To stop a patient's Clozaril^R for three days because they have elective surgery, which means it will take them months to get back to an effective dose, seems folly. One surgeon with whom I lived through putting my patient through total hell because his Clozaril^R was stopped for two days, and then he had to start over as I have outlined, suggested that if he ever had another patient on Clozaril^R he would simply order that the nasogastric tube be clamped, the patient given his Clozaril^R dose, and the tube left clamped for a couple of hours so that he could absorb his Clozaril^R. Following absorption, the tube would be unclamped and would be operational to take care of his post-op needs. I know this is something that surgeons would feel reluctant about, but I would ask them to consider it for the few patients of theirs who do take Clozaril[R]. My patient's behavior was horrendously unacceptable for a long time after his Clozaril[R] was stopped, and the patient was intolerant of Haldol and other medications which can be given by injection, so there was no easy solution to the problem.

At any rate, the psychiatrist and the surgeon should be communicating with each other before the order is written to take the patient off all psychotropic medications, since that may not only lead to a bad experience for the patient, but also problems for everybody involved, including all the surgeon's other patients on the ward.

Part III: Medication Interactions Involving Psychotropics

The first thing to say is that taking any medications while using illegal drugs is a very risky business. I know medications can cause side effects which are unpleasant, but they rarely compromise an individual so badly that the individual might die or be permanently injured, as illegal drugs often do. This chapter is about interactions between medications.

I am not going to talk about interactions between two medications both of which are prescribed by psychiatrists. These do exist, but those of us who spend all day every day prescribing know what they are and are unlikely to give our patients two medications which interact with each other in a dangerous way.

What I'm going to talk about in this chapter is interactions between a medication prescribed by a psychiatrist and a medication prescribed by another doctor. Such interactions may occur both because of ignorance about medical medications on the part of the psychiatrist and because of ignorance of psychotropics on the part of the other prescriber. Obviously a patient who goes to two different institutions for psychiatry and whatever else they have symptoms of and does not inform each provider of the existence of the other one in their lives, together with supplying a current medication list and updating that list when one of their providers changes something, is asking for trouble. I know that people don't want to admit that they are on psychotropic medications, but not to admit to your internist or family doctor or cardiologist that you are taking psychotropic medications is absolute folly. Most practitioners these days ask for a medication list when the patient first goes to them, and some are conscientious enough to ask if there are any changes in their medication since their last visit.

I think most of the problem comes from either patients' withholding information, patients not being prepared when they go and see their family doctor to be asked for a list of their psychotropic medications, or patients who don't realize that an increasing dose in something prescribed by someone other than a psychiatrist might very well affect the metabolism of something prescribed by their psychiatrist. Once again, I will encourage my readers to keep a medication history in a composition book. The genius of this idea is that you don't have to make entries every time you see the doctor. You only need to make an entry when a medication dose is change or something is discontinued or a new medication is started. You need to put down the reason for the change, what side effects you discontinued one medication to avoid (it is not good to have a patient tell you they discontinued a medication because of a drug interaction but not be able to tell you an interaction with <u>what</u> other medication at what dose), and you need to keep it clearly enough written that you know exactly when you started each one of your medications and you know what other medications have been tried but have proven unsuccessful and, in each case, for what reason.

Most people don't remember these things, which is why I am suggesting that you need to take a minute when you get home from a visit to whichever doctor who changed something, and record the change. This will save you and your providers a lot of poking around in the dark. And I'm going to be bold enough to say that we have enough variety and enough choices among medications that only twice in my entire career did I encounter someone I could not help with medicine. And our medicines are getting better and better all the time.

Now, here's something for the professions of medicine and pharmacy to work on. Pharmaceutical alerts say there is an interaction between medication X and medication Y, but they usually do not specify <u>what</u> the nature of the interaction is. If for example the existence of drug X in the body means (for instance, because it is metabolized by the same pathway as drug Y) that the metabolism of Y is a lot slower, then the logical thing to do is reduce the dose of drug Y because each molecule will hang around longer than it would do in the body of a person who is not taking drug X, and so a lower dose of Y will have a therapeutic effect because of the presence of drug X. If on the other hand drug X causes drug Y to be metabolized more rapidly, then drug Y will have to be taken at a larger dose than for a person who does not take medication X. Giving a larger dose because of the presence of another medication can be a problem because the larger dose can increase the likelihood of unpleasant side effects to the patient. Giving a smaller dose if the patient has tolerated the average dose, (when X slows down the metabolism of Y) can be very good because it will mean that the person is less likely to have a side effect from that medication, since they can do with taking less of it.

So how the drug interacts can be very important. I already told the story of being given anti-hpypertensives (medications to combat high blood pressure) to take at bedtime when I already had seven medications that I take at bedtime. I confess I did not think of asking my pharmacist were there any drug interactions, but I found out the first time I took them that something about my new blood pressure medications at peak level did not "get along" with at least one of my other medications at peak level, so that about half an hour after I took all of them together, I became extremely dizzy and fell over, hitting my head hard and bringing a standing lamp which was quite heavy down on top of me. I had the presence of mind to realize that I felt extremely dizzy for about twenty minutes, and the feeling faded straight away after that; this must have meant that the interaction that caused this side effect would occur at peak level only, since the medications were in my body 'doing their thing' for several hours, yet I did not feel this extreme dizziness for hours. It therefore occurred to me that if I separated the peak level of the blood pressure medicine in time from the peak level of the other medications, that would take care of the problem.

So what I did was take my blood pressure medications at 8 a.m., 2 p.m., 8 p.m., and 2 a.m. (waking up to do so) and take my other bedtime medications at 10 p.m. The peak of the blood pressure medication therefore would be around 8:30 but the peak of the other medications which I had been taking for quite a while would not be until 10:30, when the level of the blood pressure medicines in my system would be considerably lower. This is a good example of an adaptation to a medication interaction problem. I do not suggest paztients rearrange things on their own, but do pay attention to when a side effect starts and when it stops in relation to when you take your meds.

There are some situations in which one medication is simply not compatible with another. As a person with a newly diagnosed high blood pressure, I could not take diuretics. This is because I take lithium, and lithium carbonate is a salt just like sodium chloride. If I took a drug which would make me pee out in the urine more sodium, it would make me conserve more lithium, and this in a rather unpredictable way. Since lithium is a wonderful medication which depends on being at a steady level, and since the mental illness for which I am being treated is bipolar disorder which has a famous degree of emotional instability attached to it, taking diuretics if you're taking lithium is not a good idea.

My primary doctor and I initially had me on a beta blocker and hydralazine, neither of which is excreted through the kidneys. But we didn't arrive at a very good result with my blood pressure. It was marked in the textbook that an ACE inhibitor (a different class of drug) cannot be taken with lithium since it alters the lithium level. But the ACE inhibitor does not alter the lithium level by acting on the kidneys, it alters the lithium level because the ACE inhibitor and the part of the lithium <u>not</u> excreted by the kidneys, compete for the same liver enzyme, the lithium loses out (relatively speaking) and sticks around longer because it is 'waiting its turn' to be metabolized.

I found out that the lithium level goes up by 0.1 for every five milligrams that I might take of the ACE inhibitor. I therefore decreased my lithium by 150 milligrams for ten milligrams of the ACE inhibitor that I took, so that I was taking 750 milligrams of lithium for 10 milligrams of ACE inhibitor vs. 900 milligrams per day without the ACE inhibitor, and those worked out just fine. In other words, it is possible when you're not dealing with another medication that works through the kidneys, to change the lithium dose in such a way that the level will remain steady if you change the dose slightly. And, if I ever go off the ACE inhibitor, I may have to raise my lithium dose.

I think I have become something of an expert in this sort of thing because psychiatrists are off by themselves, often not in the same institution as other prescribers. Getting ahold of an individual from another institution is difficult, so it is up to me, if the patient tells me that they're taking a medication which would cause a medication interaction with something I want to prescribe, to adjust the dose of what I will be prescribing accordingly so that the patient will come out alright.

The exceptions that I have seen to this is at the VA and some big medical centers. This is because in the VA system, all the prescriptions written for any one patient are listed in the same place. Therefore, if I want to prescribe something for the patient and that would necessitate an alteration in dose of one of his other prescriptions, I can write a note to that doctor explaining the interaction and asking if he would be willing to write a change in the prescription he controls. Then when I next see the patient, I can just look up the prescriptions again, and if the dosage has changed, there I have my answer. Usually, other physicians are perfectly willing to be cooperative provided that what <u>they</u> are trying to do for the patient is not ignored. In other words, if for example I tell the prescriber that the anti-depressant that I'm going to be prescribing retards metabolization of the medication they prescribe such that there should be a dose reduction in the medication they prescribe, almost everybody, once you have explained to them, is perfectly willing to go along.

One could wish that other places had a completely integrated electronic system with every prescription listed with all the other prescriptions. It would make life a lot easier for the practitioners, and a lot safer for the patient.

In the absence of such a unified system, I would advise any patient who takes, say, more than half a dozen medications, to get them listed in a local pharmacy. I would suggest you might want to let them have your complete list of medications and run it by your local pharmacist if you are prescribed anything new by any one of your doctors, as to whether there is a medication interaction. If there is, I would not settle for "there is an interaction between medication X and medication Y." I would ask what is the <u>nature</u> of the interaction (which the pharmacist might have to research), because as I have been explaining in this chapter and the chapter on side effects, dosages can be adjusted so that it is possible to take two medications which interact with each other.

SHANA WIBBERLEY CLARK, M.D., DR. P.H.

Perhaps "there is a drug interaction" is useful as a screening statement, but that is not enough information to go by; you need to know at what point in the absorption, metabolism, or excretion of the medication the interaction occurs, if there is competition for a particular enzyme or a particular place on the albumin molecule, or whatever, so that more judicious prescribing can be done. There will be some medications which are absolutely not compatible with each other, but these interactions are a small minority of the interactions which take place.

CHAPTER 25

WHAT FORM DOES YOUR WEALTH COME IN?

This chapter is intended for the people who, try as they may, are just not able to support themselves and live in their own place without supervision. We falsely call this 'living independently' although no-one is truly independent. We all need each other. If you don't know what I mean, just consider that the coffee in the United States is imported from coffee-growing countries which takes the cooperation of a great many people, and unless you live on a dairy farm, you need help from the dairy industry and your local grocery store to get your milk or cream, as well as many people who grow sugar cane or sugar beets to make your sugar. There are also a great many people in trucking and other transportation who are involved, and therefore indirectly all the people who design, build, and service trucks, as well as the people who train the drivers. If you want a full discussion of this point, go to my first book, "My Money's on the Turtle".

There are, of course, people who cannot cope with all the demands of a job, including the tension, anxiety, and criticism of co-workers. There are people who cannot be responsible about spending much less money than they would like, and others who cannot keep their place decently enough so as to not get into trouble. This chapter is for the people who cannot seem to do these things but who still need to have a positive philosophical understanding of their lot in life.

Most people who are significantly mentally ill are not employed. I happen to think that the mentally ill are underemployed, and a great many more of them could be earning their own livings if we had employers who were a little more understanding; but there certainly are some people who are not up to all the demands of working, keeping their house going, and taking care of their emotional needs enough to live by themselves.

There are other people who are successful at work, and may make or have made a great deal of money, but these people often have no free time. These people may be convinced that they cannot find a few minutes to choose their spouses' anniversary presents or birthday presents themselves, and so they will hire a complete stranger to buy gifts for the people they are close to. They may indeed be rich in money, but they do not have a moment's spare time.

I would like to suggest that in contrast to such people, the mentally ill may never have much money, but they do have a lot of time at their disposal. Mentally ill people may be said to be wealthy, not in a bank account, but in time. Since there are many activities which do not cost much money, from going to museums which may have a free day to free public concerts to going to the park to going window shopping, people who have very little money can certainly have a life. People can enjoy the sunshine, the warmth of summer on their backs, sitting at a café (as long as they have the price of a lemonade). They are fortunate that they are not one of those who are perpetually "running late", looking at their watches, and dashing off to the next meeting.

Mentally ill people may have to earn the privilege of deciding where they go and when. That is, they do have to learn a degree of self-control to be out in public by themselves. This I do not regard as a bad thing. But they certainly do not need to sit at home and fret and fuss because they are unable to become captains of industry.

The key element here is to realize that just because they cannot anticipate rising on an achievement ladder that often leads to more tension, more anxiety, and even more of a feeling that their life is not their own, they should not feel inferior.

Mentally ill people are wealthy in the time that they have, and they can strive to become masters of their hours, enjoying a wonderful contentment in our very rushed and uptight world. Important here is to have the imagination to be able to find the things that are available in their communities and to allow themselves to enjoy them, instead of feeling downcast because making a fortune is not among the things they can choose as a life goal. While it is true that they won't have access to some of the things that the commercially employed can aspire to, it is also true that they can enjoy life without being compelled to be competitive, always looking out for keeping their job, engaging in clever office politics, having to get up early every single workday, and all the things that the rest of us don't like about the working world. Unoccupied time should be considered as a kind of wealth rather than a burden, as offering a possibility rather than being an endlessly boring blank. Once they make this transformation in their thought process, they can indeed be happy people. I know this because I have met quite a few.

Changing Public Attitudes

The title "Changing Public Attitudes" is a little ambiguous, in that it could be interpreted as meaning that public attitudes are already changing, or it could be interpreted as "how to change public attitudes". In this instance, I like the ambiguity, because both meanings are intended.

Public attitudes towards mental illness have changed quite a bit in the last few decades. Although there is still a stigma attached to being mentally ill, enough famous and not-so-famous people have come forward and admitted to a mental illness that the stigma is much less than it used to be. Also, I believe the Americans with Disabilities Act has been helpful in that it has obliged employers to think of finding a link between a patient's diagnosis and their current performance, before discriminatory hiring practices are applied. Merely having an illness, and taking medication for it, are not reasons not to hire someone these days; there has to be a link between that illness and job performance in the recent past in order to make refusing someone a job stick.

Early on in my career, my willingness to disclose my mental illness and take on whatever consequences might ensue did cost me some jobs. I remember one man who showed me contract to sign me on, and then when I told him of my mental illness, decided that he had an acute and immediate need to go to Boston. He got up, put on his coat and left the room, in the space of less than a minute. I do not think anyone would react that way to my mentioning that I have a perfectly controlled bipolar disorder these days.

I would like the general public to become aware that psychiatrists see not only 'crazy' people but also a great many people who are struggling with symptoms day by day, but who are by no means 'crazy'.

I remember when in the 1950's cancer was unmentionable, and it was said in the obituary that someone died "after a long illness". I have quite a number of friends who have told me over the last few years that they have had cancer, because it is no longer as stigmatized as it once was. Similarly, the question of sexual orientation has also 'come out of the closet' in recent decades. Although the question of same-sex unions, or gay marriage, has not been completely settled yet, nonetheless it is being discussed everywhere as a hot issue, which means it is not being ignored. Over the next ten to twenty years, I'm sure it will be resolved also. Mental illness is perhaps the last issue to 'come out of the closet' so to speak. How to contribute to ending stigma? People who have a psychiatric diagnosis, who are taking their medication, seeing their providers regularly, and doing well with jobs, family and social life should feel free to disclose this fact to people around them. I look forward to the day when physicians seeking licensure do not feel obliged to perjure themselves rather than to tell the truth because they are afraid of the stigma. As I have said before, I never let the fear of stigma alter my behavior. Perhaps this is because I grew up as a child very much stigmatized as "the crippled kid". The reason I put double quotes around that last phrase is because that is the term that people used when referring to me. I had to learn to become indifferent to people's reactions to my physical status, because I could not have ventured outside the house if I were going to shrink away every time someone referred to my physical deformity, which was marked in those days. Fortunately for me, I was a crippled kid who was easily at the top of the class, so while in recess I might not have too many playmates to play with, when we got back inside to our classes, I shone.

The more articles, television appearances, books, etc. are written by courageous people who are willing to admit that they have something that other people feel ashamed of, the more we will have tackled the stigma and the less difficult it will be for the average person to make the same admission. This is part of the reason why I am publishing this book under my own name, rather than a pseudonym. I am a real person, it is a true story and I want to do as much as I can to diminish the stigma of having a mental illness.

When I was working temporary contracts all over the eastern half of the United States, I used to love to say nothing to my co-workers until the last day (although the top brass of the institution knew, because I personally wrote "bipolar disorder" on my application). Then, on the last day of work in that place, I would tell the nurses that I personally had been as sick as three-quarters of the people on the unit. This would generally make their jaws drop, which still causes me to smile. The nurses would say things like "Oh, Doctor, not you!" to which I would say "Yes, me. I have been a patient in a state hospital, I have been quite ill, I have lived in a community residence for a handicapped person, etc." This gave some people something to think about; others would say to me "Oh, that's why you're so understanding of our patients."

Importance of Respecting Psychiatry in Non-psychiatric Settings

Another topic which I believe belongs in this chapter is that we have a long way to go to get psychiatry respected by non-psychiatrists. Last year I fell and broke my right arm in three pieces which necessitated surgery. Since I was born with a somewhat spastic left side and a left arm and hand which do not function very well apart from gross motor tasks, I needed to go to some rehab until I could cope with such things as toileting, washing, dressing etc. independently; I was therefore sent to a nursing home after the surgery. This particular nursing home had a whole wing which dealt with rehabilitation of people with fractures. The typical story was that Uncle Joe, aged 70, slipped on the back porch and broke his ankle.

One of the high-ups greeted me when I came to the nursing home. She told me that bubble packs had been sent of my medicines except for my psychotropics. I arrived on a Friday of a four day weekend and she told me I could not get my psychotropics until Tuesday.

I was so exhausted and worn out that I burst into tears and said "Now you are going to try to drive me crazy, and for all I know you may succeed.

I have been taking my medication for years and stopping suddenly would be very hard on my brain."

The person speaking to me then allowed as how she could take medications from other patients, and replace their supply the following week. I don't know why she didn't think of this before she told me I was going to have to do without my meds for four days.

No one would ask anyone to do without their heart medicine or their insulin for four days. It should be the same in psychiatry. I've known a bunch of people who get hospitalized for a physical condition and their psychiatric medication is not given to them in the hospital. I have also known what it is like to be called as a psychiatrist to see these people who are now fully symptomatic, having been for several days without their meds. I tell the doctor for whom I am doing the consult that this is an iatrogenic problem (that is, caused by the doctor), and that if the psychiatric patient is now causing difficulty for the service he's on, that's the consequence of cancelling the patient's psychotropic medication. But we have a great deal to do in getting the idea across to our colleagues that people <u>do need</u> their psychotropics. Putting the patient through the experience of having his symptoms come back full force because doctors do not concern themselves with their psychiatric medication is not advisable, and not what we should be doing. I think there should be a policy which says that all psychotropics are to be written or given for six days for a patient leaving facility number one and going to facility number two. Six days because there are four day weekends and that will leave two days for the receiving service to order the meds and get them from their local supplier. It is usually possible to get medication within two business days if the receiving facility has it in their thoughts that they need to do this. I have little sympathy for administrators who would allow a patient to be without their psychotropic meds and who then find out that the patient's behavior gets out of line. My sympathy lies with the patient, who because of bureaucratic indifference, has to go through this period of full-fledged symptoms.

Employment of Symptomatic Psychiatric Patients

Employment is perhaps the area in which stigma is most prevalent. It is perfectly understandable that an employer does not want to undertake the risk of hiring a mentally ill person who might behave in an unacceptable fashion, or have lots of unscheduled absences, or do something else that would upset the employer. This is perhaps especially true in competitive situations in which there are lots of applicants who do not admit to having a mental illness (though some may actually have one).

But to be legitimate grounds for refusal of employment, a connection must be established between the previous performance and mental illness. If an applicant comes with glowing references, which do not speak of unscheduled absences or weird behavior or some kind of unacceptable conduct, then there is no real reason to exclude them from employment. If doctors could be more candid when they apply for licensure about having a mental illness and it became an acceptable thing to mention, the stigma would diminish greatly. After all, most people when they achieve a certain age will have chronic symptoms of something – whether it's heartburn, or heart disease, or inflammatory bowel disease or diabetes or high blood pressure, many people do have some symptoms. People are accepted when they have a physical illness because disclosure about physical illnesses is not appropriate until the person has been hired and the time comes for the pre-employment physical. People with mental illnesses should have similar protection. After all, if their approach or behavior or something about them is bizarre, they won't get employment anyway, and will never get to the pre-employment physical. If their behavior is perfectly acceptable, their references are good etc. then why should they not be hired?

Now I am going to pose the question from the opposite tack. I'm going to talk about people who have obvious mental illnesses, yet who still may be employable in some capacity. According to a story that I heard, Tom was a person who was quite psychotic, yet he loved to walk great distances. The team found him a job to attach fliers about a new business to doorknobs throughout the community, and Tom placed so many fliers on so many doorknobs that the owner of the business actually asked the team if they had any more like him. This was a job that suited him perfectly.

From the employers' point of view, if a handicapped person is hired, they can be extremely loyal and extremely hardworking, because most of us know how difficult it might be to find another job. Therefore, we may be willing to do something extra to keep the job we have.

This is an area which needs a lot more effort. If highly functional people would admit that they see a psychiatrist, that would make it possible for those who are not quite so well-functioning to face possible discrimination towards them.

I'm going to close with a little of the story of a friend of mine who was in my medical school class in Belgium. He was an American, and had adapted extremely well to speaking French and finding himself a social life in an foreign environment. One time, figuring that it was a bit silly for two Americans to be stranded alone together and insisting on speaking French, I did get my friend to talk to me in English.

Apparently he had been mistakenly hospitalized in a psychiatric ward for two weeks of observation because he had done something which authorities found a little weird when he was young. He felt that this hospitalization was in no way justified and remained extremely angry with those who had hospitalized him, and as a matter of fact he arranged to get the right to practice in Belgium and told me, when he was close to graduation, that he never intended to return to the United States to live. So, officialdom made one mistake with him and he determined that he would never return to his home country. His parents still lived there, and they did come to Europe once to visit him, but even the fact that his family was in the States did not cause him to budge – he was not going back under any circumstances. He told me that the original deal had been that if they held him for observation and did not find his behavior abnormal they would let him go, and that is what they did, but he simply could not forgive the authorities for making a mistake and imagining he might need a short stint in a mental hospital.

Of course, he was different from me in that I knew from the beginning that I did have a mental disorder, though many things were done with me and to me which I did not agree with and which, even as a practicing psychiatrist, I do not think of as the right way to have handled my case. There are many people in positions of power over other people, who relish that power and relish the ability to make other people suffer because they have power. This is the nature of the human being, and there are far less safeguards of abuse of authority in mental health than in most courts for example – and we all know how imperfect courts are in the conclusions they draw.

My friend was able to turn away from his negative experience and basically forget about it because he did not in fact have an illness except that he had been an obstinate teenager. Most of us are not so lucky. And yet he chose to remain angry, instead of thinking of himself as blessed when, living with other mentally ill people for fifteen days, he saw the plight they were in.

In the long run I do not think being angry against those who have wronged you will advance the cause of yourself or of other patients. I can only hope that by now he has worked on this anger and it is no longer so evident. We must learn more tolerance, perhaps a little bit of relaxation about the rules concerning what behavior is acceptable and what is not.

We should learn that we are all imperfect and the person who fancies themselves as a model may also have a very limiting and crippling amount of egotism.

I think job coaching (which is getting a person a job and having another person who is very interested in keeping them on the job, who helps them get to work on time, helps smooth out minor irritations and stresses and keeps them focused on doing the work) is a very good idea, and I wish there were more job coaching programs throughout the country. I think also that as stigma lessens, the burden that a person who has a mental illness feels about having a dread secret will lessen, and this will make it easier for a lot of people to keep working. Once again, I will say that I wish that people working in mental health, including psychiatrists, would see potential in people, not just deficits. We write their strengths in a rather perfunctory way on treatment plans, but nobody puts any real energy into finding out what the patient's strengths are. I'm hoping this will change over time; we ought to take an interest in what is right with a person, not just what is wrong with them. After being the doctor for over 10,000 people I only encountered two who were so violent that I could not have described anything about what was right with them.

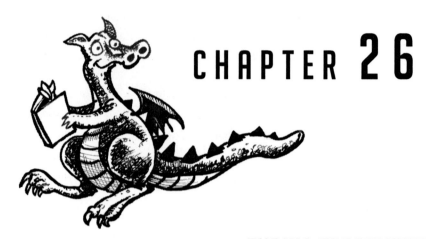

CHAPTER 26

ENDING TREATMENT

Ending Treatment with Your Prescriber

First of all, it should be said that in the case of some illnesses, people should consider themselves as probably going to take medication for life, because we have good effective treatments for most conditions which can improve the functionality of most people, but we do not have cures. In other words, psychiatric medication is <u>not</u> like an antibiotic which you take for a week or two for an infection, the infection clears up, and then you stop taking the antibiotic.

Very definitely, people with schizophrenia should consider that they are going to take medication for life, as are people with bipolar disorder. For people with depression, it used to be thought that they could stop taking their antidepressants when their symptoms improved and the depression itself was no longer in evidence. More recent research, however, shows that people who have a major depressive episode are likely to have another within a year or two if they stop their medication. Specifically, half the people who go off their medications when their symptoms wane will have another episode within a year. Given that statistic, and given that an episode of major depression is very unpleasant suffering for the patients which is very disruptive to their lives, and given also that we now have medications which are not terribly expensive for most people and which are effective without causing major side effects for many people, many patients choose to continue their medications rather than risk another episode.

For those who really don't like taking a medication for their state of mind, it is recommended that they choose a time of relatively little change in their lives to taper off their medication. Thus, if a patient is doing well and is offered and accepts a major promotion, we would not suggest he go off the medication until he is well-adjusted and doing well in his new job position. Any change, even the most positive change, can cause difficulties, tensions, conflicts, and we would not advocate a patient giving themselves something more to adjust to because they are not taking the medication they have taken for some time, until those other changes in their lives are no longer new to them. But when the patient is doing well on a particular dose of a particular medication, they can see their psychiatric prescriber only once ever several months (the limit is usually once in 6 months), or, depending on the medication regimen, the primary care doctor may be willing to take over prescribing it, so the patient sees only the primary care doctor, not mental health.

For the sake of accuracy, I will add that people with a number of other conditions may or may not have to take medication until the end of their lives. Mania particularly (changing into mania is what makes major depression in bipolar disorder different from major depression all by itself) may attenuate in older years, just as the physical body of older people slows down. But just because it is not as conspicuous to outsiders as the mania of younger ages does not mean that it would not be disruptive to the patient, and it is perhaps true that an older patient's ability to adjust to something disruptive is more limited than it was when they were younger. The fact is, we have not followed people with bipolar disorder from their forties forward to their nineties to discover how many of them still need medication as much as they did when they were younger. It is immensely expensive to find cases and follow them forward, and we do not have this information at present.

I myself am tapering off a modest dose of antipsychotic now, since, in my sixties, I just don't have the tendency to mania that I did years ago. Key is to <u>taper</u> off.

Shana Wibberley Clark, M.D., Dr. P.H.

Ending Treatment with Your Therapist

The most obvious reason to end treatment with a therapist is that the particular issue that brought the patient to the therapist has been overcome, and no other difficulty has arisen to take its place. Any patient who has been in therapy which has been successful may realize that the therapist has come to be a person who is friendly and warm and on their side as well as understanding and wise, and may not be in a hurry to stop seeing their therapist. But this is the ideal situation.

A less-than-ideal but nonetheless frequent situation is a patient whose issue that brought them to the therapy has been improved, though it is still an problem, and the therapy may have uncovered other difficulties of which the patient may not have been fully aware when they started treatment. Under these circumstances, it would be hard to recommend ending treatment.

Nonetheless, people in large clinics complain that therapists are reluctant to let them go long after, shall we say, they have stopped grieving for the spouse whose death brought them into therapy. This may be because a patient wants to get over a particular symptom or set of symptoms but the therapist has a goal of healthy functioning for all patients, and is reluctant to let go until a level of good health has been reached.

Another situation entirely is a situation in which the visits with the therapist are cut short because either the patient moves or the therapist moves or retires or dies. In other words the therapy is terminated for reasons outside of the therapeutic relationship itself.

Under these circumstances, if the separation is known in advance to be coming, I am of the conviction that therapist and patient should take some time to think about what the therapy has meant and what it has brought to the patient, both from the patient's point of view and the therapist's. The last session should be quite clearly a good-bye session and a wrap-up, so that the patient gets a chance to look back at the progress they have made since they first knew the therapist, and also so that they do not feel that the therapy has ended very abruptly, leaving them with a lot of unresolved issues and raw feelings.

It used to be said in the training of therapists that the last few minutes of any session should be spent summarizing the session and preparing the patient to go back into their own world, ready to be spending the next period of time, be it a few days, a couple of weeks, a month, away from the therapist. More recently, therapy has become so rushed that "closing time" has been eliminated from the agenda. But when the patient is contemplating never seeing this therapist again, the need to sum up and say good-bye is paramount, and so the patient should not come to the last session with the therapist with more material to discuss, if that is possible, but should come to the last session with some thoughts about how their therapy has progressed since the beginning, and how they envisage going forward. Patients who call to cancel that last appointment and to say they're not coming back are, in my view, doing themselves a considerable emotional disservice. Those of us who have been in the business for a while know that people do this, but that isn't to say we recommend it. Sometimes patients end their therapy because there is something which they should tell the therapist which they want to avoid speaking of. Remember that I said in an earlier chapter that whatever you want to avoid discussing, is the very thing you should discuss. Any negative reaction to some idea or feeling or recollection that you have should not be the reason for stopping seeing a therapist. Of course, people will be lazy and people will do things that are unwise, but once again I say the patient will suffer because of this. I still regret not discussing my sexual history, including the 1974 rape, when I was given the opportunity in Belgium.

Similarly, the patient should take financial worries which might make paying even a copay to a therapist difficult or impossible to the therapist, because there are a number of payment arrangements which it may be possible to make if the therapist knows that is the problem. To simply disappear from therapy because the patient believes they can no longer afford it, without discussing this with the therapist, is to shortchange oneself unnecessarily. If the patient takes on a new job or something such that the scheduled time with the therapist must be changed, the patient should just tell the therapist they need to change their scheduled time. Of course, for some this may provide an excuse for ending the therapy, but once again I say this is not the best way for the patient to handle the situation.

In my life, there have been times when I needed therapy very much and then there have been other times when I took what I learned from a given therapist and used it in my life and did not seem to need therapy until I reached another level of understanding which made some old problem of mine come to the fore, and I began therapy again with a new person. I was always moving around, so of course each new episode of therapy was with a new person. For a person who is not so geographically mobile, it might be an advantage to go back to one's previous therapist, because then you don't have to start a new session of therapy by discussing your old and familiar past. I would say if you go to a new therapist be careful not to get stuck in the description of something which was once very difficult but which is no longer an issue for you. It is important to maintain a certain present and future orientation in your therapy.

Getting Support

There are a number of national and regional organizations for patients and families who have to contend with a particular disorder. Some of these, such as Alzheimer's Disease Association (started by families of Alzheimer's patients) and the National Alliance for the Mentally Ill (nami.org), were originally started by parents of patients who were fed up with having their children dismissed as hopelessly mentally ill when only a few months before they had been more than averagely functional. Another somewhat newer comer to the scene is the Depression and Bipolar Support Alliance; I will caution my readers that the website for this organization is dbsalliance.org because putting in 'dbsa'.org gets one to the Development Bank of South Africa. Some organizations do not have any provider presence; others, such as dbsalliance.com, do have a provider presence to provide information for whatever questions come up, if they can get a provider to volunteer the time to the group. Having a provider present at least saves group discussions from falling into the trap of one group member quoting something they read on the internet (which can be totally incorrect) and having no-one to give the correct information.

The purpose of such groups is to a provide tips and help with navigating daily life when a family member has the illness in question. They also do an invaluable service in emotionally supporting potentially the whole family, but certainly the principle caregivers, through the discouraging parts of this experience for family members. They may also help the family members to discern whether or not a given provider is giving sage advice when he says, for example that Junior should not go back to school the next term, or whether he is just being negative, as some professionals can be about a patient's prospects.

If the groups I have just mentioned do not apply to you, put in your diagnosis on the internet and see if you can come up with a support group. The best is to use the proper medical terminology for your diagnosis without subtype, and then type in the two words 'support groups'. Also try the larger diagnostic group to which your disease belongs. In the case of depression or bipolar disorder, this would be 'Mood disorders', or 'Affective disorders'; in the case of Alzheimer's it would be 'dementia'.

Your provider may know of support groups also. I would personally be leery of a support group in which some of the patients are patients of the provider who is leading the group and some are not. One always knows one's own patients best, and there may be a bias towards helping that provider's patients, or the appearance of such bias, and that can do quite a bit of harm. The best is that either none of the patients in the group are personal patients of that provider, or that all are.

One thing I think I should warn you about support groups. Sometimes, especially in the groups where there are no providers who may have a moderating influence, a support group or a therapy group can become overtaken by a couple of strong personalities who have their own personal agenda, such as the desire to tell war stories (that is, for example, brag about how drunk and high they got) rather than provide education, support and encouragement for people to grow. A support group has the odd mission to get people to be able to function in life without the support group, which is contrary to what happens in other organizations – they perpetuate themselves. So, leaving a support group may be difficult but hopefully when a patient is ready to leave, they will know this and they will discontinue the support group as appropriate. A few people go on to start another support group or be leaders in another group in which they can share what they have learned from others, and their assistance can be most helpful.

Next, then, to the question of how the patient and family should approach speaking to people they interact with frequently and may be relatively close to. I may surprise you by saying that I think it is wise to be candid and forthright with people whom you think would be likely to find out about your family member's illness relatively quickly anyway. I am personally a little unusual in that when my bipolar illness struck me, I was in medical school, and the medical school class was a hotbed of gossip. It struck me as ironic at the time that the very people who are so careful to guard the privacy rights of patients with whom they are not associated will gobble up the juicy details of the happenings to a student colleague of theirs with great interest.

In this situation, I would not advocate cringing and trying to keep a stiff upper lip. That's what I did when I was in Columbia, and I did nothing to stop the gossiping. By the time I got to Brussels, (where my illness continued, as I had several breakdowns while there), I told the people close to me THE TRUTH. This helped decrease the gossip, because the whole point of gossiping is to be telling personal details of what is happening to someone while the person you are gossiping about is trying to conceal them. And I must say, that since the people close to me did know the truth, one or two of them took up the battle for me and pleaded my part in situations where they could have joined malicious gossipers had I not taken a fairly wide circle of people into my confidence from the beginning.

Of course, what is advisable depends a great deal on what is riding on the concealment. If we are talking about the CEO of a large company, it might cause a considerable drop in stock values if too much were known too soon. But the immediate family should be in on everything in an age appropriate manner (meaning, of course, that small children can be told "Daddy is ill" or "He is not well" without being told the details). I would even tell family members who are inclined to gossip something of the truth fairly early on, since they are inclined to gossip and will make up something anyway, and so it is better having them tell the story that you want them to tell. Frankly, I got so fed up with being the subject of malicious gossip that I once walked into a ring of the gossipers and said "So what's the latest on me, folks, huh? Am I going to die before Christmas, do you think, or what?" Being the subject of fanciful gossip does not make dealing with the real illness any easier.

Family members should perhaps have a powwow with each other as to exactly what they're going to say to others of their acquaintance. I think something which is a) simple b) direct and c) truthful is the winner, something like "Derrick has left school because he became very upset. We don't yet know what the problem really is" until the person has been fully diagnosed, in which case it might be advisable to share with a few people what the real diagnosis is. I would advise <u>not</u> giving out "juicy details" of aberrant behavior if at all possible.

One of the difficult things has to do with the medicine cabinet. I leave my pills in their bottles in my medicine cabinet with the labels, and I really don't care if someone comes to my place and tries to spy on me by seeing what I take. On the other hand, only close friends are invited to my place. More extroverted people may feel differently, in which case they can always get a lock box and keep the psychiatric patient's meds in it, so that not everybody who comes to the house can get a free look as to what medication he or she takes when they visit the bathroom.

In the second half of chapter 15, there is a section on what employers and schools should be told about someone who has recently become a psychiatric patient. The last part of <u>this</u> section will be to make a point about what the patients themselves should be feeling. While we do have some ideas about what might protect people from becoming ill (a wide circle of people they are close to, to whom they are in the habit of confiding their troubles seems to be helpful) there is no absolute recipe for preventing the onset of mental illness as such. Given that fact, the person who becomes ill has nothing to be ashamed of or to feel guilty about, unless they behave in a particularly aggressive or destructive manner when they become ill. Then it is a matter of setting right the wrongs they committed, rather than guilt which lasts for years or decades or the rest of their lives. When mental illness struck me, I did not feel ashamed or guilty. I felt dismayed, and my whole world seemed to slip away from me, but I did not feel that I personally had anything to feel sorry for. I know my mother had what she thought was yet another reason to feel ashamed of me (she already felt very ashamed of my physical handicap) but I figured that was her problem and did not feel shame just because she wanted me to. I would recommend this attitude to any patient, so that the patient and the family can focus on doing what they need to do to help the patient get better, rather than feeling badly because the problem has struck.

Shana Wibberley Clark, M.D., Dr. P.H.

How to Feather Your Recovery Nest

I have to admit here that I am not a fan of so-called personal affirmations, which are actually quite impersonal, as they were garnered from a book or a seminar or a website or somewhere such that the person who authored the affirmation does not know the person who is using it at all. I have tried saying things to myself such as "I have a beautiful soul" when the dishes are piled high in the sink, the laundry hamper is overflowing with dirty clothes and everything in my life is a complete mess, and it just seems such hypocrisy that I am not in favor of such statements.

I am, however, in favor of any positive affirmation which has to do with how the person who is affirming it sees themselves. For instance, I would say of myself that although I may be deficient in housekeeping skills, I have a great ability to be helpful to people, and so for me "I am a people person" is an affirmation of one of my strengths. Also, since I have a phenomenal auditory memory, (by formal testing scores), is "Just tell me." Because when I say it to myself it reminds me of a considerable gift that I have.

I sometimes think that the way to make someone aware of their particular gifts is to tell them to imagine a person who is average in every respect. In what way are they different from such a person? In other words, in what ways are they not average, which is to say gifted? Asking a person who feels depressed, anxious, has recently been psychotic, or is trying to recover from a mood episode or substance abuse, in what ways they are gifted may sound like telling me to say to myself as I stand in the middle of my own mess that "I have a beautiful soul" – in other words, it doesn't seem very helpful. The word "gifted" may make a person uncomfortable, where the question "In what way are you different from the average?" may not, although as far as I am concerned they are the same question.

I'm sure you've all heard the phrase "God does not make junk." The question here is, for each patient, how can they identify the ways in which they are particularly themselves, and have something to contribute to the rest of us?

Please realize that "something to contribute" can be anything from a cheerful smile to whatever is more lasting. Humble gifts are gifts nonetheless. Please remember that patient of mine who found his calling in drawing chalk portraits and scenes on the sidewalk in a big city. From his point of view, the fact that in a much-trafficked area the drawing would be gone in a couple of hours was part of its charm. And he certainly set the downtown area of Philadelphia abuzz with people wondering who had drawn that magnificent Last Supper, who drew the wonderful portrait of Dr. Martin Luther King Jr. to coincide with the Martin Luther King Jr. holiday, etc. etc. He himself did not say that he had a gift; he said it was "something worthwhile that he knew how to do."

I'm now going to return to the title of this chapter. I'm talking about your recovery nest. By that I mean that you will take little bits of many people's ideas, something you happen to read somewhere, the joke you happened to see while you were waiting in the dentist's office, what your maiden aunt told you, whatever. I would suggest that you write these down, perhaps starting from the back page of that composition book which in the front contains your medication history. I think you should garner little pieces of wisdom and things that make you smile for your recover nest every bit as seriously as a bird looking for twigs and leaves and little bits of tinsel to make their nest.

This is to help make you become a better, wiser, more seasoned person who is hopefully more understanding of other people's quandaries, which may be different from yours, but which you might comprehend are as difficult for them as yours have been for you, and in general become a more flexible, adaptable, and loving version of yourself.

One of the first things you must get under control when you are no longer completely at the mercy of your symptoms is keeping clean. There is no way around it, you must shower regularly, most of all in hot weather (I am dictating this in July). Also, use deodorant, wash your teeth, use mouthwash if you need to.

There are regular chores which all of us must do. Some of these are doing the laundry, washing the dishes, and for women at least, some kind of hair care. You do not do yourself any favors if you wear clothes with spots on them or walk around stinky. In fact, this is about the best way to silently advertise that you still are mentally ill, and it will not make you new friends. So put doing your laundry and hair care and cleaning in general on your calendar. Also, if you live by yourself, you may have to cope with paying bills, though I know there are a great many people with a significant history of mental illness who have someone else take care of that for them. Whatever you have to take care of, is something you have to do; we all do. It's like going to the bathroom; not taking care of it properly would be a social disaster. So just accept these chores as part of living; the fun part comes when all your chores are done, when you have the sequence down pat. I did not mention going to the grocery store, since I imagine hunger will get you there if nothing else, but do not forget to get cleaning materials when you're there.

Now about mini-goals. People are forever telling you that if you don't set yourself a goal, you will never know when you have reached it, or worse yet you will never even get there. I think there is some truth to this, but I also think that when we're dealing with mental illness we have to understand that there are times when getting through the day is the goal. Just arriving at the time when it is allowed and expected that one can return to bed and do nothing. Yet mini-goals do have their place too. I began using the local Y, getting there by paratransit (that is by a special bus service that exists in Rochester, New York, to help people who cannot use regular transit to get around). My reason for having difficulty for getting around is that my balance is terrible. If I get on a regular bus, the bus will stay stationary only as long as the light in front of it stays red, and soon as the light turns green, the bus charges forward and it is like a bucking bronco under my feet. The paratransit gives you a chance to pay your fare before you sit down, get seated and even get buckled in before they charge off. That's why I need them. So I began to go to the local Y in January. It is now July. I remember when I first got into the pool in January, I could just about manage to be in for fifteen minutes because I was very uncomfortable, couldn't seem to get my arms and legs to act together, and the whole thing was just awful. I now go swimming three or four times a week, and spend an hour in the pool each time. That is quite an improvement. I set myself sometime around March the goal of increasing my time in the pool from the half hour that it was then, by counting the laps that I did every day, and pushing myself, while occasionally allowing myself to have an under par day.

So while I can't say that my life has totally changed since I fell and broke my right arm into 3 pieces, or that my financial picture is improved, I can say that my exercise tolerance is up to one hour in the pool. And that makes me feel good. I can use this to help myself to feel that other parts of my life may improve shortly as well – for instance, I have nearly finished dictating this book.

It does give me satisfaction to realize that I have become able to do quite a lot of something that only a few months ago I could not do at all. I am also very slowly losing weight chiefly by asking myself every time I think of food whether I am genuinely stomach-growlingly mouthwateringly hungry now or not. If the answer is that I'm not really really hungry, then I may have a drink of water or a cup of tea, but I don't eat. My point here is that big change is brought about best and most reliably by incremental, steadily applied small change over time. Quitting smoking is brought about by every cigarette you don't smoke. Stopping drinking is brought about every time you turn down some alcohol. Is it ever easy? No, but in proportion as it is not easy, it is worthwhile.

One of the things that I usually find is very lacking given their level of general intelligence, in young people who have mental illnesses and who are recovering, is education. There is no question that a certain amount of money is very helpful in moving forward in this country, and there is also no question that formal education, be it of the book variety or the hands-on variety, is very useful in earning money. I would encourage every person under sixty who finds themselves in a financial bind to think about getting some education. This can usually be approached by the local community college and taking classes rather than enrolling immediately in a degree program, which might seem like a very audacious undertaking for somebody who is much improved but still not very sure of their mental health. Community college credits can oftentimes be transferred to other institutions of higher learning if the person so desires. And it will get you back into the discipline of having to complete an assignment on time and having to organize your work. If the person is reticent, then let them take a relatively easy class for their first term, and just one class. There are quite a lot of sources of help for paying for the tuition for the class, although if you are in the position to do so, saving up to pay for the class can be an excellent incentive to do well in that class. Be sure you pick something that you would find interesting – not what somebody else says you should take, but something that you would find absorbing, because then it will still be effort, but doing the work for it will not be an unbearable chore.

Shana Wibberley Clark, M.D., Dr. P.H.

If you're wondering what field you should go into, try thinking back to when you were a small child. Was there something that attracted you when you were in elementary school or in junior high or in high school that you never got to? Because that probably is where some of your talents lie.

The patients that I as a doctor have most difficulty helping are the ones that have settled for and settled into the status quo and although they are unhappy, they refuse to think about changing anything. If you possibly can, use your discontent with the way things are presently to make a change. Life is an adventure; and, nothing ventured, nothing gained.

When you have advanced considerably from one hundred percent helpee status, so that your own mental health symptoms are no longer the only thing you are really involved with every day, you may find that it is necessary to consciously make an effort to graduate from spending most of your time with groups of people with whom it is safe to talk about symptoms, to spending time with people who, like most of the public, have no way of responding with any ease when you mention a mental health symptom. Do not let this dismay you. I've often thought it's like a butterfly coming out of the chrysalis which the creature entered as a caterpillar.

You have the same need to grow and develop as everyone does. It may be necessary to change your church congregation or go to a different temple or mosque, if too many people are constantly reminding you (rather than your needing to remind them) of the mental health history you have.

Then you may have the difficulty of feeling a temptation to mention your mental illness status in the new congregation. I would suggest you refrain from doing this. After all, was not the whole point of your moving from the old congregation to the new to be free of too many people who are keeping you from doing what you could do because they keep reminding you of where you have come from?

Do keep working on whatever relationship you have with your God (I'm putting it that way since I realize that different people have different notions of who God is, and I'm not trying to change anyone's), but do keep seeing yourself as one creature in billions who is mysteriously connected to the others and indeed connected to every living, dead, and nonliving thing on the planet. If you have a particular fondness for trees, for sunsets, for sunrises, for birds, you can make this into a new hobby or semi-hobby. If you don't think you're up to hours and hours of just watching birds, then maybe you are up to watching flocks of migrating birds as they pass overhead in the local park. So you don't have to be a very serious hobbyist to get something out of it. If you like sailing, boats, water sports, or other things of that kind, then you can get involved in that. Try and find a way of being peripherally involved before you commit yourself to spending a definite amount of time or a definite amount of money in pursuit of such hobbies, but do explore. Find out, with time that you can spend, how you would wish to spend it.

One other area that I want to talk about is work ethic and reliability. As you transition toward the world most people live in, (most of us are not preoccupied with our state of mind moment-by-moment), you will find that one thing which distinguishes some people from others is that some people are reliable while others are not. I would encourage you to most firmly make a decision that you will be among the reliable ones, because this is how you get a good social reputation.

If you undertake to do something, mark on your calendar when it has to be done, and also mark on your personal calendar when you're going to do it, giving yourself a reasonable amount of time. If it is something such as a piece of writing which may take revising or at least looking at and reconsidering, then make sure you put enough time on your calendar to get it done well. If you tell someone that you are going to meet them at a coffee shop at nine a.m. on Monday morning, make sure you get up early enough and leave the house early enough to get there on time.

Don't ever stand anybody up, because this will not increase your confidence in yourself and if the other party has heard anything about mental illness concerning you, this may ruin things. I was recently called by someone who had met me in the community and told me that he desired to get to know me better. We made a date for coffee, and he called me at the last minute to tell me he had a reason he couldn't go. We made another date over the 'phone, and he did not call me to let me know not to go to the coffee shop to meet him. He called I think a day later to say he had been called in to work at that time, but as I pointed out to him he should, as a decent person, have called me even with a fifteen second 'phone call so that I would know not to leave the house to go to the coffee shop to meet him. There are people who say that I'm being too rigid, but I certainly am not going to be making a personal date with this person again. Not for a long time anyway, although I have no objection to running into him in the community and speaking to him if things should fall out that way.

My point is, don't be like this person. Don't forget to tell someone that you can't go and don't expect people to take a second and third chance on knowing you if you blow it the first time, especially if what happened to you the first time was not a personal emergency.

Personally, I do not undertake to do anything for someone unless I'm very sure that I can do it. I have no problem saying "No, I'm sorry, I can't do that". I think the art of saying no at the beginning is something we need to recapture. If you are treated badly by someone else, make a mental note that you will never do the same thing to another person. Use the bad things that are done to you as a way of improving your character, rather than as a way of adding to your resentments. After all, the person I'm referring to is not a bad person and has no bad intentions towards me – he's just what I call terminally disorganized.

On the other hand, realize that life is life, and if somebody does call you quickly and say, "Oh hello, I'm so sorry, I can't meet you today at two o'clock, I've been called in to work instead", and then hangs up, they are trying to remember their obligations to you in the middle of a frantic preparation for whatever the rest of the day brings them. But they did call you, and they did call you several hours in advance, not as you were on the way there. So they are a good friend. I would encourage everyone to resolve the new person they have become as they begin to emerge from the awful experience that is mental illness does not let people down, does not undertake things they can't do, does not on the other hand refuse to be helpful if it is within their capability. In other words, you can remake who you are and how you behave. So, up to you to choose, who do you want to be? And I have to say that here, most of the rewards go to the decent people. The decent, kindly, loving, accepting people.

Remember, if you are one of the lucky ones to make it out of mental illness into a regular life, don't be afraid to volunteer your time and talents to help the people who are now where you once were. I hope that every reader of this book will become one of an ever-growing army of people who are out to change the face of mental illness itself. We don't have a really good handle yet on how to prevent schizophrenia or bipolar illness or some of the other major mental illnesses, but we do know that having a sympathetic community, help that is understandable and available, is extremely important. To that end, the more people there are who have had a mental illness, or who, like me, still have one but have tamed their dragon, the more such people there are who are not afraid to talk about what happened to them and why, and are not afraid to help others who are now in the same fix, the easier it will become for the new people who fall into mental illness to find their way back out. So, readers, please, join us in this fight. Helping other people is one of the best ways to give meaning to your own life, and therefore you should keep in mind that when you help someone else, the next life you save may be your own.

CHAPTER 27

HOPES FOR THE FUTURE

I think psychiatry is already changing very rapidly, and some of the changes do not make me happy. The tendency to push for less and less one-on-one time between a patient and their provider I find very disturbing. If you see a provider for ten minutes every two months, how can you possibly develop the comfort to be able to really tell them what is on your mind, and how do they distinguish between when you are telling the truth as you know it and something less courageous because, perhaps, you are too frightened, too anxious, and too overwhelmed? The doctor patient relationship is time-honored, and even our legal system protects patients from being subjected to overly candid disclosures by doctors. In this particular regard, your doctor is rather like your priest or, if you are in a court case, your attorney. There is a privilege accorded each of those three professional relationships which does not exist for an individual otherwise, except between himself and his or her spouse. It's one of the perks of being legally married.

And yet this sacrosanct doctor patient relationship is under attack, mostly from the profit motive.

But there are a host of other problems. I cannot escape the feeling that many of my psychiatrist colleagues who worked with me throughout my career did not share my understanding of what we were about. Many of them seemed to think of themselves as better than the least of their patients. Of course we were more educated; I myself have two Master's Degrees and two Doctorates, the MD and an applied Doctorate in Public Health. But may I point out that if a physician feels better than his patients, he can never meet them in their world. He can never really understand them, and so, being estranged from what is important to them, he cannot really help them, still less can he genuinely be of service.

I read a long time ago that medical students should be required to undergo some painful procedures and be left alone for hours on end in a situation where, let us say, they can't get a bedpan and they have an uncomfortably full bladder. Something that simple, which has no real danger, but if they had any experience of having difficulty with getting their needs met, might teach them something. They could have the experience of having other people in white coats whispering about them at the end of the hall, and not know what the whispering was about. I'm sure that without doing anybody any lasting harm, we could teach medical students how to understand their patients better than we do now. I remember being to a seminar recently in which the speaker mentioned that the patients are concerned with the side effects of the medication, while the physician wants to eliminate their auditory hallucinations ("the voices") entirely. The speaker felt he had to remind his peers that the doctor and the patient did not have the same goal.

I believe we could put this differently. The doctor should be interested in helping the patient live in consensual reality, whether or not that means totally eliminating the auditory hallucinations. Just as many people with painful conditions choose to take some medicine, but less than it would take to get them pain-free, so our patients can choose to take enough medicine that they don't get into trouble, but less than the amount needed to eliminate the voices altogether. We should be far more patient oriented. I have been called the most patient-oriented physician anybody ever met, probably because I have had so many of these experiences myself.

In the VA system, veterans often get their medication from a pharmacy which is on site once it is ordered in the computer by their doctor. I remember one doctor who, told by the pharmacy that there was not in the pharmacy the supply of the medication he wanted, just told the patient come back the next day. The doctor had no idea (and made no effort to find out) that the patient had to pay a considerable cost to come from eighty miles away. I heard of this, and I pointed out the difficulty that a return visit would represent to the patient, and the psychiatrist concerned and I consulted with each other and came up with a different medicine that the pharmacy did have, and could give the patient before he went home that day. It was just by chance that I heard of this situation, and I was very polite and deferential to the doctor, but I told him very firmly that it was a great hardship for the patient to come back and spend another hundred and sixty miles' worth of gas to come back the next day. I was glad to be able to resolve the situation; providers do not think enough about what the patient has to go through to get to them.

I think it is regrettable that psychiatry is so easy for foreign doctors to get into. I don't mean that I have a prejudice against doctors from other countries or that I think they are bad. What I mean is, if a doctor comes from overseas and was a surgeon in his old country or a dermatologist or a whatever, he should not be encouraged to go into psychiatry when he finds that becoming a surgeon in this country or a dermatologist or whatever else it was will be difficult. Someone who wants to cut and wants concrete physical evidence of the need for their services and the result thereof can be very uncomfortable in a less tangible world which is psychiatry, and can have no interest in the story that the patient has to tell. Just because they had an MD in their old country does not mean they should be welcomed into psychiatry over here.

We are finally getting somewhere about the issue of parity, that is, that mental illness should be considered an insured, covered illness as much as any physical illness. But the work here is not done.

When I came back to Rochester having fallen and broken my right arm into three pieces, one of the things I had to do was find myself a psychiatrist. I heard from a friend that her psychiatrist was excellent, and I decided to go there. I did not understand at the time that my insurance that I had then as a continuation of benefits from being an employee of the State did not do business with this particular clinic. In other words, there are still pockets where an insurance company has a contract with a hospital system for physical illness but is not covered for mental illness, as I have stated in an earlier chapter. As I did say earlier, I found out after a short while which local insurance did cover that clinic, so my problem was resolved. But I still find it strange that the employees of New York State would not be able to go there, because they have the policy that all New York State employees have.

There are other things. A patient may present to an emergency room in one hospital in one city, and be sent, for insurance reasons, to another hospital far away. I think there should be a limit on how far away the patient may be placed, unless places close by are full. This is because it can be very hard for the patient's family to travel a long distance to go visit them.

I am still trying to puzzle out what happened when in 1997 I telephoned my doctor's answering service on a Sunday afternoon and told them to please let the doctor know that I was suicidal. I was being totally truthful and was literally sitting on my hands to prevent myself from taking the overdose which was so easily available to me. I said to the person who answered that I was suicidal, and the young lady in the answering service asked me how to spell 'suicidal'! I don't expect everybody who works in an answering service to be necessarily a terrific speller. But in that case, they should have a 'cheat sheet' of the words they might need to be able to spell. The reaction to a patient who states they are suicidal should be "I'll get a message to the doctor right away!" Not, "how do you spell 'suicidal'?"

The doctor made me wait over half an hour before he called me back. I thought he knew me, because he had been my psychiatrist for a few years a decade earlier. I thought he would understand I don't exaggerate; I had never called on a weekend before saying I was suicidal.

After leaving the message, I waited half an hour for him to call back, sitting on my hands in mental anguish. I finally did take a huge overdose, enough to kill 8-10 people. Three minutes later, he did call, saying he had heard I was "feeling bad'. I corrected him as to what I had said, and then realized I could say "See you next Tuesday" (our next office appointment), knowing I would be dead, or stay truthful and tell him about the overdose. I did the latter partly because I hate lying.

He then said that I should be the one to call an ambulance. Did he not realize what a liability he was opening up for himself in telling me to make the 'phone call? Could he not anticipate that if for any one of a dozen reasons I didn't manage to call the ambulance, that he would be opening himself up to a wrongful death lawsuit, because he had known I had taken a huge overdose and did nothing? I felt at the time that the whole world had gone mad, and I was hoping to leave it very soon. I told him I wasn't going to call anyone, I had already done what I needed to do. He did call an ambulance, which is why I am alive today.

Patient care means just that. It means <u>caring</u> about patients. It means more (or it should mean more) than just going through the motions.

My experience working in state hospitals has taught me that the sickest among us can learn, and can be motivated if they understand clearly the consequences of two different sets of actions. Tell someone that action one will lead to consequence one and action two will lead to a different consequence, and it is not difficult to get them interested in choosing the consequence that you would want them to choose.

But too many state hospital physicians don't bother to explain to their patients what choices the patient is facing; they would sooner be like my colleague who told a patient who was getting very upset about her family situation (the upset about this was what was keeping her in the hospital) that "we don't have time for this" because he had to go to a meeting. He delivered it to her as a rebuff. Later, when I took over that ward and had this lady as my patient, I would say to her "I can't talk about this now. I have to go to a meeting. But I would be back by noon which is when you have lunch, and I will look for you right after lunch, so we can talk about this." The actual meeting in question would be over by 11:30 but I only promised to be back by noon because I always find it better to promise less than I think I can deliver, so that if someone at the end of the meeting, such as my supervisor, wants to talk to me urgently, I could accommodate his wish without being late for my patient.

When I heard my colleague say to her that we do not have time for her, I wanted very much to ask him what he did have time for, since she was one of the patients and surely the whole hospital existed because the patients needed our time. But I felt it wiser to keep my mouth shut, and so I did.

Let me add that patients are punished for ever getting upset. But I heard him tell the rest of us one day about nearly threatening a police officer for giving him a parking ticket, and he sounded plenty upset. And the same goes for swearing. Don't tell the patients that they lose privileges over saying damn once unless you have never said damn in your life. Even so, if you have never sworn in your life, perhaps you've been extremely lucky. I tend to think that only threatening behavior or actual fighting should be sanctioned. An occasional swear word is so much part of our national fabric, on television, in film etc. that it should not be a reason to take away the poor patients' hard-earned privileges.

I will admit that I have been told that I have 'the patience of a saint' in talking to mentally ill people. I have spent my life trying to learn to be less upset, less pressured, more patient, and more loving. I think those are good goals for anyone, but I think for a mental health provider they are a must.

One would hope, not only the specially gifted and famous, but regular people can come out of the closet and admit that they take or have taken psychotropic medications or that they are consulting or have consulted a mental health professional, and that it will be no more a problem to other people to have a few days in the hospital than it would be a problem to have a week off for gall bladder surgery.

As I said before, my mental illness, which was really bad when I was in my twenties, has become no more bothersome than high cholesterol for which I take medication or a low thyroid for which I also take medication. Meaning, yes I do go to the doctor, and I do have blood work drawn and so forth, but I am in a different world from where I used to be in terms of needing everything in my life to be going just fine to be calm and content. The other day my toilet overflowed. This sort of thing used to drive me to the hospital because it would be the straw that broke the camel's back. But I told myself I would have to cope, and right away, and then mopped up the mess. My point is, when it happened I was not driven 'round the bend.

I am not beyond worries at this point, because my only income is Social Security Disability, which does not pay for life on East Avenue, in one of Rochester's expensive neighborhoods. I tried to sell my condo last year when the housing market was in crisis, and it's not a surprise that I did not succeed; but that means I <u>have</u> to pay to live here, and my income just won't cover it all. My author website is at DrSWClark.com. I hope I will succeed as an author, but at this point, I hope.

Hope is one of the great things that we can give our mental health patients. Hope, when it has reality behind it, becomes an expectation. I have repeatedly taken wards where rudeness, threatening behavior, violence, and all manner of unkindness were routine, and turned them in a matter of two or three months into the best ward in the institution. Nobody ever asked me how I did this, which made me sad. I think people sense that I expect that everybody will behave like a civilized person and I don't doubt for a minute that they are capable of it. I have met many physicians who seem to have the conviction that their patients cannot change. Therefore they write their notes with only a slight variance of last month's note which is only slightly changed from the previous month. They don't look for change and they don't see any. Out of a ward of thirty chronically mentally ill people I managed to arrange for the discharge of eighteen in eight months. This is a ward where they were used to one discharge per year.

What I am trying to convey here is that if we have positive expectations, that will go a long way to creating the result that we would like. Patients can sense who has positive expectations of them and who does not. Since everyone can learn, I tend to have positive expectations of everyone, and I hope that the profession of psychiatry will learn to be more optimistic. As for me I can say that I have become, in my early 60's, the woman I wanted to be in my early 20's, when mental illness first hit.

The last thing I will mention is new medication which might serve our patients better with less side effects. I do think this will happen because pharmaceutical companies can make a lot of money if they come up with better medications. And, there is now some research on glia, the non-neuron cells in the brain, which suggests they may contribute to neuronal control, and opens up a whole new frontier for psychiatric research.

CHAPTER 28

SUMMARY AND FAREWELL

I hope the readers of this book have derived practical benefit from it. If you would like a summary of the points I was trying to make, I will try one here.

Point 1: Mental illness is a problem which you have; it is up to you to think of this as a problem which you must solve, rather than an essential attribute of your being. How much you will need to put effort into being a mental patient depends to some extent on you. If you are willing to put in effort to solve problems from the beginning, you may achieve a much better result than if you think of your illness as a circumstance which must and will victimize you. The trick is, when you feel negative energy coming from thinking of and dealing with your mental health problems, to use that energy as fertilizer to grow solutions to your difficulties, rather than as a kind of stinky garbage to make you feel victimized. There is no human experience which may not be mined for the lessons a person can learn in dealing with the experience, or in dealing with consequences. Everything can teach you, if you are willing to learn.

Point 2: I hope you are willing to learn. Providers of care should help you with constructive suggestions as to how to better your life. These constructive suggestions may go the whole gamut from a major change in medication, to a little adjustment to the time in which they are taken so that side effects will not be a problem; but providers of care are not God, do not have a crystal ball, and do not have the right to impose upon you the life that they think you should live. If you are able to get what you want, do so. Many points have been made in this book about how to appreciate what your health care providers can do for you, and how to make best use of it, without becoming a slave to anyone.

Point 3: Timing is extremely important. By that I mean the timing of starting psychotherapy, the timing of ending it, the timing of a decision to continue or to relinquish or to resume responsibilities of work or study. You should be willing to consider any program adjustment that a person wants to suggest, even if you do not agree with them, but if you have a really good reason to disagree, it may be wise to stick to your guns.

Point 4: Be open to other points of view, even if you do not agree. Expect yourself to make progress albeit at a moderate pace, and do not tolerate getting "stuck" for a long time. Understanding what makes you get stuck may be very beneficial.

Point 5: If you do fail several times at a particular endeavor, such as living on your own, learn from your experience and be willing to set yourself a lesser hurdle (such as living in a group home or in family care -- foster care for adults)– as your next move.

Point 6: Do not lose heart – whatever progress is made is yours to keep. Do not expect a talk therapist or a doctor to have all the answers.

Point 7: Conquering a mental illness (taming your dragon) is hard work, and there is no one else who can do that work for you. The best that even providers you have known a long time and appreciated very much can do for you, is to point out in what direction you should go – but they can't do it for you. Just like walking through the valley of the shadow of death, as in Psalm 23, going through your own mental illness is something you have to do for yourself. You cannot hire a guide, or rent a cab, or find someone to take you over by helicopter. No, you have to go through it, yourself, to some extent alone. Other people can watch you go through it and may be able to offer comments which can be useful about your progress, but the task remains yours.

Point 8: If you are the family member of someone with a mental illness, realize how difficult it can be for the patient, and try, within reason, to be supportive and understanding.

Point 9: There is a fine line between being supportive and understanding and being enabling. To be supportive is to get the idea that what the person is going through is difficult and to be willing to give him credit for struggling against the difficulty. To be enabler is to expect little or nothing in the way of constructive effort on the part of the patient, so that whatever they do is tolerated, though perhaps not always with very good grace.

Point 10: The one thing that psychiatry offers is change. And we hope what we offer is constructive change, change in the direction of adaptability, flexibility, tolerance and

> acceptance of what has already happened, and a resolve not to fall into old traps.
>
> Point 11: But, as I have said before, it is your life, and you are free to make of it what you will. With this freedom comes responsibility to behave reasonably towards other people and to make use of your talents as much as you can. The idea that it is you yourself that makes the conditions of your life, and not some well-meaning physician or other provider, should be very liberating.
>
> Point 12: Do not underestimate the force of habit. There are bad habits, like smoking tobacco, or marijuana, or doing cocaine, or drinking or using other drugs, and also feeling negative about one's life and one's self, by drawing on negative incidents or continuing painful examples in which someone who should have cared did not.

Think also about the effects of good habits. Train yourself not to focus on the negative, not to hold grudges, not to hold onto envy, jealousy, pointless guilt, resentment, etc. Train your thoughts also to be quiet and be ready to cede a place to Being when thought is not required to solve a problem, to contemplate a piece of philosophy or theology, or to be used for whatever purpose you wish.

> Point 13: But tolerating chitter chatter ("monkey mind") from your mind when it is not busy can be very destructive to the soul. There are a number of ways that have been used over the centuries by a number of different cultures to quiet the mind; as with many things, first and foremost in importance is the desire to have a mind which is quiet. Only by desiring to discipline the mental processes can you arrive at having some positive energy.

Then you are waiting peacefully for your next task or undertaking, and petty gripes (or even major gripes) do not hold sway over your soul. You can change the content of your thoughts, your feelings, your moods and your impression of the meaning of life; it is up to you not to be overcome with negativity, up to you not to relinquish your hold on love and peace and joy. This is difficult, but the struggle is worth it.

I think it is perhaps wise to end with a few words about the purpose of life itself. You know we all come into the world naked, cold, wet and helpless. Of course, we do come, each of us, into a particular set of circumstances – our family, our country, our times. Perhaps one baby is born into a family which has established a large trust fund that is intended to take care of him for the rest of his days. And perhaps that person never will know want, hunger, or financial hardship of any kind.

But those who were born and who remain very wealthy have a different set of problems. There may be a number of family expectations to live up to (woe betide an artist born into a family of bankers). And I am certain, having observed closely the lives of over ten thousand people, that a life of continuous leisure without any particular mission to improve the lot of others, (or even to just improve the view from this corner, or the taste of the chicken soup for dinner) is a life that is extremely difficult for the soul. A certain amount of healthy endeavoring, trying to do something that seems worth doing, is as necessary to the human psyche, I am convinced, as food, water, clothing and shelter are to the body.

It may be, as it was in the case of Sylvie, a fellow patient with schizophrenia that I once knew, that the striving is to walk around the few acres of the grounds of the mental hospital she was in and get to know where every nest, every burrow, every bud, every cocoon was located, and to be able to see how they were all doing, and so to participate in springtime and to be able to show lovely things to others.

It may be that your striving is to keep the beautiful family home heated and lit and welcoming, as it always was. It may be that your striving is to keep your house clean and the children's clothes washed and manage to pay the mortgage and grocery bill and the electricity and heating, and still have a moment for a laugh here or there and some time to play with the kids on the weekends. It may be that your great struggle is to stay away from the temptations of cocaine or heroin or some other drug which got you in its thrall when you were too young, too innocent, and too unsuspecting to realize what was happening to you.

It may be that you have to be in prison for a long time, or even for life, as society's way to make you atone for something that you did. Perhaps the bitterest outcome is to be in prison for life for a crime you did not commit, and to have very limited resources to be able to advocate for yourself. Perhaps you have stood up for some principles or ideals which were unpopular to the regime ruling your land at the time, and so you have become a political prisoner. Perhaps your striving is to wake up every day, and to keep hope alive. Perhaps you have been the victim of some dreadful disease or of some situation, such as a war between your people and other folk that was none of your making, and you grew up to the sound of gunfire from the cradle.

Yes, we all have circumstances. With due respect to the managers of hedge funds, it is impossible to protect yourself from every adversity. In 2008 the United States saw bankruptcies of revered investment bankers, so businesses that had become household names and were identified with America's idea of itself, collapsed, and foreclosures of homes took place at an unprecedented rate, together with unemployment that topped ten percent. It is not possible to escape having bad things happen.

Some people wonder why a loving God allows bad things to happen to his children. Why does he allow death and disease and pain and sorrow? Partly, I think it is because Infinity has decided that we will all reap the consequences of whatever we have done or have allowed to be done. In other words, for example, when the German people allowed Hitler to rise to power and take control of the country, and exterminate non-Aryans, and when they individually and collectively chose to follow everything he said as their leader, then there were consequences for many many people in this world.

On an individual basis, when a governor (like New York Governor Spitzer) participates in buying services from prostitutes and so disgraces himself with his illegal activity, the consequence is obvious – he must leave office. One might contend that his children or his grandchildren did nothing evil, and so why do they have to have any consequences? Well, what we do, what we choose to do and what we choose to leave undone has grave consequences for all of us.

We people, we human beings, have a great need of all the help that we can each give to each other. Gifts and talents are dispersed among the people, and that is God's kindness. In good times, we feel loved and feel well provided for and are happy in our purpose. In bad times, it may be very hard for some of us even to believe that God still exists.

But it is the bad times that shape us, that grow our capacity. How many times has it happened that a person did not know what they were capable of until they had to be pushed to their limit, stretched to their full capability? One saying of First Lady Nancy Reagan's is: "A woman is like a teabag. She does not realize her full potential until she is put into hot water." From a plant's point of view, what matters most is the root system, which grows down unseen, unlovely, in the dark. Yet it is that root system which can support beautiful trees and branches and flowers and fruits.

All of us need all of us. To take one segment of society, (such as people with a psychiatric illness), and decide de facto that they have nothing to offer of value, can contribute nothing, can do nothing except age in institutions or group homes or wherever they may be, is not good and is not right. I told the story in an earlier chapter of a man who liked walking and was given coupons for a pizza business to hang on doorknobs. I'll bet that some of you laughed at the thought of someone who liked doing that. But if I add that this man was instrumental helping a new business in town get established, which eventually employed 21 people, perhaps you would understand his contribution better. What he did had consequences.

Furthermore, anyone, anyone on earth can get depressed, overwhelmed, over anxious – we may all have times when we are not as mentally sound as we would wish to be. Why then can we not be more accepting, more understanding, more welcoming to people with a mental illness, and see them not as flotsam and jetsam to be rejected on sight, but as human beings with potential and with surprising abilities?

You may remember the film "A Beautiful Mind." It is the story of John Nash, a schizophrenic with an extraordinary mathematical ability, who actually did win a Nobel Prize late in life for the work he had done as a young man. I feel the makers of this film understood what I'm saying when they titled it "A Beautiful Mind" instead of with a reference to being crazy or insane or something like that. Some of the most beautiful minds in the history of humankind have also been very delicate and subject to breakage when under excessive stress. Can we not think of all people who approach us, whatever their physical state and whatever their status of cleanliness or dress or superficial presentation, as people with a gift for us?

Everyone has a gift for you, whether it's a gift you'd be delighted to receive, or whether it's a lesson that you need to learn. The question is not can this person teach you something – the question is rather are you ready to learn? There are perhaps thirty million people in the United States with <u>serious</u> mental illness. I number myself among these, because although it doesn't show (I take four medications every day) it is still very much there. If I miss my meds by as much as one dose, (which has happened three times in over 40 years, and not at all, recently) my impressive functioning begins to melt. But we who have mental illnesses also have a lot to offer. We sometimes have a lot of understanding, a lot of kindness, a lot of patience – things that the so-called healthy world is rather short on. Can we not reach across the chasm that sometimes seems to divide us and just say "Hello, my friend, what can we do together today?"

Archaeologists may find a shard of fine pottery and will painstakingly go through every bit of soil looking for other shards and perhaps try to piece together the vessel that these shards once came from. They do this with love, with gentleness, with persistence. Could we not rebuild people with as much care, gentleness, persistence and focused thoughtfulness as the archeologists find for pot shards? I hope so.

If you approach any person thinking he will be stupid, dirty, uncouth and utterly uninteresting, then you will see just that. But now, approach this person as a beautiful child of God, perhaps sent unto your life with a message for you, then the beauty will become obvious, and you may be able to show that person to him- or herself as beautiful, and even convince some jaded, overworked and overstressed providers. And if that person is persuaded of their own worth, their behavior may change a great deal. For one who has an open heart and mind, many a sweet epiphany awaits.

Our deepest fear is not that we are inadequate. Our deepest fear is that we are powerful beyond measure. It is our light, not our darkness, that most frightens us. We ask ourselves, who am I to be brilliant, gorgeous, talented, fabulous? Actually, who are you not to be? You are a child of God. Your playing small does not serve the world. There is nothing enlightened about shrinking so that other people won't feel insecure around you. We are all meant to shine, as children do. We were born to make manifest the glory of God that is within us. And as we let our own light shine, we unconsciously give other people permission to do the same. As we are liberated from our own fear, our presence automatically liberates others.

Marianne Williamson